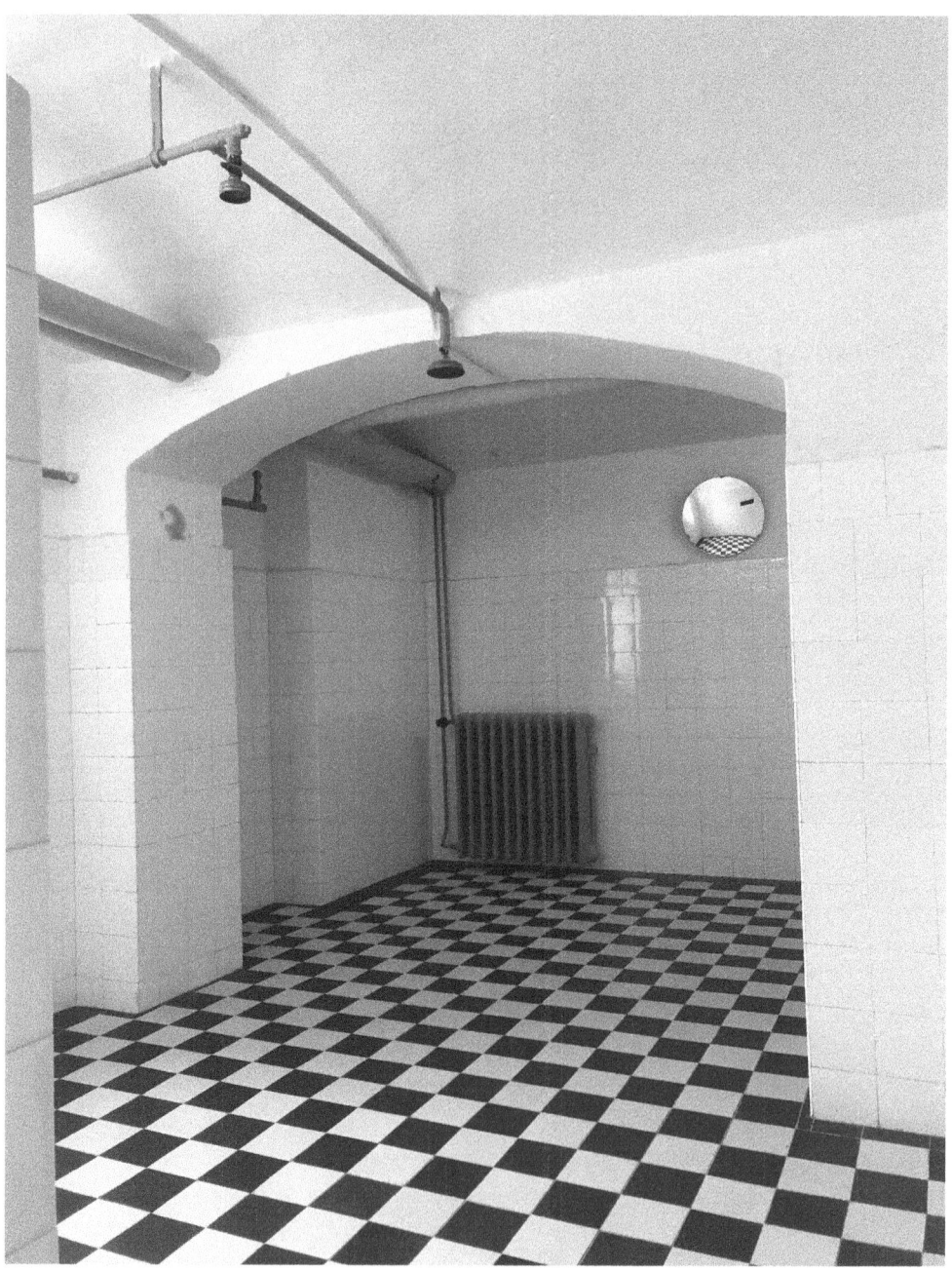

Gas chamber in the basement of the Bernburg State Sanatorium and Mental Hospital, one of six Nazi euthanasia centers. Between January 1940 and August 1941, 70,273 mentally or physically ill and other "inferior" patients were murdered, mostly with carbon monoxide gas. Psychiatric patients are still being treated at this hospital today. *Photo by Sheldon Rubenfeld*

Physician-Assisted Suicide and Euthanasia

REVOLUTIONARY BIOETHICS

Series Editor: Rachel Haliburton, University of Sudbury

Revolutionary Bioethics is a new series composed of scholarly monographs and edited collections organized around specific topics that explore bioethical theory and practice through the frameworks provided by feminist ethics, narrative ethics, and virtue ethics, challenging the assumptions of mainstream bioethics in the process. Contemporary mainstream bioethics has become ideological and repetitive, a defender of activities that bioethics was originally created to critique, and an apologist for unethical practices and policies in medicine that it once saw itself as fighting against. Taking its title from recent work being done on MacIntyre's neo-Aristotelian ethics, Revolutionary Bioethics is organized around the idea that bioethics needs to reform both its theory and practice, and its goal is to begin the conversation about what a transformed bioethics—one that is unafraid to explore new theoretical approaches, and to examine and critique current bioethical practices—might look like.

Titles in the series

Physician-Assisted Suicide and Euthanasia: Before, During, and After the Holocaust
   Edited by Sheldon Rubenfeld and Daniel P. Sulmasy, with Astrid Ley

Physician-Assisted Suicide and Euthanasia

Before, During, and After the Holocaust

Edited by
Sheldon Rubenfeld and Daniel P. Sulmasy

With Astrid Ley

LEXINGTON BOOKS
Lanham • Boulder • New York • London

Published by Lexington Books
An imprint of The Rowman & Littlefield Publishing Group, Inc.
4501 Forbes Boulevard, Suite 200, Lanham, Maryland 20706
www.rowman.com

6 Tinworth Street, London SE11 5AL, United Kingdom

British Library Cataloguing in Publication Information Available

Library of Congress Cataloging-in-Publication Data

Names: Rubenfeld, Sheldon, editor. | Sulmasy, Daniel P., 1956– editor. | Ley, Astrid,
    other.
Title: Physician-assisted suicide and euthanasia : before, during, and after the Holocaust
    / edited by Sheldon Rubenfeld and Daniel P. Sulmasy with Astrid Ley.
Description: Lanham : Lexington Books, [2020] | Series: Revolutionary bioethics |
    Includes bibliographical references and index. | Summary: "This book provides
    a history of Nazi medical euthanasia programs, demonstrating that arguments in
    their favor were widely embraced by Western medicine before the Third Reich.
    Contributors find significant continuities between history and current physician-
    assisted suicide and euthanasia and urge caution about their legalization or
    implementation" — Provided by publisher.
Identifiers: LCCN 2020028283 (print) | LCCN 2020028284 (ebook) | ISBN
    9781793609496 (cloth) | ISBN 9781793609502 (epub)
Subjects: LCSH: Assisted suicide—Moral and ethical aspects--Germany. | Medicine—
    Germany—History. | Physicians—Germany—History. | Medical ethics—History.
Classification: LCC R726 .P493 2020 (print) | LCC R726 (ebook) | DDC 179.7—dc23
LC record available at https://lccn.loc.gov/2020028283
LC ebook record available at https://lccn.loc.gov/2020028284

Dedicated to our patients —
past,
present,
and future

Contents

List of Tables

Acknowledgments

We gratefully acknowledge the numerous people who supported the Center for Medicine after the Holocaust (CMATH) and made this book a reality. We are especially grateful to Tony Rodriguez and Miriam Weiner of The Conference on Jewish Material Claims Against Germany ("Claims Conference") for their support of CMATH from its earliest days through 2019. Their support allowed us to gather scholars from the United States, Germany, Canada, and Israel to contribute to this book.

The CMATH board of directors provided indispensable support for the Physician-Assisted Suicide and Euthanasia after the Holocaust project. We thank them all: Barbara Hales, Steven Finkelman, Ben Tobor, Terry Rubin, Mary Schwartz, Tom Wheeler, Eric Pulaski, and Homer Carvajal. We also thank CMATH's many other supporters, especially Sheri Henriksen and Lise Liddell.

This book would not have been possible without the enthusiastic support and gracious hospitality of the Methodist Hospital Research Institute (MHRI) of Houston, Texas, and especially Ed Jones, its president and CEO, Mauro Ferrari, PhD, immediate past president and CEO, Marc Boom, MD, president and CEO of Houston Methodist, and Roberta Schwartz, Houston Methodist Hospital Executive Vice President, and Rebecca Hall, PhD, Director of Communications & External Relations for MHRI.

We are also grateful to Jessica Sussman of Frosch Travel who facilitated the gathering of our scholars in Berlin to exchange ideas that contributed to the development of this book.

We thank the many Lexington editors who guided this book from proposal to finished product during the Covid-19 pandemic.

We are thankful for Kathy Kobos, personal and indispensable editorial assistant to one of us (SR), for agreeing to take on this project and for her tireless devotion to getting everything just right.

We especially thank our contributors, who took time out of their busy schedules to participate in this project, which involved travel, time away from family, a commitment to experiential as well as didactic learning, free and respectful dialogue about extremely controversial topics, writing, and open responsiveness to our critiques of their manuscripts. Perhaps uniquely in academia, we shared community as well as ideas, and the outstanding contributions they produced for this volume are a testament to this model of scholarship.

Each Wednesday for the past twenty years, one of us (SR) has studied Jewish medical ethics with Rabbi Yossi Grossman of the Jewish Ethics Institute. We thank him, Ron Moses, who was there right from the first class, and all the others who have contributed to our knowledge of Jewish medical ethics, including Alan Winters, Nada Chandler, Russ Weidman, Manny Magid, Jimmy Lass, Ed Teitel, and Natalie Kravitz.

Finally, we'd like to thank our wives, Linda Rubenfeld and Lois Snyder Sulmasy, JD, who fully supported us from the very start of this project, read and critiqued drafts, shared ideas, and gracefully and genially managed without our company many days and nights.

Sheldon Rubenfeld, MD
Houston, Texas
Daniel P. Sulmasy, MD, PhD
Washington, DC
January 27, 2020
International Holocaust Remembrance Day

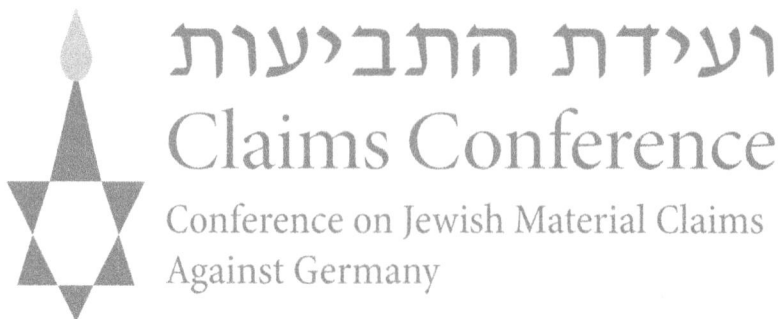

ועידת התביעות

Claims Conference

Conference on Jewish Material Claims
Against Germany

Introduction

Sheldon Rubenfeld

German medicine played a central and indispensable role in the design and implementation of the Holocaust. For nearly thirty years before Hitler became chancellor in 1933, many German physicians advocated anti-miscegenation laws (Nuremberg Laws), involuntary sterilization, and coerced euthanasia to accelerate Darwin's natural selection and to improve Germany's genetic stock. Hitler recognized the compatibility of their eugenic views with his own anti-Semitism and sanctioned these medical pioneers to carry out their "scientific" agenda. As Rudolf Hess, Hitler's deputy führer, said about the implementation of physician's reductionist, scientific, eugenic medical policies: "National Socialism is nothing but applied biology" (Lifton 1986, 31).

Nazi doctors selected and sterilized nearly 400,000 German citizens against their will, excluded "genetically unfit" couples from marrying, killed 5,000 disabled children, and designed and utilized gas chambers and crematoria during *Aktion* T4 (Action T4) to kill 70,000 German adults with disabilities and other "lives not worth living." They characterized these deaths as "mercy killings." While not all disabled patients were killed, all *Jewish* disabled patients were targeted as part of a "T4 Special Campaign," which can be considered a prelude to the Holocaust (Ley and Hinz-Wessels 2012, 155). The T4 physicians were then sent to concentration camps during *Sonderaktion* 14f13 (Special Action 14f13, or 14f13) to examine, select, and eliminate seriously ill prisoners who could not work, using the same gas chambers they had developed for the disabled. Once again, they also singled out Jews, selecting them for elimination without an examination (Lifton 1986, 135). Robert Proctor describes 14f13 as the "transition from the systematic destruction of the handicapped and the mentally ill to the systematic destruction of the ethnically and culturally marginal," adding that "The physicians responsible for administering the euthanasia operations . . . were also responsible for formulating criteria and administering the first phases of the destruction of the Jews . . ." (1988, 134–135). Subsequently, hundreds of physicians, including Josef Mengele, MD, PhD, Auschwitz's "Angel of Death," applied techniques developed in the euthanasia program to select and murder 4,500,000 Jews in bigger and better gas chambers and crematoria in death camps built for the "Final Solution of the Jewish Problem."

AN UNWELCOME HISTORY

With the worldwide adoption of German scientific medicine in the late nineteenth and early twentieth centuries, the value of the history of medicine relative to the natural sciences in medical education declined. For example, Dr. William Welch, who had studied pathology and bacteriology in Germany before becoming one of the founders of the Johns Hopkins University School of Medicine in 1889 (Johns Hopkins Medicine n.d.), was a steadfast advocate of German reductionism, viewing clinical medicine as a scientific discipline to be taught by scientists.

More importantly, the Carnegie Foundation commissioned Abraham Flexner, an educator without medical training who had studied in Germany, to report on the relative state of medical education in North America and Europe (Nevins 2010, 7–10). His 1910 "Flexner Report" accelerated the "Germanization" of American and Canadian medicine that had been under way since the end of the Civil War (Ludmerer 1985, 6). Flexner's goal was to reduce the number of Canadian and American MD or DO degree-granting, mostly apprenticeship-type schools, from 155 to 31 (Wheatley 1988, 52). By 1922, however, there still were 81 medical schools, most of which were affiliated with a university so they could practice the scientific medicine pioneered and practiced in Germany (Nevins 2010,14).

Dr. William Osler, who also studied briefly in Germany (American College of Physicians n.d.), rejected the Flexner Report and the sole reliance on science as the preferred medical education model. In a letter to the president of the Johns Hopkins University in 1911, he strongly objected to Flexner's recommendations. Because Flexner was "a man who knows the profession from the outside only," Osler viewed these errors as inevitable (1962).

Dr. Francis Peabody objected to Flexner's lack of attention to the doctor-patient relationship, writing in his oft-quoted essay that while there was a great deal of medical science for medical students to digest, the application of science to medicine is "only one limited aspect of medical practice . . . for the secret of the care of the patient is in caring for the patient" (Peabody 1927, 9–10).

Dr. Eugene Cordell, president of the Johns Hopkins Historical Club viewed the history of medicine as an antidote to the teaching of pure science to medical students, saying in 1904: "Is education to be for them merely a mastering of the dry details of anatomy, physiology, practice? Is there to be no attempt to direct motives, to strengthen conscience, to build up character? I tell you again there is danger in such a course." He concluded:

> It is probable that we may learn equally as much from the follies, omissions, and failures of the past as from its successes and achievements. Experience will always be fallacious and judgment difficult, and it is not likely that error can ever be avoided. It is well for us to realize that the future may pluck many a feather from even our ambitious wings, who plume ourselves on our attainments. (Cordell 1904, 280)

There is no greater example of medical "follies, omissions, and failures of the past" than the behavior of Germany's rational and rigorously scientific medical professionals just before and during the Holocaust. Yet, this history is almost never taught. Nor is the history of the legal, moral, and philanthropic contributions of American, Canadian, British, and other eugenicists to German eugenics taught in medical schools. These omissions are unfortunate because knowledge about Nazi medicine can lead to introspection by medical students and physicians about their own behavior and the modern medical ethos.

When doctors learn this history, they are initially stunned. Later, they attempt to cope with their new knowledge of these uncomfortable facts about medicine by disregarding this history as irrelevant to contemporary practice, or by disdainfully regarding as preposterous the idea that Nazi bioethicists offered ethical justifications for their behavior. Their reactions reiterate those of medical professionals and governments to the revelations of Nazi medical crimes at the 1946–1947 Nuremberg Medical Trial (NMT), which explains in part why most medical professionals, bioethicists, and health care policymakers remain unaware of this instructive history.

THE NUREMBERG MEDICAL TRIAL

As promised as early as 1942, the victorious allies—the United States, United Kingdom, France, and the Soviet Union—convened an International Military Tribunal to try the leading Nazi war criminals. On November 20, 1945, just six-and-a-half months after the end of World War II, in a dock built for 24 Nazis, they tried the 21 defendants who could appear in court.

Less well-known are the 12 American Subsequent Nuremberg Trials of 183 high-ranking German officials. Because of Hollywood's great 1961 film, *Judgment at Nuremberg*, the Judges' Trial is probably the most famous of all these trials. But the first trial was the Nuremberg Medical Trial or, officially, *United States of America v. Karl Brandt, et al.*, which began on December 9, 1946, and was decided on August 20, 1947.

This trial almost didn't happen for many reasons. First, the United States could not choose between prosecuting and procuring leading Nazi physicians and scientists. For example, four of the 23 defendants in the NMT were at one time or another employed by the American military (Annas and Grodin 1992, 106–107). A second deterrent was the determined effort by the German medical profession to cover up its central role in the design and implementation of the Nazi health care policies and the Holocaust. Two books by historian Paul Weindling describe the many obstacles preventing American officials from trying Nazi doctors (2004) and the heroic actions of Canadian physician John Thompson, who ultimately convinced them to proceed with the NMT (2010).

Although the lead defendant, Dr. Karl Brandt, had been the director of the Nazi euthanasia program, the focus of the NMT was Nazi medical experiments on about 25,000 human subjects (Weindling 2015) rather than the medical ethos that promoted the development and implementation of gas chambers that would ultimately claim millions of innocent Jewish victims in the Holocaust, or on the involuntary sterilizations of approximately 400,000 victims, or on the involuntary euthanasia of approximately 200,000 victims.

Michael Marrus wrote about the focus of the NMT, "Those who go to the judgment expecting a ringing statement of explanation and responsibility—a call for 'historical truth'—will certainly be disappointed" (1999, 108). He went on to say, "The indictment portrayed the accused as members of a criminal conspiracy, something like a group of gangsters who planned and carried out a bank robbery, rather than as individuals who shared a common ideology or institutional culture" (1999, 109). Marrus summed up:

> important legal and political priorities shaped the course of the trial and the presentation of evidence . . . deflected attention from the involvement of the medical profession as a whole in the Nazi enterprise . . . [and] assisted the postwar tendency of the profession to wrap itself in scientific credentials and to evade its social and ethical responsibilities. (1999, 118–119)

MYTHS ABOUT MEDICINE AND THE HOLOCAUST

The NMT also gave rise to the beliefs that Nazi science was either bad science or not really science and that Nazi doctors were not good doctors.

The omissions of the NMT enabled several groups to generate myths about medicine during the Third Reich. Many German physicians who engaged in war crimes continued to cover them up; many Jewish scholars who were forced from Germany were reluctant to admit that Nazis were capable of good science; American military authorities used the myths to disguise their recruitment of Nazi scientific and medical talent, in Operation Paperclip, for example (Jacobsen 2014); and the American public wanted to believe that similar abuses could not occur in a liberal democracy (Proctor 2000, 335–346). Western physicians today find comfort in such myths, which they use to relieve themselves of the responsibility to consider the relevance of the history of medicine and the Holocaust to contemporary medical practice and research. The following are examples of such myths and the facts that refute them:

1. *Very few German physicians supported Nazi programs or participated in Nazi medical crimes.* Yet, more than 2,700 German physicians joined the Nazi Socialist Physicians' League before Hitler became chancellor in 1933. By the time World War II ended, roughly 50 percent of physicians had joined the Nazi party and 7 percent were in the SS or *Schutzstaffel* (Protection Squad), much higher percentages than the general population or any other profession (Proctor 1988, 66).

2. *Josef Mengele, MD, PhD, who conducted his medical experiments on twins and performed selections for the gas chambers on the ramps of Auschwitz was singularly evil among the Nazi physicians.* Yet, for example, Dr. Irmfried Eberl, a physician almost no one has heard of, was initially the medical director at Brandenburg, the first of six Nazi euthanasia centers, where 9,772 people were gassed, and then became director of a second euthanasia center at Bernburg where another 8,601 people were gassed. Finally, he became commandant of the Treblinka extermination camp where he supervised the gassing of approximately 250,000 people before his dismissal for incompetence in disposing of their bodies (Lifton 1986, 123–125). If Mengele deserves the title, "Angel of Death," then what title should we reserve for Dr. Irmfried Eberl and others like him?

3. *Physicians were forced to participate in Nazi medical crimes.* There were, however, very few cases of German physicians refusing to participate in the many medical crimes of the Third Reich. Indeed, for decades prior to Hitler's election to chancellor, physicians promoted unethical programs ultimately adopted by the Nazis. At the first mass murder in a gas chamber, which took place at Brandenburg, Victor Brack, head of the euthanasia program in the Chancellery of the Führer, stated that "The syringe belongs in the hands of a physician" (see chapter 19 in this book), and Dr. Karl Brandt stressed that the gassing would be done only by doctors (Schmidt 2007, 140).

4. *Nazi physicians were incompetent.* Yet, many American physicians, such as William Welch (Johns Hopkins Medicine n.d.), William Osler (American College of Physicians n.d.), and Michael DeBakey (DeBakey 2008; 2010, 221) went to Germany to study clinical medicine and medical research. The intense competition between the United States and the Soviet Union for Nazi scientific and medical talent at the end of World War II, as compared with the relative lack of interest in Japanese talent, further disproves the notion of Nazi scientific and medical incompetence (Brody 2014).

5. *Nazi physicians were mad, and their ideas were out of the mainstream.* Yet, eugenics was not a Nazi invention. The United States was the world's leader in the eugenics movement before World War II (Friedlander 1995, 1–23). The *Journal of the American Medical Association* reported favorably on Germany's sterilization program (From Our Regular Correspondent 1933; 1934). In 1934, when Germany was sterilizing 5,000 people a month, C. M. Goethe, a leading eugenicist from California, returned from Germany and told a colleague:

> You will be interested to know that your work has played a powerful part in shaping the opinions of the groups of intellectuals who are behind Hitler in this epoch-making program. Everywhere I sensed that their opinions have been tremendously stimulated by American thought—I want you, my dear friend, to carry this thought with you for the rest of your life, that you have really jolted into action a great government of 60 million people. (Goethe quoted in Black 2003, 277)

6. *Good science and bad ethics cannot coexist.* Yet, Roelcke's careful analysis of the sulfonamide experiments in Ravensbruck concentration camp discredits this comforting belief (Roelcke 2014b). Proctor demonstrated that tobacco and cancer research was also of high quality during the Third Reich (Proctor 1999). American human subjects researchers neglected the Nuremberg Code generated by the jurists at the NMT for nearly three decades because they thought that such a code was necessary only for barbarians like Nazis but not for ethical researchers like themselves (Beauchamp 2014). Their hubris was unmasked by Henry Beecher in his 1966 *New England Journal of Medicine* article about 22 unethical human subjects research studies (Beecher 1966), by the 1972 newspaper accounts of the abuses of the Tuskegee Syphilis Study that began in 1932 under the auspices of the United State Public Health Service (Heller 1972), and by the *Final Report of the Advisory Committee on Human Radiation Experiments* that detailed the US government's exposure of thousands of its citizens to

life-threatening radiation to advance medical knowledge and safeguard national security (Faden et al. 1996).

7. *We are not Nazis, we live in a liberal democracy and, therefore, we are not capable of doing such evil.* The obvious falsity of this particularly comforting myth should speak for itself. But should anyone need convincing, one can point to the fact that while the US government was prosecuting Nazi physicians in Nuremberg, US physicians were conducting experiments in which they purposefully infected Guatemalan soldiers, prisoners, and mentally ill patients with syphilis and gonorrhea to see if penicillin could prevent or cure these infections—experiments that only came to light in 2010 (Presidential Commission for the Study of Bioethical Issues 2011).

8. *Nazi policies were legally, morally, and ethically indefensible, or perpetrators of evil acts cannot be motivated by ethical beliefs.* As described in Florian Bruns' chapter in this book, Nazi physicians were the world's leaders in medical ethics education, requiring a course for all their medical students. Indeed, one of the purposes of this book is to explore the history of euthanasia before, during, and after the Holocaust from the perspective of medical ethics. The ethics the Nazis taught was morally perverse, but they sought an intellectual justification for their biomedical policies.

BIOETHICS AFTER THE HOLOCAUST

James Rachels (1990) highlighted the moral implications of Charles Darwin's research and publications in general, while Richard Weikart in *From Darwin to Hitler: Evolutionary Ethics, Eugenics, and Racism in Germany* (2004) focused on their negative impact on traditional religious and enlightenment ethics, particularly the sanctity of human life.

Robert Jay Lifton, in *The Nazi Doctors: Medical Killing and the Psychology of Genocide*, described the Nazi philosophy of applied biology as one of:

> absolute control over the evolutionary process, over the biological future. Making widespread use of the Darwinian term "selection," the Nazis sought to take over the natural functions of nature (natural selection) and God (the Lord giveth and the Lord taketh away) in orchestrating their own "selections," their own version of human evolution. (Lifton 1986, 17)

In 1900, William Schallmayer, who together with Alfred Ploetz founded German eugenics, won the Krupp writing competition with *Heredity and Selection in the Life History of Nations*, his answer to the contest's question: "What can we learn from the theory of evolution about internal political development and state legislation?" (Weiss 1987, 69). The next year, the *American Journal of Psychology* reviewed Dr. W. Duncan McKim's *Human Heredity and Progress*:

> The dark side of human existence; the cause of human wretchedness; the defective classes; a remedy; and a consideration of objections against it, are the chief features of this book. The most striking and central idea is that artificial selection should help the elevation of the human race, partly by restricting reproduction of those organically very weak or vicious, and doing this, to use his language, "by the surest, the simplest, the kindest, and most human means of preventing reproduction among those whom we deem unworthy of this high privilege" by "a gentle and painless death." (American Journal of Psychology 1901, 275)

Well before the Nazis came to power, German academic physicians also promulgated the idea that some lives were worth less than others, as several chapters in this book demonstrate. Typical of this type of thinking was the influential 1920 book by psychiatrist Alfred Hoche and jurist Karl Binding, *Permitting the Destruction of Life Unworthy of Life* (*Die Freigabe der Vernichtung Lebensunwerten Lebens*). In their advocacy of voluntary and nonvoluntary euthanasia for selected groups, they made many statements relevant to the contemporary debate on physician-assisted suicide and euthanasia after the Holocaust. Two in particular stand out. First:

> There was a time, now considered barbaric, in which eliminating those who were born unfit for life, or who later became so, was taken for granted. Then came the phase, continuing into the present, in which, finally, preserving every existence, no matter how worthless, stood as the highest moral value. A new age will arrive—operating with a higher morality. . . . (Binding and Hoche 1920)

The moral imperative that emanated from Mt. Sinai to preserve "every existence, no matter how worthless" would be replaced by a higher Nazi morality.

In a second statement, Binding and Hoche also dismissed Hippocratic ethical values, writing, "The young physician enters practice without any legal delineation of his rights and duties—especially regarding the most important points. Not even the Hippocratic Oath, with its generalities, is operative today" (1920). With writings like these, Binding, Hoche, and others dismissed traditional Judeo-Christian Hippocratism.

In the 1920s, anti-Semitic publisher Julius Lehman sent his friend Hitler a copy of Baur, Fischer, and Lenz's textbook, *Grundriss der menschlichen Erblichkeitslehre and Rassenhygiene* (Outline of Human Genetics and Racial Hygiene) (Weikart 2004, 222). Perhaps, after reading this book, Hitler realized for the first time the potential of using the medical profession to eliminate those people he considered a danger to the *Volk* (people) and to his political ambitions. In return, the medical profession appreciated the potential to catch up with the rest of the Western world and finally implement the eugenic policies they had advocated for decades. In 1929, four years before Hitler became chancellor, doctors founded *NS-Ärztebund* (National Socialist Physicians' League); by 1933, it had 2,786 members and by 1938, it had 30,000 members (Kater 1989, 63).

Once he became chancellor, Hitler transformed the relationship between doctor and patient into one between the state and the *Volkskörper* (nation's body) and became the nation's doctor. As head of state, he empowered eager and willing medical professionals to prevent the transmission of genes from those whose lives they considered unworthy of life to the *Volkskörper* by passing eugenic sterilization and anti-miscegenation laws and by authorizing involuntary "mercy killings."

American psychiatrist Leo Alexander, a medical advisor to the NMT, wrote about the beginnings of the Nazi medical programs: "The beginnings at first were merely a subtle shift in emphasis in the basic attitude of the physicians. It started with the acceptance of the attitude, basic in the euthanasia movement, that there is such a thing as life not worthy to be lived" (Alexander 1949). After the revelations about Nazi medical crimes at the NMT, this attitude was discredited. Yet, today's advocates for physician-assisted suicide (PAS) and euthanasia also begin by making the case for accepting the attitude that "there is such a thing as a life not worthy to be lived" if a person makes an autonomous declaration to that effect, and if a physician agrees. It is, therefore, worth examining how we arrived back at the beginning.

THE BAD NAUHEIM DECLARATION AND THE WORLD MEDICAL ASSOCIATION'S DECLARATION OF GENEVA

Cultural anthropologist Margaret Mead cited the Hippocratic Oath as one of the watershed moments in human history:

> For the first time in our tradition there was a complete separation between killing and curing. Throughout the primitive world the doctor and the sorcerer tended to be the same person. He with the power to kill had the power to cure, including specially the undoing of his own killing activities. With the Greeks, the distinction was made clear. One profession, the followers of Asclepius, were to be dedicated completely to life under all circumstances, regardless of rank, age, or intellect—the life of a slave, the life of the Emperor, the life of a foreign man, the life of a defective child . . . this is a priceless possession which we cannot afford to tarnish, but society always is attempting to make the physician into a killer—to kill the defective child at birth, to leave the sleeping pills beside

the bed of the cancer patient . . . it is the duty of society to protect the physician from such requests. (Mead quoted in Levine 1972, 324–325)

While we do not know the author of the original oath, we know that it remained important in the Western world until the twentieth century and re-mained relatively unchanged until after World War II. Given the importance of the Hippocratic Oath, medicine could have resurrected, reinforced, and reaffirmed it after the NMT's revelations, but that did not happen (Frewer 2010). Before the NMT ended, delegates at a medical conference in Bad Nauheim, Germany, issued the Bad Nauheim Declaration to provide the ethical foundation for a revised professional code. Unlike the original Hip-pocratic Oath, which begins by invoking the gods and swearing by them, the declaration began with this secular statement: "I swear to practice the medical profession as a service to human beings and their health, to conscientiously carry out my medical duties and in my activity of healing to subordinate my own benefit to the well-being of the patient" (Frewer 2010, 265). Also, de-spite the history of medicine during the Third Reich, this declaration does not mention, let alone forbid, euthanasia.

Shortly thereafter, the influential World Medical Association (WMA) was founded and, in 1948, issued its Declaration of Geneva, a new formula-tion of the Hippocratic Oath, beginning with, "At the time of being admitted as a member of the medical profession I solemnly pledge myself to conse-crate my life to the service of humanity." There have since been many other new formulations of the Hippocratic Oath, such as an Oath that "Bears the Name of Hippocrates," that begins with: "I do solemnly swear, by whatever I hold most sacred" (Association of American Physicians and Surgeons n.d.). This oath was on the website of the American Association of Medical Colleges until it was abruptly removed a few years ago and replaced with the Modern, Shortened Version of the Hippocratic Oath (American Asso-ciation of Medical Colleges n.d.).

While Christianity had substituted a Christian preamble for the classical oath's reference to pagan gods (Nutton 2013, 415, n. 87; Veatch and Mason 1987), "I swear by Apollo the Physician and by Asclepius and by Health (the god Hygieia) and Panacea and by all the gods as well as goddesses, making them judges (witnesses), to bring the following oath and written covenant to fulfillment, in accordance with my power and my judgment," newer formula-tions of the oath eliminated reference to any deity.

Not only did the Bad Nauheim Declaration and the WMA Declaration omit reference to any deity, but they also failed to mention euthanasia. This omission is not surprising because the NMT failed to highlight the Nazi in-voluntary euthanasia programs, the German medical profession covered up and continues to cover up its role in the Third Reich (Roelcke 2014a), and many Nazi physicians involved in the Nazi euthanasia programs eluded prosecution and continued in their professional roles after World War II (Weinke 2014). Furthermore, once Germany gained admission to the WMA in 1951, it chose three former Nazi physicians to represent it (Seidelman 1999). From 1973–74, Dr. Ernst Fromm, a member of the SA (*Sturmabteilung* or Assault Division better known as Storm Troopers) and the SS, served as president of the WMA. In 1992, the WMA appointed as president-elect for 1993–94 Professor Dr. Hans Joachim Sewering, a member of the Nazi party and the SS who also worked at the Eglfing-Haar euthanasia, or killing, center. He was forced to step aside in January 1993 when his Nazi past was publicized outside Germany (Hohendorf 2014).

In 2011, representatives of the Center for Medicine after the Holocaust (CMATH) visited the German Medical Association where its president asked historian Robert Jütte to discuss his recently published book that was intended to set the record straight on physician involvement in the Third Reich. Volker Roelcke and Paul Weindling, two scholars traveling with CMATH, took the author to task for his superficial treatment of physician involvement in the Nazi enterprise (Roelcke 2014a, 256–258), and a raucous argument ensued. Subsequently, several scholars issued a call for the German Medical Association to issue an apology for the German medical profession's role in the Third Reich, which it did in 2012 (German Medical Association 2012, 529–530). It has since failed to deliver on its pledges, particularly its pledge to open its archives to researchers (Roelcke 2014a, 277–278).

RELIGION, TRADITION, AND BIOETHICS
IN THE UNITED STATES TODAY

Religion and traditional medical ethics might have served as bulwarks against the abuse of medical power that transpired in Germany under National Socialism. As I have shown above, it was necessary for the Nazis to push these forces to the sidelines in order to make way for their biopolitical agenda. It is, therefore, instructive to note that the role of religion and traditional medical ethics in public discourse about bioethical issues in the United States has been greatly diminished in recent decades.

In two cases in the 1960s, the Supreme Court of the United States issued 8–1 decisions, *Engel v. Vitale* and *Abington Township v. Schempp*, that greatly diminished the role of religion in the public square in general, and in the high court's judicial thinking about the beginning-of-life and end-of-life in particular (Horowitz 2018). While the court defended these decisions on the grounds that the Constitution required the state's neutrality toward religion, Potter Stewart, the lone dissenting justice in both cases, said: "And a refusal to permit religious exercises thus is seen not as the realization of state neutrality, but rather as the establishment of a religion of secularism, or, at the least, as government support of those who think that religious exercises should be conducted only in private" (374 U.S. 203 1963).

It was not surprising, therefore, that the U.S. Supreme Court's 1973 *Roe v. Wade* ruling, whose primary finding was that "A person may choose to have an abortion until a fetus becomes viable . . .," dismissed religious ethical objections in its majority opinion (410 U.S. 113 1973). The US courts have increasingly emphasized autonomy and privacy and relegated religious arguments in the public sphere.

Relying heavily on a 71-page 1943 volume, *The Hippocratic Oath: Text, Translation and Interpretation* by Ludwig Edelstein, a non-physician medical historian who was forced to flee Germany because he was Jewish (Rütten 2006), the justices also discussed the Hippocratic Oath. They dismissed the oath's opposition to abortion as "a Pythagorean manifesto and not the expression of an absolute standard of medical conduct" (U.S. Supreme Court 1973). Despite the Hippocratic Oath's venerable 2,500-year history, historians and ethicists have downplayed its importance, particularly to make room for the possibilities of abortion and euthanasia, even though more recent historical scholarship refutes their efforts (Jouanna 1999; Carrick 2001; von Staden 1996).

The Four Principles

Although the role of religious and Hippocratic ethics in medicine was gradually and inexorably diminished in the twentieth century, an acceptable alternative was not found until "The Four Principles" appeared in the 1970s.

In 1964, the WMA issued its Declaration of Helsinki: Ethical Principles for Medical Research Involving Human Subjects. As noted above, the medical profession had not yet taken the Nuremberg Code seriously and, according to Jay Katz, the WMA's watered-down declaration demonstrated that "concerns over the advancement of science began to overshadow concerns over the integrity of the person" (Katz 1992, 234). However, when a public outcry arose in response to newspaper reports about the Tuskegee Syphilis Experiments (Heller 1972), Congress passed the National Research Act of 1974, which created the National Commission for the Protection of Human Subjects of Biomedical and Behavior Research that wrote and issued the Belmont Report in 1979 with three basic principles.

The same year, two philosophers, Tom Beauchamp, one of the authors of the Belmont Report, and James Childress wrote *Principles of Bioethics*, which is a, if not the, standard textbook of bioethics. They, non-physicians like Flexner and Edelstein, rejected all previous medical ethics and replaced them with ethical principles derived from philosophy:

Although major writings in ancient, medieval, and modern health care contain a rich storehouse of reflection on the relationship between the professional and the patient, these writings are inadequate for contemporary biomedical ethics. This historical record often neglects problems of truthfulness, privacy, justice, communal responsibility, and the like. (Beauchamp and Childress 2001, 1)

They proposed a replacement for those "inadequate" writings: "To avoid a similar narrowness, we begin with philosophical reflection on morality and ethics that is remote from the history of professional ethics. Such reflection affords some distance from assumptions still evident in the biomedical sciences and health care" (Beauchamp and Childress 2001, 1; cf. Steinberg, chapter 13 in this book).

After expanding the number of basic principles from three to four—autonomy, beneficence, non-maleficence, and justice—they applied them to clinical practice and health care policy without adequately justifying their applicability beyond human subjects research. Beauchamp and Childress seem to be declaring exactly what Binding and Hoche declared in 1920: "A new age will arrive—operating with a higher morality." And so it did.

The four principles dominate contemporary bioethics and autonomy dominates the four principles, which leads to difficulties when the definitions of the three subordinate principles are dependent upon the dominant principle. To illustrate this point, consider a thought experiment in which both traditional Jewish medical ethics and Nazi medical ethics are also characterized by four principles. Life would be the dominant principle in the former and eugenics would be the dominant principle in the latter, and the definitions of beneficence, non-maleficence, and justice would differ depending upon the dominant principle. For example, PAS and euthanasia would be prohibited in a principlist system dominated by life, be optional and perhaps beneficent and just in one dominated by autonomy, and be virtually required, beneficent and just in one dominated by eugenics. This thought experiment also suggests that there is inherent danger in any principlist system with a dominant principle other than the preservation of life, as exemplified by the writings of Peter Singer.

Philosopher Peter Singer, the Ira W. DeCamp Professor of Bioethics in the University Center for Human Values at Princeton University, approaches bioethics from a utilitarian, secular perspective and favors voluntary euthanasia as well as some forms of nonvoluntary euthanasia, including infanticide in certain situations. In an article about the reception of his controversial views during a visit to Germany, "On Being Silenced in Germany," Singer wrote:

If the suggestion [. . . of my opponents] is that whenever we seek to avoid having severely disabled children, we are improperly judging one kind of life to be worse than another, we can reply that such judgments are both necessary and proper. To argue otherwise would seem to suggest that if we break a leg, we should not get it mended, because in doing so we judge the lives of those with crippled legs to be less worth living than our own. (1993, 355–356)

I find it particularly jarring that this phrase, "lives . . . less worth living . . ." was written by the son of an Austrian Jewish physician who left Vienna for Australia in 1938 after the *Anschluss*, and the grandson of three grandparents killed by Nazis (Singer 2003, 3, 5).

Regarding infanticide, Singer has also said, "It is frequently claimed . . . that it is morally wrong to base life and death decisions in the practice of medicine on the quality or kind of life in question. In this article, we shall dispute that claim . . ." (Singer 2002, 233) and, "When the death of a defective infant will lead to the birth of another infant with better prospects of a happy life, the total amount of happiness will be greater if the defective infant is killed" (Singer 1993, 186).

The widespread acceptance of philosophical principlist ethics seemed to signal the death knell for both the Hippocratic Oath and for religious medical ethics. A 1993 content analysis by Pellegrino et al. of oaths administered in 150 US and Canadian Medical Schools found that many of the core elements of the traditional Hippocratic Oath were no longer relevant. Of the contemporary oaths reviewed, only 14 percent prohibit euthanasia, 11 percent hold covenant with a deity, 8 percent foreswear abortion, 3 percent forbid sexual contact with patients, and less than 50 percent insist that the taker of the oath be held accountable for keeping the pledge (Orr et al. 1997). Seventeen years later, Pellegrino noted that contemporary revisions of the Hippocratic Oath, making it "more amenable to our contemporary ethos . . . add nothing of moral depth that might have prevented the experiments or the death camps." "What needs to be done" he added, is:

to fashion a moral philosophy to undergird the physicians' oath—one that is based in the formation of character in the physician and one that grounds the physician's ethics in the unchanging realities of the relationship between one human being, vulnerable and in distress, and another human being dedicated to helping and healing. (Pellegrino 2010, 15)

Nigel Cameron has also elaborated upon the collapse of "[Judeo-]Christian Hippocratism" and fulminated against the shift of the goal of medicine from healing the patient to relief of suffering by the patient, relatives, or society that enables physician-assisted suicide and euthanasia (Cameron 2001). Autonomy and relief of suffering are the twin engines driving PAS and euthanasia forward.

For the Hippocratic physician committed to the sanctity of life, relief of suffering cannot displace healing as medicine's mission. Healing may often relieve suffering, but not always. And when it does not, a belief in the sanctity of life prevents the Hippocratic physician from relieving suffering by ending a patient's life (Cameron 2001, 129). Similarly, Judaism, while supportive of palliative care, not only obliges physicians to heal their patients but also obliges patients to seek healing, not relief of suffering (Steinberg 2010, 214, 217).

The Medical Profession

Third party involvement with the doctor-patient relationship increased pari passu with increased health care expenditures, particularly Medicare and Medicaid. In his 1992 *Strangers at the Bedside: A History of How Law and Bioethics Transformed Medical Decision Making*, Rothman traced the transformation of the doctor-patient relationship by a third-party army of non-physicians, utilization reviewers, lawyers, government officials, and hospital administrators. Bioethicists, who are more likely to have a PhD, JD, or MA than a medical degree (Guinan 1998), are of particular interest because they possess substantial motivation and/or power to transform the medical profession, particularly its ethics. And while many non-physicians consult, advise, regulate, and legislate, they do not have "skin in the game"—they are neither responsible for making end-of-life decisions, such as PAS and euthanasia, with individual patients, nor do they implement those decisions and live with their consequences.

Kass noted that these third parties provide a new challenge to medicine:

> one that would deny autonomy to the profession because it denies the existence of a medical ethic as such. The challengers insist that what we call "medical ethics" or "the ethics of medicine" is but the application to medicine, as a particular but not unusual instance, of more universal norms of human conduct. (1985, 225).

He suggested that the challengers' "deepest reason for looking beyond medicine to external sources of ethical principles is the widely shared belief that medicine—whether regarded as a science or as an art—is in its essence morally neutral, or as our jargon has it, value free" (1985, 225). He then asked the question, "Are these prevailing opinions true?" and reflected on the answer by an explication of the traditional Hippocratic Oath, in which, Kass claimed, "the medical and the ethical are as hard to separate as the concave and the convex" (1985, 226–228).

Academic medicine has adopted the view Kass criticized. During the Third Reich, academic medicine also adopted views of a prevailing social ideology and distanced itself from its traditions. Dr. William Seidelman, a pioneering student and teacher of medicine after the Holocaust, said, "Today, we need to know more about how academic medicine and science evolved in the last century in Austria and Germany to better understand them and ourselves" (2010, 34). Others like Drs. Joseph Fins (2014), Shmuel Reis and Hedy Wald (2015), Francis Collins (2010), and Edmund Pellegrino have also encouraged medical schools to teach medicine after the Holocaust to prevent today's medical profession from making similar mistakes—"We need to know why because individual and mass defection from ethics still occurs among physicians around the world" (Pellegrino 2010, 11).

Organized medicine seems confused when dealing with pressing bioethical issues of the day such as PAS and euthanasia. Kheriaty described how the California Medical Association, a chapter of the American Medical Association (AMA), changed its position from "opposed" to "neutral" in 2015, thereby hastening the approval of California's End of Life Option Act that permits PAS (2019, 23). Several other state medical societies have also changed their position from opposition to neutrality on PAS (Kheriaty 2019, 24–25). In 2019, the AMA, at the request of the Oregon delegation, reconsidered but ultimately reconfirmed its position that "physician-assisted suicide is fundamentally incompatible with the physician's role as healer" (Kheriaty 2019, 25–26). The AMA also elected to continue using the term "physician-assisted suicide" rather than either "aid in dying" or "death with dignity." The American College of Physicians, the second largest medical association in the United States, also reaffirmed its opposition to PAS in 2017 (Kheriaty 2019, 26).

On the other hand, in 2014, the Canadian Medical Association abandoned its longstanding opposition to PAS and euthanasia and submitted a brief with its new position to the Supreme Court of Canada while it was deciding a case testing the constitutionality of laws prohibiting PAS. The court ultimately declared the laws unconstitutional, thereby enabling passage of a law permitting medical assistance in dying that included both PAS and euthanasia in 2016 (Kheriaty 2019, 26). When the WMA in 2018 responded to pressure to change its position by reaffirming its opposition to both PAS and euthanasia, Canada opted to leave the organization followed by the Royal Dutch Medical Association in 2019 (Kheriaty 2019, 27–28).

When professional medical organizations assume a neutral position on PAS and euthanasia, they are abdicating their responsibilities to both patients and physicians and abstaining on one of the fundamental ethical and political issues of the day (Sulmasy et al. 2018). Even when these organizations state their opposition to PAS and euthanasia but fail to advocate their position in the public square, they are, practically speaking, assuming a neutral position. The resulting political void is eagerly filled by the many strangers at the bedside.

Neutrality creates substantial confusion for patients. If a patient's physician does not actively oppose PAS or euthanasia, the patient might reasonably assume tacit approval, thereby encouraging the patient to choose the procedure as opposed to palliation.

Kheriaty asked a fundamental question, "Should assisted suicide and euthanasia be considered a medical issue in the first place?" (Kheriaty 2019, 34). Halevy also asked, "Why is the physician needed to assist the patient in committing suicide?" (Halevy 1994). In my experience, very few academic physicians and medical educators choose to engage with these fundamental ethical questions, let alone the difficult questions arising from the study of Nazi medicine. For example, I had great difficulty in recruiting European physicians who were willing to speak and write in favor of adult PAS and euthanasia as part of this project examining these practices in light of the Holocaust. Until such time as physicians articulate and advocate a clear position on these vital end-of-life issues, they are leaving their patients, their students, and the medical profession adrift.

PHYSICIAN-ASSISTED SUICIDE AND EUTHANASIA AFTER THE HOLOCAUST

In 2010, in an attempt to educate medical students and professionals, I founded the Center for Medicine after the Holocaust (CMATH) whose mission is "to challenge doctors, nurses, and bioethicists to personally confront the medical ethics of the Holocaust and to apply that knowledge to contemporary practice and research." But CMATH and the United States Holocaust Memorial Museum, which sponsored the extraordinary Deadly Medicine exhibit about Nazi medicine, learned from experience that getting through to physicians and bioethicists requires much more than lectures, papers, books, and exhibits (Shapiro 2013).

By trial and error, CMATH discovered that taking physicians and bioethicists to European medical sites relevant to the Holocaust can have a transformative effect on them. Prior to 2018, however, the number of participants in such trips was limited either by their lack of interest in the material and/or their inability or unwillingness to pay for the trip. CMATH, therefore, fully paid the expenses of the participants in this project and focused the academic exploration on a single aspect of medicine and the Holocaust. We recruited 11 North American and Israeli physicians, all experts in either bioethics or palliative care.

Each of the selected sites visited by the participating physicians in May 2018 was relevant to one or more of the steps that the German medical profession followed down the slippery slope displayed in figure I.1.

> Applied Biology
>> Sterilization Law
>>> Nuremberg Laws
>>>> Child Euthanasia
>>>>> Adult T4 Euthanasia
>>>>>> Wild Euthanasia
>>>>>>> 14f13
>>>>>>>> Medical Experiments
>>>>>>>>> The Final Solution

Figure I.1.   *Created by Sheldon Rubenfeld*

The sites visited were:

- The *Totgeschwiegen* (Hushed Up) exhibition at the former Karl-Bonhoeffer-Nervenklinik from which patients were selected for both compulsory sterilization and involuntary euthanasia
- The *Gedenkstätte für die Opfer der NS-"Euthanasie"* (Memorial for the Victims of Nazi Euthanasia) at Bernburg, a former psychiatric hospital that was one of the six Nazi euthanasia, or killing, centers
- The *Haus der Wannsee-Konferenz Gedenk—und Bildungsstatte* (House of the Wannsee Conference Memorial and Educational Center) where the secret Final Solution of the Jewish Question was divulged to representatives from the relevant Nazi government ministries
- The *Gedenkstätte Sachsenhausen* (Sachsenhausen Memorial and Museum) with its gas chamber, crematorium, and Medical Care and Crime exhibition about medical experiments; also, an important venue for 14f13
- The *Stiftung Denkmal für die ermordeten Juden Europas* (Memorial to the Murdered Jews of Europe) in Berlin
- The *Gedenk- und Informationsort für die Opfer der nationalsozialistischen "Euthanasie" Morde* (Memorial and Information Point for the Victims of National Socialist Euthanasia Killings) in Berlin, at the site of the offices of *Aktion* T4.

Prior to the trip the participants were given reading and viewing assignments about medicine and the Holocaust and about American eugenics. Two German scholars of medicine and the Holocaust, Drs. Gerrit Hohendorf and Astrid Ley, accompanied the American and Canadian physicians throughout the trip. Five additional European scholars lectured at a conference in Berlin on euthanasia during the Third Reich, its historical antecedents, and PAS and euthanasia in Europe today. The European scholars wrote chapters for this book and, after reflecting upon and processing their German experience for eight months, the American, Canadian, and Israeli scholars gathered for a conference at the Houston Methodist Research Institute in January 2019 to present and critique each other's papers before writing their chapters for this book.

Regarding nomenclature, there is always debate about the terminology for end-of-life choices. Two examples will demonstrate the nature of the problem. When writing about the euthanasia programs during the Third Reich, the European scholars often put quotation marks around the word *euthanasia* to indicate that euthanasia in Nazi Germany is not, in their view, the same as euthanasia in today's European nations. Similarly, some American and Canadian scholars object to the term *physician-assisted suicide* and prefer terms like *death with dignity*, *medical assistance in dying*, or *physician-assisted dying*. The reader will note each author's preference in the individual chapters.

Part I begins with two chapters by Hohendorf and one by Roelcke on the history of euthanasia and eugenics in Europe until the end of World War II, followed by Bruns' chapter on the startling fact that the Nazis required medical schools to teach medical ethics. Verhagen then tells the story of euthanasia, with a focus on infant euthanasia, in the Netherlands from the view of a protagonist. In their chapters, Sahm and Müller-Busch make the case against euthanasia in Europe.

Part II focuses on PAS and euthanasia in North America, beginning with Lerner's commentary on what we can and cannot learn from history. Quill, the first American physician to acknowledge and publish his participation in PAS, describes his approach to physician-assisted death and the importance of palliative care. Elbaum and Crawley then highlight the dangers of PAS and euthanasia for African Americans and other marginalized populations; Pearlman describes the difficulties of relying on suffering as the basis for decision-making at the end of life; and Meier focuses on the inner life of physicians, particularly countertransference, when confronted with requests for PAS. In his chapter, Steinberg objects to the fundamental doctrines underlying the principlist approach to bioethics. Downar offers his personal experience with euthanasia in Canada, making the distinction between involuntary eugenic euthanasia and voluntary euthanasia. In their chapters, Kim and Fernandes critique the concepts of human worth and utility in regard to PAS and euthanasia. Prager then describes why the best of physicians are prone to making the gravest mistakes. In his chapter, Kodish issues a spirited call for civil disobedience on the part of the medical profession in opposition to PAS in general and pediatric euthanasia in particular. The book concludes with Sulmasy's philosophical reflection on the behavior of Nazi physicians and its relevance to contemporary bioethics and medicine.

While each chapter stands on its own, the book is best appreciated by reading the chapters sequentially from beginning to end, thereby simulating the experience of the scholars in Germany.

As conveners of the project and editors of the book, Sulmasy and I had four objectives:

1. *To bring the history of medicine and the Holocaust to a new audience.* While some historians of medicine have a clear grasp of the Nazi euthanasia programs, practicing physicians and bioethicists know little if anything about medicine during the Third Reich and, if they do, their knowledge is often limited to unethical medical experiments and the Nuremberg Code.
2. *To explore this history from the perspective of biomedical ethics.* Other accounts have looked to the psychology of participating physicians but not to the underlying moral justifications for the atrocities perpetrated by the German medical profession, especially the euthanasia programs. For instance, because it has not been translated from the German, very few English speakers are aware of the Nazi medical ethics textbook by physician Rudolf Ramm who put forth serious ethical arguments for the practice of euthanasia. Involuntary euthanasia was neither the work of a lunatic fringe nor of physicians coerced by Nazis into carrying out these programs—German physicians were not pawns; rather, they thought of themselves as ethical pioneers in justifying and implementing various programs, including euthanasia.
3. *To delve into the pre-Nazi arguments for euthanasia.* These include the hermeneutical approach to medicine that was current in the early twentieth century before the Nazis took power, as well as popular ideas about technology, suffering, control, and eugenics. We sought to show how these arguments supported the development and implementation of the Nazi euthanasia programs.
4. *To explore possible continuities between the justifications that undergirded the Nazi euthanasia programs and contemporary calls for PAS and euthanasia.* Is the voluntary/involuntary distinction sufficient to mark a moral difference? Is it sufficient as a safeguard in public policy? What evidence was there of a "slippery slope" then, and can it tell us something about the use of such arguments today? Is the use of historical analogy between the present time and the Nazi period simply offensive, or can it be explored rationally? What are the limits of such a method? What can be learned?

The editors believe that that there are definite, instructive continuities between the justifications and hermeneutical approach to medicine offered for the Nazi euthanasia programs and the contemporary justifications and hermeneutical approach to medicine offered for legalization of PAS in the United States and euthanasia in Canada and Europe. While the authors and editors recognize that there are important discontinuities, to the extent that an edited volume can do so, this book argues that, at the very least, the continuities are sufficiently important that we exercise caution in legalizing PAS and euthanasia. Some will go further and suggest that the lesson to be drawn from these continuities ought to be that we prohibit legalization of PAS and euthanasia.

I conclude with a tale told by Dr. William Seidelman about a timeless symbol of medicine and its ethical spirit (Seidelman 1992, 278–279). The Greek Island of Kos is not only home to the remains of a temple to the Greek god of medicine, Aescelapius, but it is also the birthplace of Hippocrates, the father of medicine who created the paradigm of the ethical physician. On July 20, 1944, the 120 Jews of Kos were transported first to the Greek mainland and ultimately to Auschwitz, where the Jews of Hippocrates' birthplace were met on the ramp by the professional descendants of Hippocrates. Those licensed physicians made a "medical" judgment regarding all of the Jews of Kos, that they represented "useless life" and should receive the "Great Therapy of Auschwitz." They all perished ("Holocaust in Greece" n.d.).

Today on the island of Kos, its synagogue stands empty, adjacent to the ancient plane tree under the branches of which, legend has it, Hippocrates taught. These juxtaposed symbols point to the spiritual crisis of medicine arising from the Holocaust, a crisis that medicine has failed to recognize, let alone resolve (Seidelman cited in Caplan 1992). We hope our book will be one small step toward that recognition and resolution.

BIBLIOGRAPHY

Alexander, Leo. 1949. "Medical Science under Dictatorship." *New England Journal of Medicine* 241, no. 2 (July): 39–47.

American Association of Medical Colleges. n.d. "Modern, Shortened Version of the Hippocratic Oath." Accessed December 10, 2019. https://aamc-orange.global .ssl.fastly.net/production/media/filer_public/f6/a1/f6a124ce-94e7-43d2-bd96 -7bb35405b908/lessononeoath.pdf.

American College of Physicians. n.d. "Sir William Osler and Internal Medicine." Accessed December 10, 2019. https://www.acponline.org/about-acp/about-internal -medicine/sir-william-osler-and-internal-medicine.

American Journal of Psychology (The). 1901. *The American Journal of Psychology* Vol. 12, No. 2 (January). DOI: 10.2307/1412550.

Annas, George J., and Michael A. Grodin. 1992. *The Nazi Doctors and the Nuremberg Code: Human Rights in Human Experimentation.* New York: Oxford University Press.

Association of American Physicians and Surgeons. n.d. "Physician Oaths." Accessed December 10, 2019. https://www.aapsonline.org/ethics/oaths.htm#bears.

Beauchamp, Tom L. 2014. "In the Shadow of Nuremberg: Unlearned Lessons from the Medical Trial." In *Human Subjects Research after the Holocaust*, edited by Sheldon Rubenfeld and Susan Benedict, 175–194. New York: Springer.

Beauchamp, Tom L., and James F. Childress. 2001. *Principles of Biomedical Ethics*, 5th ed. New York: Oxford University Press.

Beecher, Henry K. 1966. "Ethics and Clinical Research." *New England Journal of Medicine* 27, no. 4 (June): 1354–1360. DOI: 10.1056/NEJM196606162742405.

Binding, Karl, and Alfred Hoche. (1920) 1992. *Permitting the Destruction of Life Unworthy of Life: Its Extent and Form.* Leipzig: Verlag von Felix Meiner (1920). Translated by W. E. Wright, in *Issues in Law and Medicine* 8 (Fall): 231–265.

Black, Edwin. 2003. *War Against the Weak: Eugenics and America's Campaign to Create a Master Race.* New York: Four Walls Eight Windows.

Brody, Howard. 2014. "The Origins and Impact of the Nuremberg Doctors' Trial." In *Human Subjects Research after the Holocaust*, edited by Sheldon Rubenfeld and Susan Benedict, 163–173. New York: Springer.

Cameron, Nigel M. de S. 2001. *The New Medicine: Life and Death after Hippocrates.* Chicago: The Bioethics Press.

Carrick, Paul. 2001. *Medical Ethics in the Ancient World.* Washington, DC: Georgetown University Press.

Collins, Francis S. 2010. Foreword: "This Past Must Not Be Prologue." In *Medicine after the Holocaust: From the Master Race to the Human Genome and Beyond*, edited by Sheldon Rubenfeld, xix-xxi. New York: Palgrave Macmillan.

Cordell, Eugene F. 1904. "The Importance of the Study of the History of Medicine." *Medical Library and Historical Journal*, 2, no. 4 (October): 269–282.

DeBakey, Michael. 2008. Interview of Michael DeBakey, by Sheldon Rubenfeld, May 16, 2008. Distinguished Speaker Videos. http://www.medicineaftertheholo caust.org/interview-of-dr-michael-e-debakey-may-16-2008/.

DeBakey, Michael. 2010. Afterword. In *Medicine after the Holocaust: From the Master Race to the Human Genome and Beyond*, edited by Sheldon Rubenfeld, 221–223. New York: Palgrave Macmillan.

Edelstein, Ludwig. 1943. *The Hippocratic Oath: Text, Translation and Interpretation.* Baltimore, MD: Johns Hopkins University Press.

Faden, Ruth R. (Chair), et al. 1996. *The Human Radiation Experiments: Final Report of the President's Advisory Committee.* New York: Oxford University Press.

Fins, Joseph J. 2014. "Teaching the Holocaust to Medical Students: A Reflection on Pedagogy and Medical Ethics." In *Human Subjects Research after the Holocaust*, edited by Sheldon Rubenfeld and Susan Benedict, 269–282. New York: Springer.

Flexner, Abraham. 1910. "Medical Education in the United States and Canada: A Report to the Carnegie Foundation for the Advancement of Teaching." Bulletin Number Four. New York: Carnegie Foundation.

Frewer, Andreas. 2010. "Human Rights from the Nuremberg Doctors Trial to the Geneva Declaration. Persons and Institutions in Medical Ethics and History." *Medicine, Health Care and Philosophy* 13, no. 3 (August): 259–268. DOI 10.1007/s11019-010-9247-2.

Friedlander, Henry. 1995. *The Origins of Nazi Genocide: From Euthanasia to the Final Solution.* Chapel Hill: University of North Carolina Press.

From Our Regular Correspondent. July 31, 1933. "Berlin." *Journal of the American Medical Association* 100 (July): 866–867.

From Our Regular Correspondent. January 8, 1934. "Berlin." *Journal of the American Medical Association* 102 (January): 630–631.

German Medical Association. 2012. "In Remembrance of the Victims of Nazi Medicine, Nuremberg, May 2012." *Israel Medical Association Journal* 14, no. 9 (September): 529–530.

Guinan, Patrick D. 1998. "Has Medicine Lost the Ethics Battle?" *The Linacre Quarterly* 65, no. 2 (May): 43–50. https://doi.org/10.1080/00243639.1998.11878411.

Halevy, Amir. 1994. "The Missing Link: The Physician and Assisted Suicide." *Bioethics Forum* 10, no. 2 (Spring): 14–16.

Heller, Jean. 1972. "Participating Doctor Says Syphilitics Not Told of Experiment." *Birmingham News*, July 27, 1972.

Hohendorf, Gerrit. 2014. "The Sewering Affair." In *Silence, Scapegoats, Self-Reflection: The Shadow of Nazi Medical Crimes on Medicine and Bioethics*, edited by Volker Roelcke, Sascha Topp, and Etienne Lepicard, 131–146. Göttingen, Germany: V&R unipress.

"Holocaust in Greece, The." n.d. United States Holocaust Memorial Museum website. Accessed December 11, 2019. https://www.ushmm.org/m/pdfs/20130305-holocaust-in-greece.pdf.

Horowitz, David. 2018. *Dark Agenda: The War to Destroy Christian America.* West Palm Beach, FL: Humanix Books.

Jacobsen, Annie. 2014. *Operation Paperclip: The Secret Intelligence Program that Brought Nazi Scientists to America.* New York: Little, Brown and Company.

Johns Hopkins Medicine. n.d. "The Four Founding Fathers." Accessed December 10, 2019. https://www.hopkinsmedicine.org/about/history/history5.html.

Jouanna, Jacques. 1999. *Hippocrates.* Baltimore, MD: Johns Hopkins University Press.

Kass, Leon R. 1985. *Toward A More Natural Science: Biology and Human Affairs.* New York: The Free Press.

Kater, Michael H. 1989. *Doctors under Hitler.* Chapel Hill: University of North Carolina Press.

Katz, Jay. 1992. "The Consent Principle of the Nuremberg Code: Its Significance Then and Now." In *The Nazi Doctors and the Nuremberg Code: Human Rights in Human Experimentation*, edited by George J. Annas and Michael A. Grodin, 227–239. New York: Oxford University Press.

Kheriaty, Aaron. 2019. "First, Take No Stand." *The New Atlantis: A Journal of Technology and Science*, No. 59 (Summer): 22–35.

Levine, Maurice. 1972. *Psychiatry and Ethics.* New York: George Braziller.

Ley, Astrid, and Annette Hinz-Wessels, eds. 2012. *The "Euthanasia Institution" of Brandenburg an der Havel: Murder of the Ill and Handicapped during National Socialism*. Berlin: Metropol.

Lifton, Robert Jay. 1986. *The Nazi Doctors: Medical Killing and the Psychology of Genocide*. New York: Basic Books.

Ludmerer, Kenneth M. 1985. *Learning to Heal: The Development of American Medical Education*. Baltimore, MD: Johns Hopkins University Press.

Marrus, Michael R. 1999. "The Nuremberg Doctors' Trial in Historical Context." *Bulletin of the History of Medicine* 73, no. 1 (Spring): 106–123.

McKim, W. Duncan. 1900. *Human Heredity and Progress*. London: G. P. Putnam.

National Commission for the Protection of Human Subjects of Biomedical and Behavioral Research. 1979. *The Belmont Report*. Washington, DC: U.S. Department of Health and Human Services. Accessed December 11, 2019. https://www.hhs.gov/ohrp/regulations-and-policy/belmont-report/read-the-belmont-report/index.html.

Nevins, Michael. 2010. *Abraham Flexner: A Flawed American Icon*. Bloomington, IN: iUniverse.

Nutton, Vivian. 2013. *Ancient Medicine*. New York: Routledge.

Orr, Robert D., Norman Pang, Edmund D. Pellegrino, and Mark Siegler. 1997. "Use of the Hippocratic Oath: A Review of Twentieth Century Practice and a Content Analysis of Oaths Administered in Medical Schools in the US and Canada in 1993." *Journal of Clinical Ethics* 8, no. 4 (Winter): 377–388.

Osler, William. 1962. "Sir William Osler: On Full-Time Clinical Teaching in Medical Schools." *Canadian Medical Association Journal* 87, no. 14 (October): 762–765.

Peabody, Francis W. 1927. *The Care of the Patient*. Cambridge, MA: Harvard University Press.

Pellegrino, Edmund D. 2010. "When Evil Was Good and Good Evil: Remembrances of Nuremberg." In *Medicine after the Holocaust: From the Master Race to the Human Genome and Beyond*, edited by Sheldon Rubenfeld, 11–16. New York: Palgrave Macmillan.

Presidential Commission for the Study of Bioethical Issues. 2011. "Ethically Impossible" STD Research in Guatemala from 1946 to 1948. Washington, DC: U.S. Government Printing Office. Accessed December 10, 2019. https://bioethicsarchive.georgetown.edu/pcsbi/sites/default/files/Ethically%20Impossible%20(with%20linked%20historical%20documents)%202.7.13.pdf.

Proctor, Robert N. 1988. *Racial Hygiene: Medicine Under the Nazis*. Cambridge, MA: Harvard University Press.

Proctor, Robert N. 1999. *The Nazi War on Cancer*. Princeton, NJ: Princeton University Press.

Proctor, Robert N. 2000. "Nazi Science and Nazi Medical Ethics: Some Myths and Misconceptions." *Perspectives in Biology and Medicine* 43, no. 3 (Spring): 335–346. 10.1353/pbm.2000.0024.

Rachels, James. 1990. *Created from Animals: The Moral Implications of Darwinism*. New York: Oxford University Press.

Reis, Shmuel P., and Hedy S. Wald. 2015. "Contemplating Medicine during the Third Reich: Scaffolding Professional Identity Formation for Medical Students." *Academic Medicine* 90, no. 6 (June): 770–773. doi: 10.1097/ACM.0000000000000716.

Roelcke, Volker. 2014a. "Between Professional Honor and Self-Reflection: The German Medical Association's Reluctance to Address Medical Malpractice during the National Socialist Era, ca. 1985–2012." In *Silence, Scapegoats, Self-Reflection: The Shadow of Nazi Medical Crimes on Medicine and Bioethics*, edited by Volker Roelcke, Sascha Topp, and Etienne Lepicard, 243–278. Göttingen, Germany: V&R unipress.

Roelcke, Volker. 2014b. "Sulfonamide Experiments on Prisoners in Nazi Concentration Camps: Coherent Scientific Rationality Combined with Complete Disregard of Humanity." In *Human Subjects Research after the Holocaust*, edited by Sheldon Rubenfeld and Susan Benedict, 51–66. New York: Springer.

Rothman, David J. 1992. *Strangers at the Bedside: A History of How Law and Bioethics Transformed Medical Decision Making*. New York: Basic Books.

Rütten, Thomas. 2006. "Ludwig Edelstein at the Crossroads of 1933. On the Inseparability of Life, Work, and Their Reverberations." *Early Science and Medicine* 11, no. 1(January): 50–99. doi.org/10.1163/157338206775569772.

Schmidt, Ulf. 2007. *Karl Brandt: The Nazi Doctor*. New York: Hambledon Continuum.

Seidelman, William E. 1992. "'Medspeak'" for Murder: The Nazi Experience and the Culture of Medicine." In *When Medicine Went Mad: Bioethics and the Holocaust*, edited by Arthur L. Caplan, 271–279. Totowa, NJ: Humana Press.

Seidelman, William E. 1999. "From the Danube to the Spree: Deception, Truth and Morality in Medicine." In Dokumentationsarchiv des österreichischen Widerstandes, edited by S. Ganglmair, 15–32. Freistadt: Ploechl-Druck.

Seidelman, William E. 2010. "Academic Medicine during the Nazi Period: The Implications for Creating Awareness of Professional Responsibility Today." In *Medicine after the Holocaust: From the Master Race to the Human Genome and Beyond*, edited by Sheldon Rubenfeld, 29–36. New York: Palgrave Macmillan.

Shapiro, Paul. 2013. Personal communication with Paul Shapiro, former Director of the USHMM's Center for Advanced Holocaust Studies, and Sheldon Rubenfeld, July 2013.

Singer, Peter. 1993. *Practical Ethics*. Cambridge, UK: Cambridge University Press.

Singer, Peter. 2002. *Unsanctifying Human Life*. Malden, MA: Blackwell.

Singer, Peter. 2003. *Pushing Time Away: My Grandfather and the Tragedy of Jewish Vienna*. New York: HarperCollins.

Steinberg, Avraham. 2010. "Jewish Medical Ethics and Risky Treatments." In *Medicine after the Holocaust: From the Master Race to the Human Genome and Beyond*, edited by Sheldon Rubenfeld, 213–220. New York: Palgrave Macmillan.

Sulmasy, Daniel P., Ilora Finlay, Faith Fitzgerald, Kathleen Foley, Richard Payne, and Mark Siegler. 2018. "Physician-Assisted Suicide: Why Neutrality by Organized Medicine is Neither Neutral Nor Appropriate." *Journal of General Internal Medicine* 33, no. 8 (August): 1394–1399. doi: 10.1007/s11606-018-4424-8.

U.S. Supreme Court.1963. *School District of Abington Township, Pennsylvania v. Schempp*. 374 U.S. 203 (1963). https://www.law.cornell.edu/supremecourt/text/374/203#writing-USSC_CR_0374_0203_ZD.

U.S. Supreme Court. 1973. *Roe v. Wade*. 410 U.S. 113 (1973). Accessed December 11, 2019. https://cdn.loc.gov/service/ll/usrep/usrep410/usrep410113/usrep410113.pdf.

Veatch, Robert M., and Carol G. Mason. 1987. "Hippocratic vs. Judeo-Christian Medical Ethics: Principles in Conflict." *The Journal of Religious Ethics* 15, no. 1 (Spring): 86–105.

von Staden, Heinrich. 1996. "'In a Pure and Holy Way': Personal and Professional Conduct in the Hippocratic Oath?" *Journal of the History of Medicine and Allied Sciences* 51, no. 4 (October): 404–437.

Weikart, Richard. 2004. *From Darwin to Hitler: Evolutionary Ethics, Eugenics, and Racism in Germany*. New York: Palgrave Macmillan.

Weindling, Paul J. 2004. *Nazi Medicine and the Nuremberg Trials: From Medical War Crimes to Informed Consent*. New York: Palgrave Macmillan.

Weindling, Paul J. 2010. *John W. Thompson: Psychiatrist in the Shadow of the Holocaust*. Rochester, NY: University of Rochester Press.

Weindling, Paul J. 2015. *Victims and Survivors of Nazi Human Experiments: Science and Suffering in the Holocaust*. New York: Bloomsbury Academic.

Weinke, Annette. 2014. "Judging Medical Crimes in Divided Germany." In *Silence, Scapegoats, Self-Reflection: The Shadow of Nazi Medical Crimes on Medicine and Bioethics*, edited by Volker Roelcke, Sascha Topp, and Etienne Lepicard, 87–99. Göttingen, Germany: V&R unipress.

Weiss, Sheila Faith. 1987. *Race Hygiene and National Efficiency: The Eugenics of Wilhelm Schallmayer*. Berkeley: University of California Press.

Wheatley, Steven C. 1988. *The Politics of Philanthropy: Abraham Flexner and Medical Education*. Madison: University of Wisconsin Press.

Part I

THE HISTORY AND CURRENT STATUS OF PHYSICIAN-ASSISTED SUICIDE AND EUTHANASIA IN EUROPE

Chapter One

On a Slippery Slope

The Historical Debate on Euthanasia in Germany

Gerrit Hohendorf

Euthanasia was not a National Socialist invention. In this chapter, I will first depict the history of the term *euthanasia*, and then the development of the slippery slope from mercy killing at the end of the nineteenth century to the National Socialist annihilation of "life unworthy of living" (von Engelhardt, 2010; Benzenhöfer 1999, 77–108; Hohendorf 2016).

EUTHANASIA IN ANTIQUITY

The term *euthanasia*—Greek for *good death*—probably was first used in the fifth century BCE by the Greek comic poet Cratinus (Benzenhöfer 1999, 13–76). In the second century BCE, Pollux quoted Cratinus, ". . . but it would happen to those, to be deathly ill, as Herodotus died with difficulty, whereas Cratinus spoke of a good death," indicating that in Greek antiquity, a good death meant dying easily as opposed to a difficult death from a terminal illness (Benzenhöfer 1999, 15). The ancients also characterized the time of death as either favorable or unfavorable. Thus, when the Greek comic poet Menander (342–292 BCE) used the term *euthanasia*, he meant "to depart by a good death" at the right moment, before age and illness make life unbearable (Benzenhöfer 1999,16).

And so a good death belongs to the worthy ambitions of the Hellenistic Stoic philosophers, as expressed on this anonymous fragment from the third century BCE: "Having a good age as well as a good death means namely to live toward decline at the right time, with whatever age, but dying a good death means expiring in the right way with whatever death" (Benzenhöfer

1999, 18). According to Stoic philosophy, whose goal is imperturbability and serenity in the face of all that can befall one in life, a good death means not so much a specific time or mode of death, but rather the manner in which the wise person anticipates death (Dowbiggin 2005, 8).

The death of Caesar Augustus, portrayed by historian Suetonius in an idealized form, was considered an exemplary good death. Augustus, overcome with diarrhea on a journey through the south of Italy, died easily and painlessly in the arms of his wife, surrounded by his friends (Benzenhöfer 1999, 20–21).

Euthanasia can also indicate an honorable death in battle, thereby avoiding the ignominy of falling into the hands of the enemy. Greek historian Polybius (200–115 BCE) gave an account of Spartan king Cleomenes, who was captured in Alexandria and, after escaping a failed uprising, took his own life so as not to fall into the hands of his enemies (Benzenhöfer 1999, 18–19).

Although we generally know little about the medical treatment of incurably ill or dying people in ancient medicine, the term *euthanasia* had no specific medical meaning in antiquity; it was not linked to the question of medical treatment of dying people or ending of life by physicians, whether it be in the form of killing on request or in the form of assisted suicide. Benzenhöfer noted that in the *Corpus Hippocraticum*, the collection of Greek medical texts from the fourth century BCE attributed to legendary physician Hippocrates, there were differing views on whether physicians should treat incurably ill people. On the one hand, because of the limited scope of medical art and the potential harm to one's reputation, treating them was considered unwise. Other texts, like the piece "On the Diseases," explicitly called for medical care for incurably ill people and, in their treatment, attending to the "greatest possible benefit," indicating that there were already approaches for palliative treatment of incurably ill people and care for the dying in ancient times (1999, 39).

The Hippocratic Oath takes an unambiguous stand on the question of medically assisted suicide: "Neither will I administer a poison to anybody when asked to do so, nor will I suggest such a course" (Hippocratic Oath 1923). However, the history of the development, prevalence, and binding character of the moral obligations formulated in the Hippocratic Oath in ancient medicine is not clear. The text was certainly not penned by the historical figure Hippocrates, and its origin can be traced at the earliest to the Hellenistic period in the third century BCE (Edelstein 1943). The fact that a Hippocratic medical community explicitly distanced itself from physician-assisted suicide and abortion confirms that both procedures occurred in antiquity. For example, in 65 CE, physician Statius Annaeus assisted his friend Lucius Seneca with his suicide (which perhaps is better described as a self-administered death sentence ordered by Nero). Seneca was a Stoic philosopher who justified suicide under certain conditions. In his seventieth letter to Lucilius, he wrote:

> The best thing which eternal law ever ordained was that it allowed to us one entrance into life, but many exits. Must I await the cruelty either of disease or of man, when I can depart through the midst of torture, and shake off my troubles? This is the one reason why we cannot complain of life; it keeps no one against his will. (Seneca 1920; Benzenhöfer 1999, 35)

Plato, in contrast to Aristotle, also considered suicide permissible under certain, narrow constraints, namely when God deems it necessary, meaning when a situation has become hopeless due to illness or fate (Plato's "Phaedo" 1871, 379–468). Plato's Socrates further rejects medical treatment to prolong unnecessarily the wretched lives of the weak and infirm who are no longer useful to the community in the ideal state, saying that Asclepius, the god of healing, did not attempt to cure

> bodies which disease had penetrated through and through he would not have attempted to cure by gradual processes of evacuation and infusion: he did not want to lengthen out useless lives, or to raise up puny offspring to an enfeebled sire;—if a man was not able to live in the ordinary way he had no business to cure him; this was all in the interest of the state. (Plato, "The Republic, III" 1871, 234; Benzenhöfer 1999, 29)

Plato also advised that only the offspring of the best should be raised, ". . . for this is the only way of keeping the flock in prime condition . . . but the offspring of the inferior, or of the better when they chance to be deformed, they will conceal in some mysterious, unknown place" ("The Republic, V," 1871, 290–291; Benzenhöfer 1999, 31–32). Plato's eugenic policy prescriptions provide justification for the Spartan infanticide described by Roman writer Plutarch (75 CE):

> Offspring was not reared at the will of the father, but was taken and carried by him to a place called Lesche, where the elders of the tribes officially examined the infant, and if it was well-built and sturdy, they ordered the father to rear it, and assigned it one of the 9000 lots of land; but if it was ill-born and deformed, they sent it to the so-called Apothetae, a chasm-like place at the foot of Mount Taygetus. (Benzenhöfer 1999, 14)

Although Plutarch's report may be unreliable (Grubbs and Parkin 2013, 83–88), contradictory trends in dealing with illness and disabilities were present in antiquity. While some philosophers opposed suicide and euthanasia, and the Hippocratic Oath rejected both physician-assisted suicide and euthanasia, there were simultaneous efforts to link end-of-life decision-making to criteria of curability and beginning-of-life decision-making to the perception of a baby's health or infirmity soon after birth. Both at the beginning and at the end of life, the perceived usefulness of each individual for society was decisive.

EUTHANASIA IN THE MIDDLE AGES

While euthanasia elicited contradictory responses from philosophers in antiquity, it played no role in the Christian medieval tradition, as death itself had nothing good about it and must be overcome. According to the *ars moriendi* tradition, the dying person, accompanied by a minister and strengthened by the sacraments of confession, the Eucharist, and the last rites, may resist the demonic temptations of the hour of death, confess their deadly sins, and persevere in the faith (Reinis 2010). By believing in *Christus medicus*, the savior, an ailing person in the Middle Ages could share in Christ's suffering and, in this way, attain everlasting life. Suicide as an escape from earthly suffering was denied believers at least since the time of Augustine—life and death lay not in the hands of the medical profession, but in God's hands alone (Decher 1999, 29–40).

In the Jewish tradition as well, human life was and is considered of incomparable valuable. *Halakhah* (Jewish law) forbids interference in the natural process of dying. The life of the dying person should neither be shortened nor artificially prolonged. Citing ancient rabbinic sources, Dr. Abraham S. Abraham summarized Judaism's position:

> It is also forbidden to hasten his death, for example, when the period of dying is long drawn out, it is forbidden to remove the pillow or cushion from under him because it is said that the feathers of certain fowl cause a prolongation of dying. Similarly, he should not be moved from where he is lying. However if there is something external to the patient or on his body that prevents his soul from leaving him, it may be removed, since by doing so one does not do a positive action to shorten his life, but merely removes an impediment to his dying" (Abraham 2003, 319, 326–327).

With the advent of the Renaissance and Humanism, attitudes toward death, suffering, and incurable illness changed. Physical suffering was no longer understood as participation in the suffering of Christ and a path to everlasting life. On the contrary, a few philosophers argued that people could end their own lives when they suffered unbearably and became a burden to themselves (and society). For example, the Scottish enlightenment philosopher David Hume (1777) justified suicide as an act of human freedom. Thomas More's position is unclear but could be interpreted as a plea for self-administered euthanasia of the incurable sick. In *Utopia*, his popular satirical novel published in 1516, he described an ideal society:

> I have already told you with what Care they look after their Sick, so that nothing is left undone that can contribute either to their Ease or Health: And for those who are taken with fixed and incurable Diseases, they use all possible ways to cherish them, and to make their Lives as comfortable as may be: They visit them often, and take great pains to make their time pass off easily: But when any is taken with a torturing and lingering Pain, so that there is no Hope either of Recovery or Ease, the Priests and Magistrates come and exhort them, that since they are now unable to go on with the Business of Life, and are become a Burden to themselves, and to all about them, so that they have really out-lived themselves, they would no longer nourish such a rooted Distemper, but would choose rather to die, since they cannot live, but in much Misery; being assured that if they either deliver themselves from their Prison and Torture, or are willing that others should do it, they shall be happy after their Death. (1737, 94–95; see also Benzenhöfer 1999, 61–66)

In 1605, English statesman and philosopher Francis Bacon both revitalized the ancient term *euthanasia* and differentiated *euthanasia exterior*, easing the process of dying as a duty of the physician, from *euthanasia interior*, a person's mental preparation for dying in a spiritual context. While not urging that physicians should end patients' lives deliberately, Bacon's euthanasia called on physicians to make the passage from this life to the next as gentle as possible, using analgesics when necessary (1605/1904, 163; Roelcke 2006, 34–35; Benzenhöfer 1999, 66–69). Bacon's euthanasia exterior did not, however, find a place in the medical literature of the early modern era.

EUTHANASIA IN EARLY MODERN TIMES

Death in early modern times was often preceded by unbearable suffering characterized, for example, by pain, nausea, vomiting, and shortness of breath. Because many people died alone, penniless, and homeless, without support from their family or friends, the wish for an easy death is all too understandable (Stolberg 2011, 96–103). In his 1723 dissertation "De mortis cura," Georg Christoph Detharding spoke of a *euthanasia palliative*, a manner of death preferred by the dying (and by bystanders) in which they "would not have a difficult end, go to sleep etc." and could "die gently" (1723, 84–85; Stolberg 2011, 43). In the seventeenth and eighteenth centuries, the notion of *euthanasia medica*, or a gentle death provided by physicians, gained favor, including withholding unnecessary and senseless treatments and prescribing analgesics such as nightshade, hemlock, henbane, and above all, laudanum, or a tincture of opium (Stolberg 2011, 52–53; Schilling 2011; Nolte 2010). In contrast, because prognosis was unpredictable, around 1723 Dr. Hans Heinrich Helcher insisted that physicians fight for their patients' lives to the end (Stolberg 2011, 57–67, 77–83).

In 1794, Leiden medical professor Nicolaus Paradys spoke of *euthanasia naturalis*, the "art of making death as easy, as bearable as possible." If the terminal nature of the disease was certain and death was imminent, then life-extending medication could be suspended and all efforts could be made to ease death. In addition to easing the dying process with medication, spiritual support should be provided to achieve "such necessary peace of mind," a prescription that sounds very much like contemporary palliative care (Paradys 1796, 571; Roelcke 2006, 36–37). Even though physicians of that age may have been confronted with patient requests for euthanasia (in the contemporary sense of deliberately hastening death as an act of mercy), their published stance toward these wishes was clearly negative until the end of the eighteenth century (Stolberg 2011, 73–74).

In the first half of the nineteenth century, two German physicians, Karl Georg Theodor Kortum and Christian Ludwig Mursinna, admitted to euthanizing incurable, suffering patients (Stolberg 2007, 2008). Faced with his consumptive patient's struggle with death, Kortum wrote in 1800, "and is there anything left to wish for such a sick person other than a quick resolution, as gentle as possible? [. . .] A moderate dose of poppy juice, e.g., 20 drops *Laudanum liq.*, infallibly shortens such agony by extinguishing the weak vital flame entirely, and it is, in my opinion, morally permitted in such cases" (quoted in Stolberg 2011, 157).

EUTHANASIA IN GERMANY BEFORE WORLD WAR I

In 1895, Adolf Jost, a young philosophy student who gained attention as a psychologist with his studies on memory and learning, published *The Right to Die* in which he connected the right of the individual to end his life to pity for those with hopeless suffering, whether they were able or unable to request euthanasia (Schmuhl 1992; Schwartz 1998; Hohendorf 2013; Grosse-Vehne 2005; Grübler 2007):

> When we see someone with an incurable illness writhing in his bed in unspeak-
> able pain, with the bleak prospect of languishing for perhaps months more, with
> no hope of recovery, when we walk through the rooms of an asylum and see the
> madman or the paralytic with all the sympathy of which man is capable, then

despite all absorbed preconceptions the thought must enter our heads, do these people not have a right to die, does human society not have a duty to give them as painless a death as possible? (Jost 1895, 6; Lorey 1908, 183f)

Jost promoted a utilitarian, objective, and quantitative assessment of the value of a human life to society. If the value of a human life is negative, then the state can utilize the right to die for those lives that have no use to either the individual or society. Jost suffered from encephalitis and died in 1908 in the Sorau Mental Hospital.

Also in 1895, physician and eugenicist Alfred Ploetz wrote in *Grundlinien einer Rassenhygiene Teil 1* (*The Basics of Racial Hygiene, Part 1*): "If [despite all regulations of human breeding] it turns out that a newborn is a weak and defective child, the council of physicians which decides on the living right in society will carry out a gentle death, let's say with a little dose of morphine" (1895, 144). Social Darwinists of the late nineteenth century devalued the lives of adults with incurable illnesses when they no longer produced any profit for society; only healthy people who excelled in the daily "struggle for life" should have a right to exist, while those of minor value should disappear from the *Volkskörper* (the nation's body). For example, Ernst Haeckel in 1870 was, according to Weikart (2004, 146), among the earliest advocates of eugenics, infanticide, and killing the unfit in *The Natural History of Creation*. In his 1904 *Die Lebenswunder* (*The Wonders of Life*), Haeckel advocated voluntary mercy killing of incurably ill people who requested it and involuntary mercy killing of the mentally insane who were allegedly artificially kept alive in asylums without any profit for society (1904, 134).

In 1913, Haeckel's *Monistenbund* (*Monist League*), which advocated a secular world view based on natural law, hosted an intense debate about euthanasia (Burleigh 1994, 13). Its weekly journal, *Das Monistiche Jahrhundert* (*The Monistic Century*), published Roland Gerkan's legislative proposal: "Anyone who has an incurable illness has the right to be assisted to die [. . .]." Gerkan was suffering from lung disease and felt useless: "Allied to all this is the painful awareness that I am a heavy burden on my family. Although the sacrifices of time, capacity for work and money were gladly given to me with loving devotion—I nevertheless remain a harmful parasite" (Gerkan 1913, 173). By choosing the term *parasite*, Gerkan echoed Friedrich Nietzsche in his 1889 *Götzendämmerung* (*Twilight of the Idols*):

The sick man is a parasite of society. In certain cases it is indecent to live any longer. It should receive deep contempt from society to vegetate in cowardly dependency upon physicians and their practices after the meaning of life and the right to live have gone. It should be the duty of the physicians to impart this contempt [. . .]. (Nietzsche 1889, 108)

Thus, by the turn of the twentieth century, in certain secular and Social Darwinist circles, the right to die applied equally to patients capable of requesting euthanasia and to patients incapable of making the request—especially defective newborns and the institutionalized, incurably mentally ill—in which case the state could mandate death based upon the value of a life determined by its biological and economic utility to society. On an emotional level, the right to die was motivated by a pity that concealed contempt for suffering. Nonetheless, the German legislature and the medical profession prohibited "killing on request." For example, Martin Mendelsohn, a Berlin professor of medicine and nursing, wrote in 1898 in the well-known *Encyclopedia of Therapy*: "The strict prohibition of shortening life on request makes perfect euthanasia in a significant way difficult. But even though pity and empathy may urge the physician [. . .] never ever may the alleviation of suffering be carried out at the expense of life."

ANNIHILATING LIFE UNWORTHY OF LIVING IN THE WEIMAR REPUBLIC

The debate on euthanasia changed radically after World War I. In 1920, noted criminal lawyer Karl Binding and well-known psychiatrist Alfred Hoche posed and answered this question in *Die Freigabe der Vernichtung lebensunwerten Lebens* (*The Permission to Annihilate Life Unworthy of Living*): "*Are there human lives that have lost the quality of legal protection so much that their continuation has permanently lost all value for the living being and for society?*" (Binding and Hoche 1920, 27, 51; 2006, 26, 48; italics in original; Naucke 2006).

Binding began his sophisticated juridical argumentation with an individual's right to die—because man is sovereign over his life, the state may not prohibit suicide, a choice whose moral legitimation depends on the value the life to be ended has for either the individual or for society. Binding postulated that there exist lives unworthy of living both from the subjective perspective of the individual who wants to end his irremediable suffering and from the objective perspective of society that wants relief from the burden of these unproductive and costly lives. In consequence, these lives do not deserve the protection the state normally guarantees its citizens and their termination is, according to Binding, a "duty of lawful pity" (1920, 30–31). By conceptualizing certain lives as life unworthy of living, Binding and Hoche encouraged not only voluntary euthanasia for patients with an incurable illness or who awaken from an unconscious state to a nameless misery, but also nonvoluntary euthanasia of the "mentally dead" who lead a "ballast existence" in institutions (1920, 30–31). Hoche added psychiatric support for this negative anthropology of a large institutionalized subpopulation: they lack self-consciousness; the "mentally dead" have no relationship to people around them; they are incapable of productive work; and they fully depend on public support and care. In sum, they have neither the will to live nor to die, and so killing them would not be wrong or illegal (1920, 51–59).

Many influential lawyers and academic physicians in the Weimar Republic discussed Binding and Hoche's controversial essays (Schwartz 1998, 626–631; Hohendorf 2013, 53–63). For example, eugenicist physician and geneticist Fritz Lenz, who was a follower of Ploetz, co-edited the *Archives for Racial and Social Biology* from 1913 to 1933, held the first professorship in eugenics in Germany, and welcomed the writing of Binding and Hoche as a sign that the individualistic philosophy of life that demands the maintenance of the individual against his will and against his interest may be overcome (Lenz 1920, 1048). Some psychiatrists like Hans Haenel supported the annihilation of "incurable idiots" (1923). In 1923, Borchardt, the town councilor of Liegnitz in Silesia, proposed legislation based on Binding and Hoche's writing that entitled not only relatives but also the local council caring for the poor to apply for the annihilation of life unworthy of living (Borchardt 1922).

On the other hand, psychiatrist Johannes Bresler, the editor of the widely read *Psychiatric and Neurological Weekly*, defended the right to live of the "incurable mentally insane" (1920, 289–290), as did the influential German lawyer Ludwig Ebermayer. According to Ebermayer, no one should have the right to decide upon the existence of a human being, even if its life was useless (Ebermayer 1920, 599–604; 1922, column 1655). Some medical and juridical authors supported physician-assisted dying on request by the patient but rejected the killing of the incurable mentally ill. Surprisingly, these authors seldom questioned the negative anthropology of the so-called "mentally dead."

Aroused by Binding and Hoche's paper, Dr. Ewald Meltzer, Director of the Katharinenhof, a Protestant institution for mentally handicapped children and adolescents in Saxony, conducted a survey in the early 1920s of parents of children in his care. Citing Binding and Hoche and several theologians, he asked parents if they would consent to a painless shortening of their child's life if it were established by experts that the child was incurably mentally defective. The answers, intended as a refutation of Binding and Hoche's proposals, astonished Meltzer. Of the 162 parents responding to the question, 119 answered "yes" while only 43 answered "no." Among the "no" responses, only 20 refused to countenance the painless killing of their child in any circumstances (Meltzer 1925, 83–88). It is striking that parents answering "yes" often cited personal and societal economic reasons for euthanizing their children. A letter from a miner to Meltzer expressed this candidly: "Our society has so far shown no comprehension of the suffering of these poor mentally incurables. [. . .] Are these mentally dead not a burden on the state and society as well as on their family?" (Meltzer 1925, 93). Some parents also opined that the "release" of the children was an act of mercy (Meltzer 1925, 89).

While the killing of severely disabled newborns was not the particular focus of Binding and Hoche, and racial hygiene was not the starting point of their argument, economics played a crucial role in aggregating the eugenic purification of the *Volkskörper* with the annihilation of life unworthy of living, especially institutionalized children. Also, Social Democrat eugenicists like Oda Olberg or Julius Tandler in Vienna integrated the medical killing of disabled newborns in their vision of a socialist society (Schwartz 1998, 634–637; Schwarz 2017, 207–208). Thus, euthanasia of disabled newborns can be considered the gateway to the annihilation of life unworthy of living (Schwartz 2001).

The legal debate on mercy killing and assisted dying did not lead to legislation during the Weimar Republic (Grosse-Vehne 2005, 71–85). Killing on request remained prohibited by law with no exception for physicians performing euthanasia because, according to Schumann, the majority of lawyers reacted unfavorably to Binding and Hoche's proposals, especially the annihilation of the mentally insane (Schumann 2005, 55–58). The term *life unworthy of living*, however, remained a point of reference in the debate on assisted dying until the 1960s (Ehrhardt 1965, 2, 47) and served as the ideological and legal justification for killing the sick under National Socialism. Indeed, one of the employees in the Führer's Chancellery testified after the war that their euthanasia programs had nothing to do with National Socialism because they were based on the ideas of people such as Karl Binding and Alfred Hoche who were not Nazis (Benzenhöfer 2005, 131). It is important to note that the economic crises and social misery in the last years of the Weimar Republic intensified the debate and radicalized proposals. In 1932, the aforementioned Meltzer wrote: "But the question [of 'annihilation of life unworthy of living'] catches our attention more urgently nowadays as in the years of food shortage in the time after the war" (1932, 584–585). In the same year, Dr. Berthold Kihn, the Erlangen lecturer of psychiatry and later a participant in *Aktion* T4, the centrally organized Nazi euthanasia program, calculated the cost of caring for the mentally ill and feebleminded at 150 million Reichsmarks per year. Referring to Binding and Hoche, he asked "whether by sacrificing life unworthy of living could our people not be freed from a large proportion of such ballast existences" (Kihn 1932, 395). The acceptance of Binding and Hoche's terminology that devalued the lives of institutionalized patients partially explains the readiness of a large proportion of German psychiatrists to ultimately tolerate, if not actively support, the National Socialist annihilation of life unworthy of living, as Kihn wrote in 1932:

> It is really a different question whether the general population looks after pensioners and old people, who in previous years have done their bit and who share the fate of growing old with us all, or whether the state perpetuates existences that have never done anything other than eat, shout, tear their clothes and soil their bed. (Kihn, 1932, 394, 3n)

By the end of the Weimar Republic, when the right of the incurable mentally ill to live was threatened in a legal and social sense, its severe austerity measures in psychiatric institutions and diminished social services raised questions about continuing expenditures on so-called "inferior people" and "parasites."

MERCY KILLING: THE DOUBLE-EDGED LEGITIMATION OF NATIONAL SOCIALIST EUTHANASIA

At the 1929 Nuremberg rally, Adolf Hitler announced that the annihilation of "life unworthy of living" was compatible with national socialist population policy: "If Germany was to get a million [new] children a year and was to remove 700,000–800,000 of the weakest people, then the final result might even be an increase in strength. . . . As a result of our modern sentimental humanitarianism we are trying to maintain the weak at the expense of the healthy" (quoted in Lankheit 1994, 345–354). Nonetheless, hoping to avoid an open discussion of euthanasia and the annihilation of life unworthy of living that might lose the support of German Christians, National Socialists did not adopt legislation for the termination of human life (Grosse-Vehne 2005). Yet, pity for the incurably ill and the idea of a right to die for those who wanted to end their physical suffering played a decisive role in the legitimation and marketing of the annihilation of life unworthy of living.

Although Hitler chose to await the long-planned war against the outer enemies of Germany before implementing his euthanasia policy, a proposal for a law that was to be implemented after the victorious end of the war was discussed in 1940:

> § 1 One suffering from an incurable illness, heavily burdening himself or others or leading certainly to death, can, with his express request and assent from a specially authorized physician, receive euthanasia from a physician.

> § 2 The life of a person who is in need of continuous custody due to incurable mental illness and who is not capable of survival in life, can be imperceptibly, painlessly terminated prematurely by medical measures. (Roth and Aly 1984, 108)

The passing of this law was postponed to avoid a public discussion about euthanasia during the war. Nevertheless, in the National Socialist state, euthanasia became a self-evident option both for the individual who no longer wanted to suffer from an incurable illness, and for the institutionalized incurable mentally ill in whom a wish for death could be assumed. Thus, "mercy killing" became a euphemism for the first National Socialist campaign of mass murder, the covert *Aktion* T4. For their part, physicians were convinced that they were participating in a comprehensive work of salvation and acting out of pity. As Dr. Karl Brandt, Hitler's personal physician and administrator of the euthanasia program, testified at the Nuremberg Medical Trial, euthanasia was not at all about eliminating a person, ". . . but rather it was about freeing him from the suffering that lay upon him . . . and the question of humanity, what is more humane, to help such a being to find a quiet end, or to continue to nurse and bother him, this answer is there, to be sure, even if one doesn't voice it" (quoted in Dörner, Ebbinghaus, and Linne 2000).

LEARNING FROM HISTORY: IS THERE SUCH A THING AS GOOD MEDICAL KILLING?

In my opinion, the historical debate on euthanasia in Germany and the legitimation of the annihilation of life unworthy of living under National Socialism clearly demonstrate a dangerous shift from the presumed right to die of the incurably ill to the medical killing of those incapable of requesting an assisted death. The strong motive of deliverance from suffering, a deadly and contemptuous form of pity, facilitated the medical killing of those lives presumed to have no social and economic value in Nazi Germany. This profound change illustrates a slippery slope that began with the right to die and ended with the extermination of life unworthy of living (Hohendorf 2013, 191–216; Hohendorf 2014, 296–302; Guckes 1997), a possibility Christoph Wilhelm Hufeland, Goethe's physician and director of the Charité hospital in Berlin, presciently raised in 1806:

> [The physician] should and may do nothing other than preserve life; whether it may be happy or unhappy, whether it may have value or not, does not concern him, and if he ever presumes to take such considerations into account in his work, the consequences are unforeseeable and the doctor becomes the most dangerous man in the country. (Hufeland 1837, 502)

Acknowledgment: The author is very grateful to Laurie Ann Johnson, Dachau, Germany, for translating parts of this paper.

BIBLIOGRAPHY

Abraham, Abraham S. 2003. *Nishmat Avraham: Medical Halachah for Doctors, Nurses, Health-Care Personnel and Patients. Vol. II: Yoreh Deah*. Brooklyn, NY: Mesorah Publications.

Bacon, Francis. (1605) 1904. *The Physical and Metaphysical Works. Advancement of Learning and Novum Organum*, edited by Joseph Devey, 1904. London: G. Bell and Sons.

Benzenhöfer, Udo. 1999. *Der gute Tod? Euthanasie Und Sterbehilfe in Geschichte Und Gegenwart*. Munich: C. H. Beck.

Benzenhöfer, Udo. 2005. "Bemerkungen Zur Binding-Hoche-Rezeption in Der NS-Zeit." In *'Die Freigabe Der Vernichtung Lebensunwerten Lebens.' Beiträge Des Symposiums Über Karl Binding Und Alfred Hoche Am 2. Dezember 2004 in Leipzig*, edited by Ortrun Riha, 114–133. Schriftenreihe Des Instituts Für Ethik in Der Medizin Leipzig e. V. 7. Aachen: Shaker.

Binding, Karl, and Alfred Hoche. 1920. *Die Freigabe Der Vernichtung Lebensunwerten Lebens. Ihr Mass Und Ihre Form*. Leipzig: Meiner.

Binding, Karl, and Alfred Hoche. 2006. *Die Freigabe Der Vernichtung Lebensunwerten Lebens. Ihr Mass und Ihre Form*, Juristische Zeitgeschichte Taschenbücher 1. Berlin: Berliner Wissenschaftsverlag.

Borchardt. 1922. "Die Freigabe Der Vernichtung Lebensunwerten Lebens." *Deutsche Strafrechtszeitung* 9, no. 7, column 206–210.

Bresler, Johannes. 1920. "*Karl Bindings 'Letzte Tat Für Die Leidende Menschheit,'*" *Psychiatrisch-Neurologische Wochenschrift* 22, no. 35: 289–290.

Burleigh, Michael. 1994. *Death and Deliverance: 'Euthanasia' in Germany, c. 1900 to 1945*. New York: Cambridge University Press.

Decher, Friedhelm. 1999. *Die Signatur Der Freiheit. Ethik Des Selbstmords in Der Abendländischen Philosophie*. Lüneburg: Klampen.

Detharding, Georg Christoph. 1723. *Disputatio Inauguralis Medica de Mortis Cura*. Rostock: Adlerus.

Dörner, Klaus, Angelika Ebbinghaus, and Karsten Linne, eds. 2000. *Der Nürnberger Ärzteprozess 1946/47. Wortprotokolle, Anklage- Und Verteidigungsmaterial, Quellen Zum Umfeld*. Microfiche-Edition, German Edition. München: De Gruyter Saur.

Dowbiggin, Ian. 2005. *A Concise History of Euthanasia: Life, Death, God, and Medicine*. Lanham, MD: Rowman & Littlefield.

Ebermayer, Ludwig. 1920. "Die Freigabe Der Vernichtung Lebensunwerten Lebens." *Leipziger Zeitschrift Für Deutsches Recht* 14: 599–604.

Ebermayer, Ludwig. 1922. "Erwiderung Gegen Borchardt." *Deutsche Medizinische Wochenschrift* 48: column 1655.

Edelstein, Ludwig. 1943. *The Hippocratic Oath: Text, Translation and Interpretation*. Bulletin of the History of Medicine Supplements No. 1. Baltimore: Johns Hopkins University Press.

Gerkan, Roland. 1913. "Euthanasie." In *Das Monistische Jahrhundert 2/2*, edited by Wilhelm Ostwald, vol. 7, 169–173. Leipzig: Unesma.

Grosse-Vehne, Vera. 2005. *Tötung Auf Verlangen: 'Euthanasie' Und Sterbehilfe.* *Reformdiskussion Und Gesetzgebung Seit 1870*, Juristische Zeitgeschichte Abt. 3, Beiträge Zur Modernen Strafgesetzgebung vol. 19: 86–108. Berlin: Berliner Wissenschaftsverlag.

Grubbs, Judith Evans, and Tim Parkin, eds. 2013. *The Oxford Handbook of Childhood and Education in the Classical World.* New York: Oxford University Press.

Grübler, Gerd, ed. 2007. *Quellen Zur Deutschen Euthanasie-Diskussion 1895–1941.* Geschichte in Quellen 2. Berlin: LIT.

Guckes, Barbara. 1997. *Das Argument Der Schiefen Ebene. Schwangerschaftsabbruch, Die Tötung Neugeborener Und Sterbehilfe in Der Medizinethischen Diskussion.* Medizinethik 9. Stuttgart: Fischer.

Haeckel, Ernst. 1904. *Die Lebenswunder. Gemeinverständliche Studien Über Biologische Philosophie. Ergänzungsband Zu Dem Buche über die Welträthsel.* Stuttgart: Kröner.

Haenel, Hans. 1923. "'Darf der Arzt töten?'163. Sitzung Der Forensisch-Psychiatrischen Vereinigung Zu Dresden Am 22. Juni 1922." *Allgemeine Zeitschrift Für Psychiatrie Und Psychisch-Gerichtliche Medizin* 97: 438–442.

Hippocratic Oath. 1923. *Hippocrates.* Edited by William H. S. Jones. The Loeb Classical Library 147. London, New York: Heinemann; Putnam. Accessed September 20, 2018. https://www.loebclassics.com/view/hippocrates_cos-oath/1923/pb_LCL147.299.xml.

Hohendorf, Gerrit. 2013. *Der Tod Als Erlösung Vom Leiden. Geschichte Und Ethik Der Sterbehilfe Seit Dem Ende Des 19. Jahrhunderts in Deutschland.* Göttingen: Wallstein.

Hohendorf, Gerrit. 2014. "The National Socialist Patient Murders between Taboo and Argument: Nazi Euthanasia and the Current Debate on Mercy Killing." In *Nazi Ideology and Ethics*, edited by Wolfgang Bialas and Lothar Fritze, 275–303. Newcastle upon Tyne: Cambridge Scholars Publishing.

Hohendorf, Gerrit. 2016. "Death as a Release from Suffering—The History and Ethics of Assisted Dying in Germany since the End of the 19th Century." *Neurology, Psychiatry and Brain Research* 22, no. 2 (2016): 56–62.

Hufeland, Christoph Wilhelm. 1837. *Enchiridion medicum oder Anleitung zur medicinischen Praxis. Vermächtniss einer fünfzigjährigen Erfahrung*, 3rd edition. Herisau: Literatur-Comptoir.

Hume, David. 1777. "Of Suicide." London.

Jost, Adolf. 1895. *Das Recht Auf Den Tod. Sociale Studie.* Göttingen: Dieterich'sche Verlagsbuchhandlung.

Kihn, Bertold. 1932. "Die Ausschaltung Der Minderwertigen Aus Der Gesellschaft." *Allgemeine Zeitschrift Für Psychiatrie Und Psychisch-Gerichtliche Medizin* 98.

Lankheit, Klaus A., ed. 1994. *Hitler–Reden Schriften Anordnungen–Februar 1925–Januar 1933: Zwischen den Reichstagswahlen. Juli 1928–September 1930: BD III / Teil 2: Maerz 1929–Dezember 1929.* München: Saur.

Lenz, Fritz. 1920. "Die Freigabe Der Vernichtung Lebensunwerten Lebens. Von Prof. Dr. jur. et phil. Karl Binding Und Prof. Dr. med. Alfred Hoche." *Münchner Medizinische Wochenschrift* 67, no. 36: 1048.

Lorey, Wilhelm. 1908. "Adolf Jost." In *Mathematisch-Naturwissenschaftliche Blät-
ter 5*. Berlin: Verband mathematischer und naturwissenschaftlicher Vereine an
deutschen Hochschulen.

Meltzer, Ewald. 1925. *Das Problem Der Abkürzung 'Lebensunwerten Lebens.'* Halle
upon Saale: Carl Marhold Verlagsbuchhandlung.

Meltzer, Ewald. 1932. "Die Frage Des Unwerten Lebens (Vita Non Iam Vitalis) Und
die Jetztzeit." *Psychiatrisch-Neurologische Wochenschrift* 34, no. 48: 584–591.

Mendelsohn, Martin. 1898. "Euthanasie." In *Encyklopaedie Der Therapie* vol. 2,
edited by Oskar Liebreich, 245–250. Berlin: Hirschwald.

More, Thomas. (1516) 1737. *Utopia*, translated by Gilbert Burnet 1737. Dublin:
Oxford University Press.

Naucke, Wolfgang. 2006. "Einführung: Rechtstheorie Und Staatsverbrechen." In *Die
Freigabe Der Vernichtung Lebensunwerten Lebens. Ihr Mass Und Ihre Form*, edited by Karl Binding and Alfred Hoche, 5–71. Juristische Zeitgeschichte Taschenbücher 1. Berlin: Berliner Wissenschaftsverlag.

Nietzsche, Friedrich. 1889. *Götzen-Dämmerung Oder Wie Man Mit Dem Hammer
Philosophiert*. Leipzig: Naumann.

Nolte, Karin. 2010. "Ärztliche Praxis Am Sterbebett in Der Ersten Hälfte Des 19.
Jahrhunderts." In *Ärztliches Ethos im Kontext, Historische, Phänomenologische
Und Didaktische Analysen*, edited by Walter Bruchhausen and Hans-Georg Hofer,
39–57. Bonn: V&R Unipress.

Paradys, Nikolaus.1796. "Rede Von Nikolaus Paradys, Professor in Leyden, Über
Das, Was Die Arzneiwissenschaft Vermag, Den Tod Leicht Und Schmerzlos
Zu Machen." Translated by Johann Georg Klees. *Neues Magazin für Aerzte* 18:
560–72.

Plato. 1871. "Phaedo." In *The Dialogues of Plato*, edited by and translated by Benjamin Jowett, vol. 1, 379–468. Oxford: Oxford University Press.

Plato. 1871. "The Republic. Part III." In *The Dialogues of Plato*, edited by and translated by Benjamin Jowett, vol. 1, 209–245. Oxford: Oxford University Press.

Plato. 1871. "The Republic. Part V." In *The Dialogues of Plato*, edited by and translated by Benjamin Jowett, vol. 1. Oxford: Oxford University Press.

Ploetz, Alfred. 1895. *Die Tüchtigkeit Unsrer Rasse Und Der Schutz Der Schwachen.
Ein Versuch Über Rassenhygiene Und Ihr Verhältnis Zu Den Humanen Idealen,
Besonders Zum Socialismus.* Grundlinien Einer Rasssen-Hygiene 1. Berlin: Fischer.

Plutarch, Lucius Mestrius. n.d. *Lycurgus.* translated by John Dryden. Accessed September 26, 2018. http://classics.mit.edu/Plutarch/lycurgus.html.

Reinis, Austra. 2010. "Ars moriendi. Ritual- Und Textgeschichte." In *Sterben Und
Tod. Geschichte—Theorie—Ethik. Ein Interdisziplinäres Handbuch*, edited by
Héctor Wittwer, Daniel Schäfer, and Andreas Frewer, 159–169. Stuttgart and
Weimar: J. B. Metzler.

Roelcke, Volker. 2006. "'Ars moriendi' Und 'euthanasia medica': Zur Neukonfigura-
tion Und Ärztlichen Aneignung Normativer Vorstellungen Über Den 'Guten Tod'
Um 1800." In *Sterben Und Tod Bei Heinrich Von Kleist in Seinem Historischen
Kontext*, edited by Lothar Jordan, 29–44. Beiträge Zur Kleist-Forschung 18. Würzburg: Königshausen u. Neumann.

Roth, Karl Heinz, and Götz Aly. 1984. "Das 'Gesetz Über Die Sterbehilfe Bei Unheilbar Kranken.' Protokolle Der Diskussion Über Die Legalisierung Der Nationalsozialistischen Anstaltsmorde in Den Jahren 1938–1941." In *Erfassung Zur Vernichtung. Von Der Sozialhygiene Zum 'Gesetz Über Sterbehilfe,'* edited by Karl Heinz Roth, 101–179. Berlin: Verlagsgesellschaft Gesundheit.

Schilling, Katharina. 2011. *Ach Gieb Mir Doch Nur Etwas Luft. Du Hast Der Luft So Viel! Palliativmedizin im Frühen 19. Jahrhundert.* Duisburg, Köln.

Schmuhl, Hans-Walter. 1992. *Rassenhygiene, Nationalsozialismus, Euthanasie: Von Der Verhütung Zur Vernichtung 'Lebensunwerten Lebens'; 1890–1945.* 2nd edition. Kritische Studien Zur Geschichtswissenschaft 75. Göttingen: Vandenhoeck und Ruprecht.

Schumann, Eva. 2005. "Karl Bindings Schrift 'Die Freigabe Der Vernichtung Lebensunwerten Lebens.' Vorläufer, Reaktionen Und Fortwirken in Rechtshistorischer Perspektive." In *'Die Freigabe Der Vernichtung Lebensunwerten Lebens.' Beiträge Des Symposiums Über Karl Binding Und Alfred Hoche Am 2. Dezember 2004 in Leipzig,* edited by Ortrun Riha, 35–67. Schriftenreihe Des Instituts Für Ethik in Der Medizin Leipzig e. V. 7. Aachen: Shaker.

Schwartz, Michael. 1998. "'Euthanasie'-Debatten in Deutschland." *Vierteljahrshefte Für Zeitgeschichte 46,* no. 4: 617–665.

Schwartz, Michael. 2001. "Einfallstore Der 'Euthanasie.' Deutsche Debatten Über Die 'Vernichtung Lebensunwerten Lebens' 1895–1945." In *Jahrbuch Der Juristischen Zeitgeschichte 2,* edited by Thomas Vormbaum, 131–52. Berlin: Berliner Wissenschafts-Verlag.

Schwarz, Peter. 2017. *Julius Tandler. Zwischen Humanismus Und Eugenik.* Wien: Edition Steinbauer.

Seneca, Lucius Annaeus. 1920. *Moral letters to Lucilius (Epistulae morales ad Lucilium).* Translated by Richard Mott Gummere, Letter 70: On the Proper Time to Split the Cable, no. 14 and 15. A Loeb Classical Library edition, vol. 2. Harvard University Press. Accessed September 25, 2018. https://en.wikisource.org/wiki/Moral_letters_to_Lucilius/Letter_70.

Stolberg, Michael. 2007. "Active Euthanasia in Pre-Modern Society, 1500–1800: Learned Debates and Popular Practices." *Social History of Medicine 20,* no. 2 (August): 205–221.

Stolberg, Michael. 2008. "Two Pioneers of Euthanasia around 1800." *Hastings Center Report 38,* no. 3 (May–June): 19–22.

Stolberg, Michael. 2011. *Die Geschichte Der Palliativmedizin. Medizinische Sterbebegleitung 1500 Bis heute.* Frankfurt am Main: Mabuse-Verlag.

von Engelhardt, Dietrich. 2010. "Euthanasie in Geschichte Und Gegenwart–Im Spektrum Zwischen Lebensbeendigung Und Sterbebeistand." *Vorträge Und Abhandlungen Zur Wissenschaftsgeschichte,* 187–212. Stuttgart: Wissenschaftliche Verlagsgesellschaft.

Weikart, Richard. 2004. *From Darwin to Hitler: Evolutionary Ethics, Eugenics, and Racism in Germany.* New York: Palgrave Macmillan.

Chapter Two

International and German Eugenics from ca. 1880 up to the Post–World War II Period

Medical Expertise—Political Ambition— Relations to Euthanasia in the Nazi Context

Volker Roelcke

The relationship between eugenics and euthanasia in the Nazi context has long been a topic of intense debates. This chapter will summarize the history of international and German eugenics and consider its implications in view of the historical evidence on the systematic patient killings during the Nazi period.

Eugenics may be defined as an international social movement characterized by a specific configuration of aims, means, actors, and justifications to improve the biological quality of a population. The methods to achieve this aim are educational, legal, and physical interventions in human reproduction. Both the aim and the applied methods are justified by scientific expertise. The history of eugenics is closely linked with the history of medical genetics, the political ambitions of biomedical scientists, and the public authority of the corresponding sciences. The main actors who pursued eugenic programs were professionals such as physicians, statisticians, lawyers, and teachers. In the first decades of the twentieth century, eugenics played a significant part in shaping government policies, depending, however, on the specific socio-economic, cultural, and religious configurations in varying national contexts (Levine 2017). Eugenics in the Nazi context represented one particular manifestation of this broader historical movement.

The following overview of international and German eugenics is structured in three parts:

1. The beginnings of organized eugenics, including the formation of eugenic associations
2. Eugenically motivated medical genetics and its cooperation with state social policies, with the most radical manifestation in Nazi Germany

3. Considerations on the relation between eugenics and the systematic patient killings ("euthanasia") in the Nazi context.

THE INTERNATIONAL BEGINNINGS
OF ORGANIZED EUGENICS

The term *eugenics* was coined by the British mathematician Francis Galton
around 1880. In his highly influential 1883 book *Inquiries into Human Faculty and its Development*, Galton defined eugenics as "a new field of enquiry"
that aimed at the "improvement of the race" (1883, 24). The well-being of the
population, or the race in Galton's own wording, was the utmost priority of
eugenics as he defined it: "Eugenics is the study of the agencies under social
control that improve or impair the racial qualities of future generations either
physically or mentally" (Galton 1883, 17).

Galton was a distinguished scholar in the field of statistics (Bulmer 2003).
He introduced core statistical concepts such as "regression," "standard deviation," and "regression to the mean." He also co-initiated and edited the
highly influential journal *Biometrika* and was knighted in 1909. Together
with some of the leading British intellectuals of the time, he co-founded the
Eugenics Educational Society in 1907 and served as its first president. The
Society campaigned for sterilization and marriage restrictions in Britain. It
also organized the first International Eugenics Conference in 1912. In 1926,
it was renamed the Eugenics Society (Mazumdar 1992).

In 1895, approximately a decade after Galton had coined the term *eugenics*, the German physician Alfred Ploetz introduced the largely synonymous
term *Rassenhygiene*, or *racial hygiene*. Inspired by Ernst Haeckel, the German Social Darwinist, he argued that this new field of both scientific enquiry
and political action should respond to the process of counter-selection, which
he perceived as the result of modern civilization and social policies. The idea
was that while the process of natural selection led to an improvement of the
biological qualities of a race, measures such as sick insurance and welfare
programs subverted such beneficial natural processes and instead enabled the
unfit to survive and to reproduce. To counteract this process, racial hygiene
should organize human reproduction according to scientific knowledge in the
realm of biology, and in particular, in hereditarian studies. In 1904, Ploetz,
together with a number of like-minded physicians such as Ernst Rüdin and
Fritz Lenz, founded the *Archiv für Rassen- und Gesellschaftsbiologie (Archives for Racial and Societal Biology)* and, in 1905, the *Gesellschaft für
Rassenhygiene* (Society for Racial Hygiene) (Weingart, Kroll, and Bayertz
1988; Weindling 1989).

At least during the first three decades of the twentieth century, the terms *eugenics* and *racial hygiene* were used in a widely overlapping sense, frequently synonymously, with Germans and Scandinavians preferring the term *racial hygiene*. However, the precise semantic content of both terms, *eugenics* and *racial hygiene*, was the subject of constant dispute and discussion, even within associations for eugenics and racial hygiene. Independent of the specific variations in details, the shared core content of the terms in all their usages was the link between a scientifically authorized stock of knowledge with the objective of political application. According to the understanding of the actors in this field, science and politics were inseparably entwined with each other: the political objective of improving the biological quality of a given population motivated research programs and scientifically authorized medical actions. In a complementary fashion, science provided the terms and theories that were to be used to interpret contemporary social and political problems and to develop rational approaches to resolve them. It was the responsibility of scientists as well as the state to implement social technologies derived from scientific knowledge to solve social problems like dissocial behavior, poverty, the spread of disease, prostitution, alcoholism, and criminality (Galton 1904; Ploetz 1911).

Eugenic thinking found fertile breeding ground around the beginning of the twentieth century and in the following decades. This time was marked by intense concerns about degeneration, that is, the idea that alcohol, syphilis, and—as already stated—the elimination of natural selection through modern hygiene and medical care would lead to a deterioration of the collective genetic material in a given population, be it a state or a nation.

In this context, in the years immediately after 1900, the first eugenic organizations were founded. One year after the already mentioned (German) Society for Racial Hygiene had convened in Berlin in 1905, the American Breeders' Association, founded in 1903, established a eugenics section devoted to human breeding. Further associations with similar objectives soon followed, such as the Eugenics Education Society in England in 1907 (Mazumdar 1992), the Swedish Society for Racial Hygiene in 1909 (Broberg and Roll-Hansen 1996), the American Eugenics Association in 1911 (Black 2003), *Société Eugénique* (Eugenic Society) in France in 1912 (Carol 1995), and the Czechoslovakian Eugenic Society in 1915 (Turda and Weindling 2007).

In Germany, the United States, and other national contexts, eugenic measures were propagated by representatives across the political spectrum, from socialists and communists to liberals, conservatives, and right-wing nationalists (Dowbiggin 1997; Kline 2001; Weiss 2010). The ideas were also propagated by Protestants, Catholics, and Jews, by social reformers as well as by anti-democratic elitists and backward-oriented aristocrats (Weindling

1989; Kline 2001; Leon 2013). The advocates of eugenic programs included geneticists, anthropologists, psychiatrists, and social hygienists, as well as lawyers, sociologists, and politicians. Eugenic ideas and measures were also endorsed by internationally renowned scientists like Charles Richet and Alexis Carrel, Nobel laureates in Physiology or Medicine (Lepicard 2019). Even the Catholic Church, as documented in the Pope's 1930 encyclical, took a positive stance on eugenic objectives to improve the biological quality of populations, for example by marriage counseling, although it rejected so-called "negative" methods, especially sterilizations and eugenically justified abortions (Lepicard 1998).

In view of the broad appeal of and support for the eugenic movement in all political groups and religious confessions, it is inappropriate to construct images of the past suggesting that eugenics was the result of one specific political or religious agenda, such as National Socialism, or progressivism. From the fact that an individual or a group with a particular background supported eugenic programs, it may not be concluded that eugenics in general was the result of that specific intellectual background. For example, the fact that progressive politicians such as Theodore Roosevelt supported eugenics (Kline 2001, 11; Black 2003, 99, 209; Comfort 2012, 49) does in no way justify the generalized assumption that eugenics was simply the result of progressivist activism, since right-wing nationalists propagated eugenic agendas as well (Weingart, Kroll, and Bayertz 1988; Kühl 2002; Spiro 2009). Similarly, the fact that prominent eugenicists in Germany and France were Catholics, such as Eugen Muckermann (Weindling 1989; Schmuhl 2008) or Alexis Carrel (Lepicard 2019), does not allow the conclusion that eugenics was a corollary of twentieth-century Catholic thought.

While the eugenics-racial hygiene movement shared a general goal—to biologically purify and strengthen a given population—it also harbored considerable internal differences, not least of which was the precise understanding of the concept of race. While one group of eugenicists made the presumed specific genetic attributes of a given population the standard for their racial concept, another group postulated instead that the totality of genetic material in a defined geographic space should be designated as race. This differentiation more or less corresponded to the distinction between *Systemrasse* and *Vitalrasse*, concepts that had been formulated by Alfred Ploetz shortly after the turn of the century (Essner 2002, 40–75; Ploetz 1911; the terms have repeatedly been translated as *system race* and *vital race*, e.g., in Turda and Quine 2018, 18).

The first, narrower understanding of the concept of race was frequently linked to the presumption that the "Nordic" race had distinct genetic characteristics, suggesting that eugenic measures should be directed primarily toward the preservation and improvement of this Nordic race. In the German context, this was a core idea for such protagonists as Alfred Ploetz and Fritz Lenz, in Sweden for Hermann Lundborg, and in the United States for Harry Laughlin, the superintendent of the Eugenics Record Office in Cold Spring Harbor (Weingart, Kroll, and Bayertz 1988; Weindling 1989; Black 2003; Comfort 2012).

The diverse fronts on this issue remained in flux, not only among German scientists, but also among their British, Scandinavian, and American colleagues and certainly among politicians. In the German context, this controversy was not settled when the Nazi government took over in 1933 and was only resolved around 1936 when the narrower concept of race took center stage (Essner 2002, 40–75).

EUGENICALLY MOTIVATED MEDICAL GENETICS AND ITS CLOSE COOPERATION WITH STATE SOCIAL POLICIES

The eugenics movement heavily relied on scientific knowledge from contemporary genetics, but also from the social sciences and statistics. Eugenics derived its legitimacy and its public standing from these scientific fields. In a complementary fashion, a considerable number of geneticists were motivated by eugenic objectives. Examples include the American Nobel laureate Hermann J. Muller and the British population geneticist Ronald A. Fisher. Thus, the history of eugenics cannot be explained without the history of genetics, and vice versa (Koch 2004; Comfort 2012; Roelcke 2019). A core feature of this close interrelation is the fact that in the early twentieth century, eugenic motivations were constitutive for the newly emerging research institutions in the realm of human genetics.

In 1905, the Francis Galton Laboratory for the Study of National Eugenics was founded in association with University College London; Galton himself provided the funds for an endowed professorship in eugenics at University College. In Oslo, Norway, the Vinderen Laboratory was set up in 1906. In 1910, with funding from the Carnegie Foundation, Charles Davenport founded the Eugenics Record Office in Cold Spring Harbor, New York, and appointed Harry Laughlin as its superintendent. Davenport later became the first president of the International Federation of Eugenic Organizations (Broberg and Roll-Hansen 1996; Bulmer 2003; Comfort 2012; Kühl 2002).

In 1917, the eugenically inspired Genealogical-Demographic Department (*Genealogisch-Demographische Abteilung*) opened at the German Institute for Psychiatric Research (*Deutsche Forschungsanstalt für Psychiatrie*) in Munich, making it the world's first research institution for the field of psychiatric genetics. It was substantially funded by the American-Jewish philanthropist James Loeb, but also received resources from public institutions, such as the state of Bavaria (Roelcke 2002, 2006). Additional state-sponsored research institutions emerged, such as the Institute for Racial Biology in Uppsala (1922), the National Eugenics Research Institute in Prague (1923), and the Institute for Human Genetics in Copenhagen (1938) (Broberg and Roll-Hansen 1996).

Starting in the mid-1920s, genetic research with eugenic objectives was supported in Germany with funds from the most important institutions for research funding at the time. In 1928, the elitist Kaiser Wilhelm Society (*Kaiser Wilhelm Gesellschaft*), predecessor of today's Max Planck Society, founded the Kaiser Wilhelm Institute for Anthropology, Human Genetics and Eugenics in Berlin. The building and infrastructure of the new institute were jointly funded by the Reich, the Prussian state, and, to a smaller extent, by private sponsorship from various German sources raised by the Catholic eugenicist Eugen Muckermann; the operating costs were covered by the Kaiser Wilhelm Society (Schmuhl 2008). By 1924, the German Institute for Psychiatric Research had also been integrated into the Kaiser Wilhelm Society. Due to the rise in public and political interest in eugenics, the budget of the Genealogical-Demographic Department, its eugenically grounded genetics department, was tripled in 1928 (Roelcke 2006).

The efforts of eugenicists to convince the public and state authorities of the necessity of eugenic practices, culminating in sterilization laws, was quite successful, especially in the United States, Scandinavia, and Germany. Beginning in Indiana in 1907, followed by California, Connecticut, and Washington in 1909, a growing number of American states legalized sterilization of those of supposedly minor biological value, in particular the mentally "defective," who were perceived as a threat to the prosperity of the population. However, until the early 1920s, most of these laws had limited effect, as documented in Laughlin's book *Eugenical Sterilization in the United States* (1922). Laughlin asserted that most state laws were highly flawed, being either too poorly crafted to be constitutional—indeed, many were ruled unconstitutional by state courts—or too confusing in their wording to be used efficiently. To remedy these flaws, Laughlin proposed a "Model Eugenical Sterilization Law" (Black 2003; Comfort 2012). In 1924, Virginia passed a law derived from Laughlin's model, which the US Supreme Court declared constitutional in the case of *Buck v. Bell* in 1927 (Kline 2001; Black 2003). This decision prompted additional states to either bring their statutes in line with *Buck v. Bell* or pass new sterilization laws, resulting in many more eugenic sterilizations through the period of World War II. By 1930—clearly before the Nazi government was in power—more than twenty American states, as well as two Canadian provinces (Alberta and British Columbia) had such laws. Altogether, in the United States, eugenic sterilization laws in more than 30 states resulted in the sterilization of over 64,000 mentally ill and developmentally disabled patients by the time these laws went into general disuse in the mid-1970s (Lombardo 2008, appendix C).

In Europe, the Swiss canton Vaud introduced a sterilization law in 1928; it remained in effect until 1985 (Meier 2004). In 1929, Denmark became the first European country to implement a eugenically motivated sterilization law on a national level. The other Scandinavian states, as well as the Baltic states followed in the early and mid-1930s. In Sweden, for example, a sterilization law was implemented in 1935 and remained in force until 1976. Under this law, approximately 63,000 individuals were sterilized, about one-third of them against their will (Broberg and Roll-Hansen 1996).

Prior to 1933, European eugenicists looked to the United States for the formulation and implementation of such laws, but after the Nazi takeover, both Scandinavian and American eugenicists regularly referred in a positive way to the—as they saw it—particularly coherent and strict implementation of the law in Germany (Kühl 2002). In July 1933, the newly elected Nazi government passed the German Law for the Prevention of Hereditary Ill Offspring (*Gesetz zur Verhütung erbkranken Nachwuchses*). Beginning in January 1934, more than 360,000 individuals were sterilized after registration and a formal review procedure by the newly established hereditary health courts (Weindling 1989; Ley 2004). Various medical associations had lobbied for such a law during the Weimar Republic in the late 1920s and early 1930s, but they had failed to make it a constitutive part of state health and social policies. The law finally adopted by the Nazi regime essentially followed an already existing blueprint, which in large parts had been drafted by medical protagonists of the eugenic movement (Weindling 1989; Schmuhl 2008). Therefore, it is incorrect to assume that the Nazi sterilization law was simply the consequence of state intrusion in medical affairs, and in the rights of those directly affected. Rather, medical initiative and expertise were constitutive for both the origins and the implementation of so-called "hereditary health care" (*Erbgesundheitspflege*), the program of racial hygiene as propagated and practiced during the Nazi regime (Weindling 1989; Schmuhl 2016).

The intrinsic link between eugenics and human genetics, as well as the close relationship between high profile representatives of the eugenic-genetic field and eugenically motivated state policies is exemplified by Ernst Rüdin. He was the director of the Genealogical-Demographic Department in Munich and one of the protagonists of the eugenic movement both in Germany and internationally, who enjoyed a stellar international reputation as a scientist in the 1930s. For instance, in 1934, the English reference work on human genetics called him the world's leading figure in the field of psychiatric genetics (Roelcke 2002). In the early and mid-1930s, those physicians now regarded as the founders of the national schools of psychiatric genetics in the United States, Great Britain, and Scandinavia, namely Franz Kallmann (New York), Eliot Slater (London), and Erik Stromgren (Stockholm/Lund), came on scholarships to work with Rüdin in Munich (Roelcke 2019). And as late as summer 1939, on the eve of World War II, Rüdin was invited to be a plenary speaker at the International Genetic Congress in Edinburgh (Roelcke 2002).

From the beginning of his career, Rüdin's work was inspired by eugenic objectives. He was unwavering in his belief that his research would create a scientific foundation for health and social policy measures on the basis of biological laws, and that the collective welfare of the people, the nation, or the race had a higher priority than the welfare of any individual, a value hierarchy shared by almost all eugenicists of his time. Starting in 1905, the *Gesellschaft für Rassenhygiene*, co-founded by Rüdin, advocated excluding those "genetically burdened" from reproduction. In 1930, Rüdin succeeded Davenport as president of the International Federation of Eugenics (Kühl 2002). When the sterilization law was passed by the Nazi government in 1933, Rüdin co-authored the extensive official commentary on the law, together with Arthur Gütt, head of the department of health affairs in the Reich Ministry of the Interior, and the lawyer and SS-member Falk Ruttke (Weindling 1989; Schmuhl 2016). Altogether, beginning around 1900, Rüdin's scientific activities had been motivated by the political agenda of eugenics. Even after he began to collaborate closely with the Nazi state, Rüdin and his institute continued to enjoy great prestige in the international scientific community. Rüdin's career demonstrates that German eugenicists were by no means internationally isolated before the outbreak of World War II, in spite of close cooperation with the Nazi regime (Kühl 2002; Roelcke 2002, 2019).

After 1945, many countries still had sterilization programs, including all the Scandinavian states and numerous "Third World" countries (Broberg and Roll-Hansen 1996; Kline 2001; Bashford and Levine 2010; Levine 2017). Eugenic motivations for sterilizations, however, were largely discredited internationally due to their radical manifestations during the Nazi regime. The practice of sterilization was now justified with arguments from population policy, family planning, and social welfare, in fact quite often from the same experts who previously had held leading positions in eugenic organizations (Connelly 2008).

The historical analysis of the Nuremberg Medical Trial of 1946–1947 also reveals a certain ambivalence on the part of American judges and physicians, or at least no clear rejection of eugenic objectives and practices. Judged by their choices of defendants and crimes and their decision to focus on forced human subjects research in concentration camps, eugenic sterilization and euthanasia played only a marginal role in the trial (Marrus 1999; Lepicard 2007). Indeed, given the continuing existence of eugenic organizations and sterilization laws after 1945, the widespread practice of sterilization in many Western countries including the United States, and the close international nexus of eugenicists and geneticists, moral condemnation of the National Socialist sterilization program and corresponding juridical indictments and sentencing were unlikely outcomes of the trial.

ON THE RELATIONSHIP BETWEEN EUGENICS, RACIAL HYGIENE, AND EUTHANASIA IN THE NAZI CONTEXT

The exact relationship between eugenics and euthanasia in the sense of the systematic killing of those "not worthy to live" has been the subject of intense debates. While these two movements were largely separate in their original motivation and reasoning, they soon converged in the programmatic statements of key figures in the eugenics movement. To clarify their commonalities and differences, it is helpful to examine the core ideas and justifications for the movements' specific agendas.

The idea of euthanasia in the sense of medically legitimated killing by physicians of those "not worthy to live" was associated with a reinterpretation of the previously existing concept of euthanasia that originated in antiquity. From the late eighteenth until the second half of the nineteenth century, this term referred to physical and psychological support for the dying individual but, explicitly, without any measures to shorten his or her life. Beginning in the 1870s, with the decline of religion's public authority and the rise of the sciences, human life became accessible to interventions targeting its very nature, culminating in the possibility of its termination based on the judgment of medical experts. This shift and the associated new options of terminating life relied on three central presuppositions and justifications: (1) the elimination of the exceptional status of the human being in cosmology and its integration in the broader order of nature; (2) the alleged compassion for the (supposedly) suffering individual; and (3) the (explicit or implicit) argument for relief of the economic burden on families and society supposedly caused by those suffering from "life unworthy of living." In addition to physicians, the primary propagators of this agenda included writers, lawyers, and philosophers (Hohendorf 2013).

Eugenics, on the other hand, which emerged in parallel at the end of the nineteenth century, was similarly based on three core assumptions: (1) human life may be evaluated according to biological criteria (again presupposing the integration of the human being into the order of nature); (2) the biological quality of human populations is determined by the reproductive rates and the hereditary health of their members; and (3) the impact of civilization and social institutions ("contra-selection") leads to an imminent biological deterioration of populations ("degeneration"). As a result of these assumptions, it was argued that scientifically grounded interventions in human reproduction could counteract perceived threats to human populations and political entities. By evaluating the biological quality of human life and the impact of this quality on health and performance of a given population, the eugenics discourse was also associated with an explicit or implicit economic assessment. The primary propagators of this agenda were physicians, biologists, and statisticians.

Both eugenics and euthanasia have in common the medical and biological evaluation of human life, as well as an explicit or implicit economic rationality. They differ in regard to the compassion argument (euthanasia) and the goal of a biological optimization of populations (eugenics). While important representatives of the euthanasia tradition in the late nineteenth and early twentieth centuries, such as Adolf Jost, Roland Gerkan, Karl Binding, and Alfred Hoche, placed a strong emphasis on the economic argument, they did not refer to a goal of biologically optimizing the population by intervening in reproduction. Conversely, the protagonists of eugenics like Francis Galton, Eugen Muckermann, and Eugen Fischer, did not link compassionate killing with economic arguments. One might claim, as does Weikart (2004, 146), that the German Social Darwinist Ernst Haeckel who proposed killing disabled newborns in his book *Natürliche Schöpfungsgeschichte* (*Natural History of Creation*) (1870) represents an early example of convergence between euthanasia and eugenics. Closer examination, however, suggests that such an argument is anachronistic and inappropriate. As described above, around 1870, eugenics existed neither as a term nor as a program. In fact, in his book, Haeckel only made a short reference to the Spartan custom of abandoning severely handicapped newborns, and suggested that this practice might, in the long run, have a positive effect on the "human stock." Thus, the idea is rather marginal in Haeckel's book, and not part of a systematic program of applying scientific knowledge in order to improve the biological quality of human populations, which is the core of eugenics. Nevertheless, by 1900, Alfred Ploetz, the founding figure of German racial hygiene, and William Duncan McKim, an American eugenicist, independently brought the two strands of argument together (Hohendorf 2013; Dowbiggin 2003). In the 1930s, the previously mentioned French-American Nobel laureate Alexis Carrel propagated both eugenics and euthanasia of the "unfit" outside Nazi Germany (Lepicard 2019).

After 1933, in the Nazi context, practically all the central figures involved in the planning and implementation of "mercy" killing were also propagating a eugenic agenda. Representative leaders were the aforementioned Ernst Rüdin, who also acted as the president of the German Association of Neurology and Psychiatry, Kurt Pohlisch and Carl Schneider, university professors of psychiatry, and Hans Heinze and Paul Nitsche, directors of psychiatric asylums (Schmuhl 2016). Rüdin not only offered justifications for the killing program but was also involved in the planning and implementation of research designed to provide a scientific foundation for the selection of the victims of euthanasia. For him and other prominent psychiatrists, euthanasia was an integral component of a comprehensive reform program to reorganize society according to biological principles (Roelcke 2002, 2012; Schmuhl 2016).

However, there were also prominent advocates of eugenics and forced sterilization, such as Gottfried Ewald, professor of psychiatry and neurology in Göttingen, and Hans Roemer, director of the Illenau psychiatric asylum in Baden, who explicitly rejected killing patients. In 1940, while the killings were carried out, Roemer opposed the extermination program in a lengthy memorandum addressed to the Interior Ministry of Baden, albeit with little success (Beyer 2013; Roelcke 2013; Schmuhl 2016).

Thus, the historical evidence clearly documents that the relation between eugenics and euthanasia is rather complex. Eugenics and euthanasia had different historical roots and a somewhat different rationale. Whereas eugenics had as its goal the biological improvement of the population by means of scientific knowledge, euthanasia had at its core an intrinsic combination of mercy and economics aimed at reducing the purported burden of suffering on the individual as well as society. Also, unlike eugenicists, euthanasia advocates did not really base their position and agenda on scientific knowledge and further research in the realm of genetics; instead, they relied on the alleged high professional integrity of physicians to justify the decision to terminate human life.

In their trajectories, these movements in part overlapped—a number of eugenicists also advocated euthanasia, and many proponents of euthanasia were eugenicists. But significantly, not all eugenicists approved of euthanasia, and not all advocates of euthanasia were eugenicists. In the final analysis, this means that there are no intrinsic and inevitable links between eugenics and euthanasia. But certainly, eugenics, with its assumption that it is possible to judge the biological quality of human beings and with its contemporary authority as a science, strongly contributed to the plausibility and acceptance of the idea of euthanasia.

BIBLIOGRAPHY

Bashford, Alison, and Philippa Levine, eds. 2010. *The Oxford Handbook of the History of Eugenics*. New York, Oxford: Oxford University Press.

Beyer, Christof. 2013. "Gottfried Ewald und die 'Aktion T4' in Göttingen." *Der Nervenarzt* 84, no. 9 (September): 1049–55.

Black, Edwin. 2003. *War against the Weak: Eugenics and America's Campaign to Create a Master Race*. New York: Four Walls Eight Windows.

Broberg, Gunnar, and Nils Roll-Hansen, ed. 1996. *Eugenics and the Welfare State. Sterilization Policy in Denmark, Sweden, Norway, and Finland*. East Lansing: Michigan State University Press.

Bulmer, Michael. 2003. *Francis Galton: Pioneer of Heredity and Biometry*. Baltimore: Johns Hopkins University Press.

Carol, Anne. 1995. *Histoire de l'eugenisme en France: Les médecins et la procréation, XIXe–XXe siècle*. Paris: Seuil.

Comfort, Nathaniel. 2012. *The Science of Human Perfection: How Genes Became the Heart of American Medicine*. New Haven: Yale University Press.

Connelly, Matthew. 2008. *Fatal Misconception: The Struggle to Control World Population*. Cambridge, MA: Harvard University Press.

Dowbiggin, Ian. 1997. *Keeping America Sane: Psychiatry and Eugenics in the United States and Canada*. Ithaca: Cornell University Press.

Dowbiggin, Ian. 2003. *A Merciful End: The Euthanasia Movement in Modern America*. Oxford: Oxford University Press.

Essner, Cornelia. 2002. *Die "Nürnberger Gesetze" oder Die Verwaltung des Rassenwahns 1933–1945*. Paderborn: Schöningh.

Galton, Francis. 1883. *Inquiries into Human Faculty and its Development*. New York: Dutton 2nd ed. n.d (1st ed. 1883).

Galton, Francis. 1904. "Eugenics: Its Definition, Scope and Aims," *Sociological Papers* X, no. 1 (July): 43–99.

Haeckel, Ernst. 1870. *Natürliche Schöpfungsgeschichte* [*Natural History of Creation*], 2nd edition. Berlin: Reimer.

Hohendorf, Gerrit. 2013. *Der Tod als Erlösung vom Leiden. Geschichte und Ethik der Sterbehilfe seit dem Ende des 19. Jahrhunderts in Deutschland*. Göttingen: Wallstein.

Kline, Wendy. 2001. *Building a Better Race: Gender, Sexuality, and Eugenics from the Turn of the Century to the Baby Boom*. Berkeley: University of California Press.

Koch, Lene. 2004. "The Meaning of Eugenics: Reflections on the Government of Genetic Knowledge." *Science in Context* 17, no. 3 (September): 315–31.

Kühl, Stefan. 2002. *The Nazi Connection: Eugenics, American Racism, and German National Socialism*. New York: Oxford University Press.

Laughlin, Harry. 1922. *Eugenical Sterilization in the United States*. Chicago: Psychopathic Laboratory.

Leon, Sharon. 2013. *An Image of God: The Catholic Struggle with Eugenics*. Chicago: University of Chicago Press.

Lepicard, Etienne. 1998. "Eugenics and Roman Catholicism. An Encyclical Letter in Context: Casti connubii, December 31, 1930." *Science in Context* 11, no. 3–4 (Autumn-Winter): 527–44.

Lepicard, Etienne. 2007. "Trauma, Memory, and Euthanasia at the Nuremberg Medical Trial, 1946–1947." In *Trauma and Memory. Reading, Healing, and Making Law*, edited by Austin Sarat, Nadav Davidovich, and Michal Alberstein, 204–24. Stanford: Stanford University Press.

Lepicard, Etienne. 2019. *"L'Homme, cet inconnu" d'Alexis Carrel (1935): Anatomie d'un succès, analyse d'un echéc*. Paris: Classiques Garnier.

Levine, Philippa. 2017. *Eugenics: A Very Short Introduction*. Oxford: Oxford University Press.

Ley, Astrid. 2004. *Zwangssterilisationen und Ärzteschaft. Hintergründe und Ziele ärztlichen Handelns 1934–1945*. Frankfurt / Main: Campus.

Lombardo, Paul A. 2008. *Three Generations, No Imbeciles: Eugenics, The Supreme Court, and Buck vs. Bell*. Baltimore: Johns Hopkins University Press.

Marrus, Michael R. 1999. "The Nuremberg Doctors' Trial in Context." *Bulletin of the History of Medicine* 73, no.1 (Spring): 106–23.

Mazumdar, Pauline. 1992. *Eugenics, Human Genetics, and Human Failings: The Eugenics Society, Its Sources and Its Critics in Britain*. London: Routledge.

Meier, Marietta. 2004. "Zwangssterilisationen in der Schweiz." *Traverse—Zeitschrift für Geschichte/Revue d'Histoire* 11: 130–46.

Ploetz, Alfred. 1911. "Die Begriffe Rasse und Gesellschaft und einige damit zusammenhängende Probleme." *Schriften der Deutschen Gesellschaft für Soziologie* 1: 111–36.

Roelcke, Volker. 2002. "Programm und Praxis der psychiatrischen Genetik an der Deutschen Forschungsanstalt für Psychiatrie unter Ernst Rüdin." *Medizinhistorisches Journal* 37 (January): 21–55.

Roelcke, Volker: 2006. "Funding the Scientific Foundations of Race Policies: Ernst Rüdin and the Impact of Career Resources on Psychiatric Genetics, ca. 1910–1945." In *Man, Medicine, and the State: The Human Body as an Object of Government Sponsored Medical Research in the 20th Century*, edited by Wolfgang U. Eckart, 73–87. Stuttgart: Steiner.

Roelcke, Volker. 2012. "Ernst Rüdin: Renommierter Wissenschaftler—radikaler Rassenhygieniker." *Der Nervenarzt* 83, no. 3 (March): 303–10.

Roelcke, Volker. 2013. "Hans Roemer (1878–1947): Überzeugter Eugeniker, Kritiker der Krankentötungen," *Der Nervenarzt* 84, no. 9 (September): 1064–68.

Roelcke, Volker. 2019. "Eugenic Concerns, Scientific Practices: International Relations in the Establishment of Psychiatric Genetics in Germany, Britain, the US and Scandinavia, ca. 1910–1960." *History of Psychiatry* 30, no. 1 (March): 19–37.

Schmuhl, Hans-Walter. 2008. *The Kaiser-Wilhelm-Institute for Anthropology, Human Heredity and Eugenics, 1927–1945*. Dordrecht: Springer.

Schmuhl, Hans-Walter. 2016. *Die Gesellschaft Deutscher Neurologen und Psychiater im Nationalsozialismus*. Berlin: Springer.

Spiro, Jonathan Peter. 2009. *Defending the Master Race: Conservation, Eugenics, and the Legacy of Madison Grant*. Burlington: University of Vermont Press.

Turda, Marius, and Paul Weindling, eds. 2007. *"Blood and Homeland": Eugenics and Racial Nationalism in Central and Southeast Europe, 1900–1940*. Budapest/ New York: Central European University Press.

Turda, Marius, and Marie Sophia Quine. 2018. *Historicizing Race*. London: Bloomsbury.

Weikart, Richard. 2004. *From Darwin to Hitler: Evolutionary Ethics, Eugenics, and Racism in Germany*. New York: Palgrave Macmillan.

Weindling, Paul. 1989. *Health, Race, and German Politics between National Unification and Nazism, 1870–1945*. Cambridge: Cambridge University Press.

Weingart, Peter, Jürgen Kroll, and Kurt Bayertz. 1988. *Rasse, Blut und Gene: Geschichte der Eugenik und Rassenhygiene in Deutschland*. Frankfurt am Main: Suhrkamp.

Weiss, Sheila. 2010. *The Nazi Symbiosis: Human Genetics and Politics in the Third Reich*. Chicago: University of Chicago Press.

Chapter Three

Euthanasia in Nazi Germany

Children's Euthanasia Program, Aktion T4, and Decentralized Killing

Gerrit Hohendorf

THE LIFE OF ADELHEID BLOCH AND THE
DESTRUCTION OF LIFE UNWORTHY OF LIVING

Adelheid was the youngest child in a Jewish family from Konstanz, Germany. She was born in 1908 and raised with an older brother and two half-siblings from her father's first marriage in a sheltered and well-to-do family. Adelheid was musical, and despite impaired language and mental development from encephalitis when she was one-and-a-half-years old, music remained her means of expression even when she lacked the words. In 1916, Adelheid's parents placed her in a reformatory school to encourage her mental development. She "continuously [repeated] a peculiar series of sounds," especially when she became restless or afraid of something, but she understood simple things and helped out in the ward until 1921. Then she started to destroy her toys, tear her clothing, and pluck flowers from their pots. Adelheid calmed down for a while, played with the other children, and enjoyed the company of others. In 1923, she attacked an attendant and was transferred, first to an asylum in Eichberg and later to one in Wiesloch. The physicians and nurses in these asylums only saw the 15-year-old girl's deficits, and labeled Adelheid as "incurable," an "inferior idiot," and "merely vegetating." In their view, Adelheid no longer had any human qualities, like a body without a soul. On August 8, 1938, Dr. Gregor Overhamm, the senior physician at Wiesloch, noted in Adelheid's file that she "continues to be horribly difficult a[nd] disruptive. Life unworthy of living!" (Federal Archives Berlin n.d., R 179/22496). During the November 1938 pogrom against Jews, Adelheid's father was arrested and severely mistreated, and her family was forced to emigrate without 30-year-old Adelheid.

On June 25, 1940, Adelheid was transferred to the Grafeneck asylum and murdered in its gas chamber (Hohendorf 2009, 24–29; Federal Archives Berlin n.d., R 179/22496).

National Socialists did not invent the concept of "life unworthy of living" (Hohendorf 2013a; see also chapter 1 in this book). In 1920, influenced by Germany's defeat in World War I, renowned lawyer Karl Binding and well-known Freiburg psychiatrist Alfred Hoche published *Die Freigabe der Vernichtung lebensunwerten Lebens* (*The Permission to Annihilate Life Unworthy of Living*). They wrote, "*Are there human lives which have lost their status of being a legally protected interest to such a degree that their continuation has permanently lost any value both for the bearers of these lives and for society?*" (Binding and Hoche 1920; italics in original text).

The concept "destruction of life unworthy of living" was not actualized during the Weimar Republic. On the other hand, eugenics (racial hygiene, or *Rassenhygiene* in German), became the leading and exclusive scientific foundation of health and population policy during the Third Reich (Weindling 1989; Weingart, Kroll and Bayertz 1988; Weiss 2010) as discussed in chapter 2 in this book. The main goal of the National Socialist state was to strengthen the German *Volkskörper* (nation's body) primarily by eliminating all human beings who either did not live up to the idealized physical and mental standards of the Aryan Race and/or did not contribute sufficiently to society. The implementation of this policy began with the 1933 eugenic Sterilization Law for the "the prevention of hereditarily diseased offspring," which resulted in the involuntary sterilization of up to 400,000 people with specified mental, neurological, and physical impairments in the German Reich between 1934 and 1944 (Bock 2010; Benzenhöfer and Ackermann 2015).

Even if early National Socialist propaganda did not openly call for the physical destruction of mentally ill and physically disabled people, it depicted them as "ballast existences" and "useless eaters" (Makowski 1996) with little if any value to society. In the Darwinian "struggle for life," they lost their right to exist, and, furthermore, providing them with medical care was not consistent with the preservation and strengthening of the *Volkskörper* (Schmuhl 1992). It seemed logical, therefore, to release these existences from their suffering and to free society from their burden, a postulation that became more respectable and acceptable once the Great Depression began in 1929.

Living conditions in mental hospitals and nursing homes worsened during the 1930s as a consequence of drastic financial austerity measures in social care and psychiatric treatment, and of abandonment of reforms such as early discharge, family care, and outpatient treatment (Siemen 1987; Faulstich 1998; Burleigh 1995, 11–92). Shortages of food, clothing, heating, nursing staff, and medical care had dire effects on the physical and mental health of the many patients in neuropsychiatric institutions. They often lived without hope for either recovery or return to society in overcrowded dormitories with bad hygienic conditions, suffering from weight loss and infectious diseases, especially tuberculosis. As reported in 1936 by the director of the Sonnenstein asylum, Prof. Hermann Paul Nitsche, who later became a central figure in the *Aktion* T4 euthanasia program, conditions steadily worsened:

> The main difficulty [. . .] is that there are more and more of those run-down patients who are difficult to treat and who tend toward restlessness and to mess things up in all wards. The cases of violence against the nursing staff und injuries of them have severely increased again. One has to work increasingly with sedatives and has to take the extraordinary double-edged sanction of isolation. (quoted in Faulstich 1998, 194–195)

Subsequently, patients became the "run-down existences" and "final states" that racial hygienists claimed they were, especially when they did not respond to violent therapeutic measures such as insulin or electric shock therapy (Hohendorf 2013b). These bothersome, incurable, and economically useless patients were then killed by National Socialist health care policy makers, physicians, and nurses who had created the "intolerable suffering" that was used to justify murder.

EUTHANASIA AND WAR

In October 1939, Adolf Hitler signed this document and backdated it to September 1, 1939:

> Reichsleiter Bouhler and Dr. med. Brandt are charged with the responsibility of enlarging the authority of certain physicians to be designated by name in such a manner that persons who, according to human judgment, are incurable can, upon a most careful diagnosis of their condition of sickness, be accorded a mercy death. (Federal Archives Berlin 1939, R 3001/24209)

The backdating of the document to the first day of World War II had a symbolic meaning (Schmuhl 1992, 180–181)—the German invasion of Poland was not only the start of an "outward war," but also an "inward war" against allegedly "worthless" people unfit for socially useful work. With deadly consequences, the National Socialists waged this war against "inferior people" in the German Reich and in areas annexed both before and after World War II began.

In the autumn of 1939, *SS-Sonderkommandos*, or special command units of the SS (*Schutzstaffel*, or Protection Squads), were shooting or gassing to death thousands of institutionalized Polish patients as well as German patients who had been deported to occupied Poland from Pomerania and East

Prussia. In the forest of Spengawsken between September 1939 and January 1940, one such unit led by Kurt Eimann murdered between 1,600 and 2,000 patients from the Konradstein Hospital near Gdansk. At the instigation of the *Gauleiter* of Pomerania, Franz Schwede-Coburg, German physicians selected about 1,400 German patients from Pomeranian asylums who were shot in a forest near Neustadt in the west of Gdansk by Eiman's unit and buried in mass graves in November and December 1939 (Riess 1995).

Another special unit under Herbert Lange was responsible for the murders of patients in the annexed Polish territory of Wartheland, initially with an improvised gas chamber in Fort VII in Poznań, but then with mobile carbon monoxide gas chambers. This unit, for example, murdered mainly Jewish and Polish patients from the Dziekanka (Tiegenhof) institution from December 1939 to June 1941 (Riess 1995, 273–354; Schwanke 2014), and approximately 1,550 patients from East Prussian institutions who were selected at the request of the local *Gauleiter* Erich Koch between May to June 1940 and then sent to the transit camp of Soldau (Topp et al. 2008). Excluding victims of starvation and neglect, approximately 16,000 Polish psychiatric patients were killed during the German occupation of Poland (Jaroszewski 1993, 226–227).

The Wehrmacht exploited the resources of the occupied territories of the Soviet Union. In cooperation with the Wehrmacht, *SS-Einsatzkommandos* (company-sized subunits of battalion-sized *SS* special action groups called *Einsatzgruppen*) murdered more than 17,000 Soviet psychiatric patients by mass executions, thereby enabling the Wehrmacht to take over these "liberated" hospitals (Winkler and Hohendorf 2018). Initially, they killed patients unable to work and all Jewish patients, based upon anti-Semitic, anti-Slavic, and anti-Bolshevist concepts of the enemy, the ideology of "life unworthy of living," and the stigmatization of psychiatric patients as a perceived threat to security. In a second step, they murdered the surviving patients. The killing methods included starvation, freezing, bombing, poisoning, shooting, and gassing, either by mobile gas vans or by immobile gas chambers. The murder of psychiatric patients was closely connected to the annihilation of the Jewish population, which was the main task of the *SS-Einsatzgruppen* and *SS-Einsatzkommandos* (Klein and Angrck 1997).

On a visit to the psychiatric hospital of Novinki near Minsk in August 1941, Heinrich Himmler instructed Arthur Nebe, the head of *Einsatzgruppe* B, and his chief chemist, Albert Widman, to find a more efficient method of killing psychiatric patients. They first tried explosives, but this proved to be unsafe for the perpetrators as well as inefficient and gruesome. When they arrived at the psychiatric hospital in Mogilev, Widman and Nebe, with the help of a Wehrmacht physician, selected 30 to 35 patients for a trial gassing with engine exhaust fumes in a provisory gas chamber in one of the hospital buildings.

Some weeks later, probably on October 1, 1941, *Einsatzkommando* 8 killed approximately 800 patients in the same way (Winkler and Hohendorf 2018, 154–159). After the gassing, Prieb, the interpreter for *Einsatzkommando* 8, justified the procedure to the hospital staff: "They [the Germans] also practice this kind of annihilation in Germany, since the annihilated patients are of no use to anybody, neither to themselves, nor to others, and this category of people is only to be destroyed" (quoted in Winkler and Hohendorf 2010, 96). In January 1942, *Einsatzkommando* 8 transported the emaciated, surviving patients to a nearby village, Novo Pashkovo, forced them to undress in extremely cold weather, and shot them to death. Subsequently, the Wehrmacht converted Mogilev Psychiatric Hospital into a military hospital and appropriated its medical and domestic staff (Winkler and Hohendorf 2018, 159–161).

HITLER'S CHANCELLERY

In the German Reich itself, the euthanasia campaign was organized by the Führer's Chancellery (*Kanzlei des Führers*), which handled unsolicited requests from citizens, including requests to euthanize mentally and/or physically disabled family members. To fulfill these requests, leading German psychiatrists and pediatricians helped establish in early 1939 two bureaucracies: the Children's Euthanasia Program and *Aktion* T4 for the registration, selection, and annihilation of asylum patients. To conceal their true missions, Hitler's Chancellery chose euphemisms for these bureaucracies, the Reich Committee for the Scientific Registration of Serious Hereditary and Constitutional Illnesses and the Charitable Foundation for Institutional Care, respectively. In April 1940, the Chancellery located some of its offices in a mansion at *Tiergartenstrasse* 4 in Berlin (Hinz-Wessels 2016), thereby giving the name "T4" to the bureaucracy of *Aktion* T4. It was not until after World War II that *Aktion T4* came to mean the killing of psychiatric patients, including men, women, and children, in 1940 and 1941 in specialized euthanasia centers equipped with gas chambers. The T4 organization cooperated closely with the Reich's Ministry of Interior that was responsible for health care and the corresponding administrative authorities of asylums in the German states and Prussian provinces (Burleigh 1995, 99ff; Friedlander 1995; Hohendorf et al. 2016).

THE CHILDREN'S EUTHANASIA PROGRAM

The Reich Committee for the Scientific Registration of Serious Hereditary and Constitutional Illnesses was responsible for the euthanasia of children

(Topp 2004; Benzenhöfer 2008; Kaelber 2012). As early as August 1939, the Reich Ministry of the Interior ordered physicians and midwives to register mentally and physically disabled children less than three years old with the Reich Committee. Three pediatric experts—Professor Werner Catel, director of the Leipzig University Children's Hospital, Professor Hans Heinze, a child and adolescent psychiatrist, and pediatrician Dr. Ernst Wentzler—selected patients for admission to *Kinderfachabteilungen* (special children's wards) run by the Reich Committee. The children not yet in institutional care were identified and admitted with the help of the local public health departments. The institutionalized children were registered with the Reich Committee by the institution's physician.

Parents were told their children would receive the best possible treatment in the special children's wards but, after a period of observation, they learned that their child had died. In most cases, an enabling letter from the Reich Committee authorized a child's involuntary euthanasia or "special treatment," but physicians in the wards had considerable discretion regarding which children would live or die, usually from an overdose of tranquilizers administered by nurses. In March 1941, the age limit for the children's euthanasia program was raised from three to 14 years of age, including those children who were already in nursing care institutions or reformatories, and they now fell under the responsibility of the "Reich's Committee" (Klee 1985, 103; Mitscherlich and Mielke 1960, 211–212; Archives of the District of Upper Bavaria n.d., patient file no. 10 346). Between 1939 and 1945, roughly 7,000 children registered by the Reich Committee were murdered in approximately 30 special children's wards in the German Reich, Poland, and Czechoslovakia, and an unknown number were also murdered either in the special children's wards without being registered, in *Aktion* T4, or in the decentralized euthanasia described later in this chapter (Hohendorf and Rotzoll 2004).

Consider, for example, Wilhelmine Haussner, who was born in 1927 and developed encephalitis after a vaccination that resulted in impaired mental development and constant motion. Her parents placed Wilhelmine in a nursery school in Schönbrunn, a Catholic nursing home near Dachau, where she was content. Her parents and siblings visited her frequently. As part of a campaign to relocate residents of church institutions to state institutions, Wilhelmine was transferred on May 23, 1941, to the pediatric ward at Eglfing-Haar where she was classified as an "inferior idiot." The Reich Committee had already marked Wilhelmine for death, and she was killed on November 7, 1942, by an overdose of luminal, a tranquilizer. Shortly beforehand, her mother received this letter from Director Pfannmüller: "After a prolonged catarrh of the upper respiratory tract, your daughter has also contracted pneumonia. The girl's condition is critical. We are informing you so that that you can still visit the

diplomatic efforts to halt or modify the euthanasia campaign, the courageous public sermon of Clemens Count von Galen, the Bishop of Münster, on August 3, 1941, led to the cessation of the gassing of institutional patients. Apparently, Adolf Hitler did not want to weaken the already battered morale of the German population by continuing the killings (Faulstich 1998, 271–288).

According to internal T4 statistics, 70,273 institutional patients were murdered in the six killing centers between January 1940 and August 1941, and this "disinfection" saved 880 million Reichsmarks over the next eight years (National Archives and Records Administration n.d., Case 000-12-463, 4). In regions that were included in *Aktion* T4 early on, such as Baden, Württemberg, Bavaria, and Austria, more than half of all institutional patients were murdered (Faulstich 1998, 569–581).

One group of patients had no chance of survival within the T4 program. Approximately 2,500 institutionalized Jewish psychiatric patients were murdered solely because they were Jewish, regardless of the selection criteria applied to non-Jewish patients. Starting in the spring of 1940, Jewish patients were brought together in certain collective institutions in the various states and provinces, such as Eglfing-Haar in Bavaria, before being transferred to a T4 killing center (Hinz-Wessels 2013).

DECENTRALIZED EUTHANASIA

There is a widely held misconception that the National Socialist killing of patients was separated into two or more consecutive phases, the centrally managed patient killing in the six T4 euthanasia centers followed by decentralized killing ordered by local personnel. These decentralized killings were often referred to as "wild euthanasia" by researchers to characterize their unregulated and random nature (von Tiedemann, Hohendorf, and von Cranach 2018b, 169–171). In fact, documentation from the T4 administrative offices confirm that physicians from individual institutions were killing patients with medication before and during *Aktion* T4 (Federal Archives Berlin 1942, R 96 I/16). For example, as early as 1939/1940, psychiatrist Hermann Paul Nitsche, who subsequently became medical director of the T4 medical department, prescribed food deprivation of the so-called "run-down" ill people in Saxony during *Aktion* T4 (Faulstich 1998, 480–485). Regional health department heads in individual provinces such as Württemberg and in the state of Saxony prompted institutional physicians to kill incurably ill patients with medication after *Aktion* T4 officially ended. A few institutional physicians, like Alfred Schulz in Gross Schweidnitz, followed these demands (Faulstich 1998, 356, 499–502, 519–520).

Similarly, the November 30, 1942, order by the Bavarian Ministry of the Interior "to take effect immediately that those inmates of mental hospitals and nursing homes who perform useful labor or are in therapeutic treatment [. . .] be better cared for both quantitatively and qualitatively at the expense of the rest of the inmates" was a veiled directive for continuation of euthanasia by starvation (von Tiedemann, Hohendorf, and von Cranach 2018a, 111). Thereafter, the institution provided a meatless and fat-free "E-Kost" (deprivation diet) to patients seen as useless and decrepit so that they would die of starvation within a few months. Eglfing-Haar mental hospital established two hunger houses where more than about 440 patients died by the end of the war (von Tiedemann, Hohendorf, and von Cranach 2018a, 110–117). A survivor reported her experiences in the summer of 1945: "In here you don't get enough, after all, because it is a jail where they want to kill you. You're a loony bin lady. You don't need anything. They say, you need more sleeping draft, then you don't need to eat so much" (Schmidt 1983, 139).

In a study of the 1,321 fatalities of Munich patients in the Eglfing-Haar asylum between September 1, 1939, and July 1945, my colleagues and I documented that only 471 patients died from natural causes, while 850 were euthanized either by starvation, sedatives, individual neglect characterized by withholding necessary medical treatments, or systemic neglect characterized by abhorrent general conditions such as poor hygiene, overcrowding and, especially, rampant institution-acquired infections such as tuberculosis (von Tiedemann, Hohendorf, von Cranach 2018a; 2018b).

Those regions where the heads of institutions and the *Gauleiter* held particularly anti-patient and anti-psychiatric attitudes during *Aktion* T4 were especially enthusiastic about killing patients after the end of the program. Even before T4 was operational, Fritz Bernotat, the head of institutions in the Wiesbaden district in the Prussian province of Hesse as well as a member of the SA and the SS, said: "Just strike [the patients] dead, then they're gone!" (Sandner 2003, 320). In 1942, he reactivated the defunct Hadamar extermination center near Limburg with the approval of the Frankfurt *Gauleiter* Jakob Sprenger. Retired psychiatrist Adolf Wahlmann implemented Bernotat's instructions to kill patients by medication—gas was no longer being used—when space became scarce. Consequently, Hadamar personnel killed an additional 4,500 patients before the end of World War II, including those transferred from other regions whose subsistence costs were reimbursed as long as they were alive (Sandner 2003, 607–653).

Between 1942 and 1945 in the Pomeranian institution Meseritz-Obrawalde, an estimated 10,000 people died, most of them from areas threatened by air raids (Beddies 2002). Health departments and the *Gauleiters* of threatened cities transferred older, chronically ill people from institutions in densely populated areas to surrounding mental hospitals and nursing homes, which were already overcrowded from dual use as reserve military hospitals. With space at a premium, the T4 administration and Dr. Herbert Linden, Reich Commissioner for Mental Hospitals and Nursing Homes, transferred the elderly and the chronically or mentally ill on short notice to make hospital beds available for other civilians who were either victims of bombings or suffering from an acute, limited illness. After these vulnerable patients were transferred to institutions far away from areas being bombed, willing, local physicians euthanized them, thereby making space for more and more transports. In the early summer of 1943, Karl Brandt, now General Commissioner of Military Medical Services and Public Health with extensive special executive powers, ordered the transfer of 23,000 mentally ill people from heavily bombed industrial centers of the Rhineland and Westphalia provinces to provide more medical resources for patients with somatic illnesses. As it turned out, only about 8,000 psychiatric patients from the Rhine Province and about 2,800 from Westphalia were transferred (Faulstich 1998, 386, 410; Süss 2003, 327–339; Walter 1996).

The T4 office attempted to gain more control over the euthanasia process by recruiting additional institutional physicians to administer lethal dosages of luminal and morphine-scopolamine and, secondly, by providing sufficient medication to the receiving institutions in middle and east Germany and the occupied territories in the East to complete their task. While Karl Brandt gave verbal support for these administrative changes, he rejected the resumption of patient killing on the large scale of *Aktion* T4 (Süss 2003, 355–366). As far as it is known, at least 28,000 patients were transferred in 1943 and 1944 from regions threatened by air raids to asylums in Hesse, Bavaria, Austria, central Germany (Thuringia, the province of Saxony, the state of Saxony), and the eastern territory of the Reich (Pomerania, Warthegau, General Government); approximately 85 percent of the transferred patients did not survive the war (Faulstich 1998, 620–624).

The best estimate of the number of patients killed in the years of decentralized euthanasia by starvation, medications, and neglect is between 90,000 and 110,000 (Faulstich 2000, 225–226). Finally, in the last years of the war, mentally ill forced laborers and those suffering from tuberculosis were killed systematically in designated asylums within the framework of the T4 organization (Klee 2010, 299–305).

HEALING AND KILLING

How do we explain why doctors who are supposed to heal chose to kill, especially when they were neither ordered nor forced to do so? Many were convinced they were taking part in a great "work of salvation" (Lifton 1986). They thought that the elimination of useless and incurable asylum patients would provide more money and staff to patients who could be cured. For many psychiatrists in the Nazi period, destroying and healing were very closely connected (Schmuhl 1994). In a 1943 memorandum for the reform of German psychiatry, leading Nazi psychiatrists wrote:

> But also the measures of euthanasia will find even more understanding and approval, once it is established and known that in every case of mental illness, all possibilities for healing the patients, or at least improving their conditions enough so that they are brought to economically valuable work, be it in their profession, or another form, will be exhausted. (National Archives and Records Administration n.d., 126, 423–424)

Some psychiatrists and asylum staff claimed after the war that they had only participated in order to prevent worse from happening (Schmuhl 2016, 393; Leipert 1991, 113–117). Some denied knowing the fate awaiting the patients transferred from their institutions, and many claimed they had acted with compassion for those lives unworthy of living (see chapter 1 in this book). Be that as it may, physicians certainly lost their feeling of empathy for the patients entrusted to them and, incomprehensibly, chose to murder them (von Cranach 2013).

AFTER THE WAR

Doctors continued to murder patients in Kaufbeuren for weeks after the end of World War II and stopped only when American officers visited the asylum and conducted investigations (Friedlander 1995). Many other institutionalized patients died from neglect and malnourishment even after the war. The perpetrators often remained in their positions and continued their careers as if nothing had happened. Although some perpetrators were called to account in front of German and American courts, interest in investigating the murders and persecuting the murderers came to a virtual standstill in the 1950s (Hohendorf 2013a, 132–140).

The voices of the survivors and the victims' relatives were not heard, and they have yet to receive adequate compensation. Dedicated citizens, historians, and psychiatrists have been working for about 25 years to come to terms with and educate the world about the euthanasia murders. Many families now speak about their murdered relatives, and many psychiatric hospitals display plaques and memorials. In particular, the six former killing centers—Brandenburg, Grafeneck, Sonnenstein, Hartheim, Hadamar, and Bernburg, a site visited by the North American authors of this book, and *Tiergartenstrasse 4* in Berlin, where the organizers of the patient murders had their office—have outstanding educational memorials (Stiftung Denkmal für die ermordeten Juden Europas n.d.; Foundation Memorial to the Murdered Jews of Europe n.d.).

BIBLIOGRAPHY

Aly, Götz. 2013. *Die Belasteten: 'Euthanasie' 1939–1945. Eine Gesellschaftsgeschichte*. Frankfurt am Main: Fischer.

Archiv der Stiftung Liebenau. Letter from Helene M. (1902–1940) to her father, dated 1 October 1940, transcript, Archiv der Stiftung Liebenau.

Archives of the District of Upper Bavaria, Munich. n.d. Archival holding Eglfing-Haar, patient file no. 10 346.

Archives of the District of Upper Bavaria, Munich. 1942. Archival holdings Eglfing-Haar, Letter signed by director Hermann Pfannmüller to the mother of Wilhelmine Haussner, November 2, 1942. patient file no. 7,800.

Bader, Helmut. 2014. "Martin Bader. 'Mein Name Ist in Giengen Und Umgebung Gut Bekannt.'" In *Das Vergessen Der Vernichtung Ist Teil Der Vernichtung Selbst, Lebensgeschichten Von Opfern Der nationalsozialistischen 'Euthanasie*, 3rd edition, edited by Petra Fuchs, Maike Rotzoll, Ulrich Müller, Paul Richter, and Gerrit Hohendorf, 105–122. Göttingen: Wallstein.

Beddies, Thomas. 2002. "Die Heil- Und Pflegeanstalt Meseritz-Obrawalde im Dritten Reich." In *Brandenburgische Heil- Und Pflegeanstalten in Der NS-Zeit*, edited by Kristina Hübener, 231–258. Berlin: be.bra wissenschaft verlag.

Benzenhöfer, Udo. 2008. *Der Fall Leipzig (Alias Fall 'Kind Knauer') Und Die Planung Der NS-'Kindereuthanasie.'* Münster: Klemm & Oelschläger.

Benzenhöfer, Udo, and Hanns Ackermann. 2015. *Die Zahl Der Verfahren und Der Sterilisationen Nach Dem Gesetz Zur Verhütung Erbkranken Nachwuchses*. Münster: Klemm & Oelschläger.

Binding, Karl, and Alfred Hoche. 1920. *Die Freigabe Der Vernichtung Lebensunwerten Lebens: Ihr Mass Und Ihre Form*. Leipzig: Meiner.

Bock, Gisela. 2010. *Zwangssterilisation Im Nationalsozialismus: Studien Zur Rassenpolitik Und Geschlechterpolitik*, 2nd ed. Münster: Verlagshaus Monenstein und Vannerdat.

Burleigh, Michael. 1995. *Death and Deliverance: 'Euthanasia' In Germany 1900–1945*. Cambridge: Cambridge University Press.

Crawford, Zacherey. 2015. "The Administration of Death: Karl Brandt, Philipp Bouhler, Victor Brack, and Leonardo Conti." *Western Illinois Historical Review*, Vol VII, Spring: 59–85.

Faulstich, Heinz. 1998. *Hungersterben in Der Psychiatrie 1914–1949: Mit Einer Topographie Der NS-Psychiatrie*. Freiburg im Breisgau: Lambertus.

Faulstich, Heinz. 2000. "Die Zahl Der 'Euthanasie'-Opfer." In *'Euthanasie' und Die Aktuelle Sterbehilfe-Debatte. Die Historischen Hintergründe Medizinischer*

Ethik, edited by Andreas Frewer and Clemens Eickhoff, 218–234. Frankfurt am Main: Campus.

Federal Archives Berlin. n.d. R 179/22496, patient file of Adelheid Bloch.

Federal Archives Berlin. 1939. Adolf Hitler's authorization decree for euthanasia. R 3001/24209.

Federal Archives Berlin. 1942. R 96 I/16, planning report for Baden by [Robert] Müller from September 15, 1942.

Foundation Memorial to the Murdered Jews of Europe. n.d. "Memorial and Information Point for the Victims of National Socialist 'Euthanasia' Killings." website. Accessed August 11, 2019. https://www.stiftung-denkmal.de/en/memorials/memorial-and-information-point-for-the-victims-of-national-socialist-euthanasia-killings.html.

Friedlander, Henry. 1995. *The Origins of Nazi Genocide: From Euthanasia to the Final Solution.* Chapel Hill: University of North Carolina Press.

Gruchmann, Lothar. 1984. "Ein Unbequemer Amtsrichter Im Dritten Reich: Aus Den Personalakten Des Dr. Lothar Kreyßig." *Vierteljahrshefte für Zeitgeschichte* 32, no. 3 (July): 463–488.

Heidelberg University Archives. 1943. Letter from Mathilde N. to Prof. Johann Duken, director of the Heidelberg Children's Hospital from July 6, 1943. Archival holdings Kinderklinik Acc. 15/01 L-II, patient file Christel N. Prot.-No. 1648/1943.

Hessian Main Capital Archives Wiesbaden. Letter from Albert F. to Eichberg State Mental Hospital, Abt. 430/1 Nr. 11074.

Hinz-Wessels, Annette. 2013. "Antisemitismus Und Krankenmord: Zum Umgang Mit Jüdischen Anstaltspatienten Im Nationalsozialismus." *Vierteljahrshefte für Zeitgeschichte* 61, no.1 (January): 65–92.

Hinz-Wessels, Annette. 2016. "From Banker's Villa to The Memorial and Information Point for the Victims of National Socialist 'Euthanasia' Killings." In *Tiergartenstrasse 4. Memorial and Information Point for The Victims of National Socialist 'Euthanasia' Killings*, edited by Foundation to the Murdered Jews of Europe, 34–43. Berlin: Stiftung Denkmal für die ermordeten Juden Europas.

Hinz-Wessels, Annette, Petra Fuchs, Gerrit Hohendorf, and Maike Rotzoll. 2005. "Zur Bürokratischen Abwicklung Eines Massenmords; Die 'Euthanasie'-Aktion Im Spiegel Neuer Dokumente." *Vierteljahrshefte für Zeitgeschichte* 53, no. 1 (January): 79–107.

Hohendorf, Gerrit. 2009. "Adelheid B. '. . . Wiederholt Fast Beständig Eine Eigentümliche Folge von Tönen.'" In *Tödliche Medizin: Rassenwahn Im Nationalsozialismus*, edited by Margret Kampmeyer, 24–29. Göttingen: Wallstein-Verlag.

Hohendorf, Gerrit. 2013a. *Der Tod Als Erlösung Vom Leiden: Geschichte Und Ethik Der Sterbehilfe Seit Dem Ende Des 19. Jahrhunderts in Deutschland.* Göttingen: Wallstein-Verlag.

Hohendorf, Gerrit. 2013b. "Therapieunfähigkeit Als Selektionskriterium. Die 'Schocktherapieverfahren' Und Die Organisationszentrale Der Nationalsozialistischen 'Euthanasie' in Der Berliner Tiergartenstraße 4, 1939–1945." In *'Heroische Therapien': Die Deutsche Psychiatrie Im Internationalen Vergleich, 1918–1945*, edited by Hans-Walter Schmuhl, and Volker Roelcke, 287–307. Göttingen: Wallstein Verlag.

Hohendorf, Gerrit. 2014. "Leopoldine S. '... Scheint Sie Doch Zeitlich in Einer Ganz Anderen Welt Zu Sein.'" In *Das Vergessen Der Vernichtung Ist Teil Der Vernichtung Selbst, Lebensgeschichten Von Opfern der Nationalsozialistischen 'Euthanasie'* 3rd edition, edited by Petra Fuchs, Maike Rotzoll, Ulrich Müller, Paul Richter, and Gerrit Hohendorf, 267–273. Göttingen: Wallstein.

Hohendorf, Gerrit, and Maike Rotzoll. 2004. "'Kindereuthanasie' in Heidelberg." In *Kinder in Der NS-Psychiatrie*, edited by Thomas Beddies and Kristina Hübener, 125–148. Berlin: be.bra wissenschaft verlag.

Hohendorf, Gerrit, Christof Beyer, Jens Thiel, Maike Rotzoll. 2016. "The Murder of Patients in National Socialism: An overview." In *Tiergartenstrasse 4. Memorial and Information Point for the Victims of National Socialist 'Euthanasia' Killings*, edited by Foundation Memorial to the Murdered Jews of Europe, 10–33. Berlin: Stiftung Denkmal für die ermordeten Juden Europas.

Jaroszewski, Zdzislaw, ed. 1993. *Die Ermordung Der Geisteskranken in Polen: 1939–1945*. Warschau: Wydawnictwo Naukowe PWN.

Kaelber, Lutz. 2012. "Child Murder in Nazi Germany: The Memory of Nazi Medical Crimes and Commemoration of 'Children's Euthanasia' Victims at Two Facilities (Eichberg, Kalmenhof)." *Societies* 2, no. 3 (June): 157–94.

Klee, Ernst, ed. 1985. *Dokumente Zur 'Euthanasie.'* Frankfurt am Main: Fischer Taschenbuch.

Klee, Ernst. 2010. *'Euthanasie' Im NS-Staat: Die 'Vernichtung Lebensunwerten Lebens,'* 3rd edition. Frankfurt am Main: Fischer.

Klein, Peter, and Andrej Angrick. 1997. *Die Einsatzgruppen in Der Besetzten Sowjetunion, 1941/42: Die Tätigkeits- Und Lageberichte Des Chefs Der Sicherheitspolizei Und Des SD*. Publikationen der Gedenk- und Bildungsstätte Haus der Wannsee-Konferenz Bd. 6. Berlin: Edition Hentrich.

Leipert, Matthias. 1991. "'Euthanasie' Und 'Widerstand' Von Ärzten in Der Rheinprovinz 1939–1945." In *Psychiatrie im Abgrund. Spurensuche Und Standortbestimmung Nach Den NS-Psychiatrie-Verbrechen*, edited by Ralf Seidel and Wolfgang Franz Werner, 110–124. Rheinprovinz 6. Köln: Rheinland-Verlag, Bonn: Habelt.

Lifton, Robert Jay. 1986. *The Nazi Doctors: Medical Killing and the Psychology of Genocide*. London: Macmillan.

Lutz, Petra. 2006. "Mit Herz Und Vernunft. Angehörige Von 'Euthanasie'-Opfern im Schriftwechsel Mit Den Anstalten." In *'Moderne' Anstaltspsychiatrie im 19. Jahrhundert. Legitimation Und Kritik*, edited by Heiner Fangerau and Karin Nolte, 143–167. Medizin, Gesellschaft und Geschichte 26. Stuttgart: Steiner Verlag.

Makowski, Christine Charlotte. (1996). *Eugenik, Sterilisationspolitik, "Euthanasie" und Bevölkerungspolitik in der nationalsozialistischen Parteipresse*. Husum: Matthiesen Verlag.

Mitscherlich, Alexander, and Fred Mielke, eds. 1960. *Medizin Ohne Menschlichkeit: Dokumente Des Nürnberger Ärzteprozesses*. Frankfurt am Main: Fischer.

National Archives and Records Administration, College Park, MD, US Army Europe, Records of the Judge Advocate General, War Crimes Branch, Records Relating to Medical Experiments, Record Group 549, Stock Area 290, Row 59, Compartment 17, box 2, folder 10, pp. 126, 420–427, Rüdin, de Crinis, C. Schneider, Heinze,

Nitsche, Gedanken und Anregungen betr. die künftige Entwicklung der Psychiatrie, here pp. 126, 423–424.

National Archives and Records Administration, College Park, MD. n.d. Record Group 549, Records of the US Army Europe, Judge Advocate Division War Crimes Branch. War Crimes Case Files Cases not Tried, Case 000-12-463, Box 490–491.

Riess, Volker. 1995. *Die Anfänge Der Vernichtung 'Lebensunwerten Lebens.' In Den Reichsgauen Danzig-Westpreußen Und Wartheland 1939/40.* Frankfurt/Main: Lang.

Rotzoll, Maike, Petra Fuchs, Paul Richter, and Gerrit Hohendorf. 2010a. "Die nationalsozialistische 'Euthanasieaktion T4.' Historische Forschung, individuelle Lebensgeschichten und Erinnerungskultur." *Der Nervenarzt* 81, no. 11 (Nov): 1326–1332.

Rotzoll, Maike, Gerrit Hohendorf, Petra Fuchs, Paul Richter, Christoph Mundt, and Wolfgang U. Eckart, eds. 2010b. *Die Nationalsozialistische 'Euthanasie'-Aktion T4'Und Ihre Opfer: Geschichte Und Ethische Konsequenzen Für Die Gegenwart.* Paderborn, München, Wien, Zürich: Schöningh.

Sandner, Peter. 2003. *Verwaltung Des Krankenmordes: Der Bezirksverband Nassau im Nationalsozialismus.* Historische Schriftenreihe des Landeswohlfahrtsverbandes Hessen Hochschriften vol. 2. Giessen: Psychosozial-Verlag.

Schmidt, Gerhard. 1983. *Selektion in Der Heilanstalt 1939–1945.* Frankfurt am Main: Suhrkamp.

Schmuhl, Hans-Walter. 1992. *Rassenhygiene, Nationalsozialismus, Euthanasie: Von Der Verhütung Zur Vernichtung 'Lebensunwerten Lebens,' 1890–1945,* 2nd ed. Kritische Studien zur Geschichtswissenschaft 75. Göttingen: Vandenhoeck und Ruprecht.

Schmuhl, Hans-Walter. 1994. "Reformpsychiatrie und Massenmord." In *Nationalsozialismus Und Modernisierung,* 2nd edition, edited by Michael Prinz, and Rainer Zitelmann, 239–266. Darmstadt: Wissenschaftliche Buchgesellschaft.

Schmuhl, Hans-Walter. 2016. *Die Gesellschaft Deutscher Neurologen Und Psychiater im Nationalsozialismus.* Berlin, Heidelberg: Springer.

Schwanke, Enno. 2014. *Die Landesheil- Und Pflegeanstalt Tiegenhof: Die Nationalsozialistische 'Euthanasie' in Polen Während Des Zweiten Weltkrieges.* Frankfurt am Main: Peter Lang Internationaler Verlag der Wissenschaften.

Siemen, Hans-Ludwig. 1987. *Menschen Blieben Auf Der Strecke: Psychiatrie Zwischen Reform Und Nationalsozialismus.* Gütersloh: Van Hoddis.

Stiftung Denkmal für die ermordeten Juden Europas. n.d. "Gedenk- und Informationsort für die Opfer der Nationalsozialistischen 'Euthanasie'- Morde." Accessed August 11, 2019. https://www.t4-denkmal.de/.

Süss, Winfried. 2003. *Der 'Volkskörper' im Krieg: Gesundheitspolitik, Gesundheitsverhältnisse Und Krankenmord im Nationalsozialistischen Deutschland 1939–1945.* München: Oldenbourg.

Topp, Sascha. 2004. "Der 'Reichsausschuß Zur Wissenschaftlichen Erfassung Erb- und Anlagebedingter Schwerer Leiden.' Zur Organisation Der Ermordung Minderjähriger Kranker im Nationalsozialismus 1939–1945." In *Kinder in Der*

NS-Psychiatrie, edited by Thomas Beddies and Kristina Hübener, 17–54. Berlin: be.bra wissenschaft verlag.

Topp, Sascha, Petra Fuchs, Gerrit Hohendorf, Paul Richter, and Maike Rotzoll. 2008. "Die Provinz Ostpreussen Und Die Nationalsozialistische 'Euthanasie': SS-'Aktion Lange' Und 'Aktion T4.'" *Medizinhistorisches Journal* 43, no. 1 (February): 20–55.

von Cranach, Michael. 2013. "Handlungsmotivation der NS-Euthanasieärzte." In *Theory of Mind. Neurobiologie Und Psychologie sozialen Verhaltens*, 2nd edition, edited by Hans Förstl, 253–262. Heidelberg: Springer.

von Tiedemann, Sibylle, Gerrit Hohendorf, and Michael von Cranach. 2018a. "Dezentrale 'Euthanasie' in der Heil- und Pflegeanstalt Eglfing-Haar." In *Gedenkbuch Für Die Münchner Opfer Der Nationalsozialistischen 'Euthanasie'-Morde*, edited by Michael von Cranach, Annette Eberle, Gerrit Hohendorf, and Sibylle von Tiedemann, 169–192. Göttingen: Wallstein.

von Tiedemann, Sibylle, Gerrit Hohendorf, and Michael von Cranach. 2018b. "Die Ermittlung der Opfer der dezentralen 'Euthanasie.'" In *Gedenkbuch Für Die Münchner Opfer Der Nationalsozialistischen 'Euthanasie'-Morde*, edited by Michael von Cranach, Annette Eberle, Gerrit Hohendorf, and Sibylle von Tiedemann, 169–192. Göttingen: Wallstein.

Walter, Bernd. 1996. *Psychiatrie Und Gesellschaft in Der Moderne: Geisteskrankenfürsorge in Der Provinz Westfalen Zwischen Kaiserreich Und NS-Regime.* Paderborn: Schöningh.

Weindling, Paul. 1989. *Health, Race and German Politics Between National Unification and Nazism, 1870–1945.* Cambridge: Cambridge University Press.

Weingart, Peter, Jürgen Kroll, and Kurt Bayertz. 1988. *Rasse, Blut Und Gene: Geschichte Der Eugenik Und Rassenhygiene in Deutschland.* Frankfurt am Main: Suhrkamp.

Weiss, Sheila Faith. 2010. *The Nazi Symbiosis: Human Genetics and Politics in the Third Reich.* Chicago: University of Chicago Press.

Winkler, Ulrike, and Gerrit Hohendorf. 2010. "'Nun Ist Mogiljow Frei Von Verrückten.' Die Ermordung Der PsychiatriepatientInnen in Mogilew 1941/42." In *Krieg Und Psychiatrie 1914–1950*, edited by Babette Quinkert, Philipp Rauh, and Ulrike Winkler, 75–103. Göttingen: Wallstein.

Winkler, Ulrike, and Gerrit Hohendorf. 2018. "The Murder of Psychiatric Patients by the SS and the Wehrmacht in Poland and the Soviet Union, especially in Mogilev, 1939–1945." In *Mass Violence in Occupied Europe*, edited by Alex Kay and David Stahel, 147–170. Bloomington: Indiana University Press.

Chapter Four

Ethics and Ideology for Future Doctors

How Nazi Values Were Taught in the German Medical Curriculum 1939–1945

Florian Bruns

Why did all too many physicians in Nazi Germany allow themselves to fulfill the murderous Nazi policy toward Jews, mentally disabled patients, or persons deemed "hereditarily ill"? How was it possible that people morally committed to the Hippocratic tradition of *primum nil nocere* (first do no harm) disregarded the personal integrity and dignity of human beings? The confusion gets even greater when we consider that Nazi Germany, of all countries, was one of the first to introduce a compulsory course of lectures in medical ethics into its medical curriculum (Bruns and Chelouche 2017). Though many would call the phrase "Nazi medical ethics" an oxymoron, its dismissal would be a mistake. Nazi ideology did indeed incorporate a system of moral values, even if we reject it and its premises today (Proctor 2000; Reich 2001; Weikart 2009). Nazi society was loaded with moral meanings derived from racial ideology, and the Nazi paradigm was saturated with moral terminology, including terms like defilement (of the race), treason (of the people), sin (against the blood), or, positively connoted: fidelity, honor, and decency. After the war, most of the doctors who had participated in acts of violence, forced sterilizations, or murder under the guise of euthanasia, not only felt no guilt but also believed in the moral correctness of their conduct. They displayed anything but a bad conscience (Bialas 2013). For example, many of the Nazi doctors in the Nuremberg Medical Trial who were found guilty of performing deadly human experiments invoked ethical arguments in their own defense, such as a crude form of utilitarianism (Caplan 2010).

Until recently, relatively little has been published on Nazi efforts to introduce their morality into the medical curriculum. Drawing on previously published findings on Nazi medical ethics in Germany (Bruns 2009), this chapter intends to demonstrate that Nazi-influenced medical ethics was an integral part of the curriculum at German medical schools between 1939 and 1945. The compulsory lecture course entitled *Ärztliche Rechts- und Standeskunde* (Medical Law and Professional Studies, or MLPS) was taught at all medical faculties in Germany during World War II. I will focus on three aspects:

1. Why did the Nazis introduce medical ethics into the curriculum?
2. Who taught these lectures?
3. What topics were addressed?

Answers to these questions rely on primary as well as secondary sources, including the standard textbook on MLPS, *Ärztliche Rechts- und Standeskunde*, written by Dr. Rudolf Ramm, "the leading Nazi medical ethicist" (Proctor 1992, 17; Ramm 1942). Course catalogs of all the medical faculties under German control from 1939 to 1945 were used to identify lecturers on medical ethics. Their biographies and political backgrounds were pieced together from documents and membership files relating to the *Nationalsozialistische Deutsche Arbeiterpartei*, or NSDAP (National Socialist German Workers' Party) and the *Reichsärztekammer* (Reich Physicians' Chamber) held at Germany's Federal Archives. I also used documentation from the archives of the de Gruyter publishing company held in the Berlin State Library, and the archives of the former Friedrich-Wilhelm-University in Berlin (today Humboldt-University) where Rudolf Ramm taught MLPS from 1940 to 1945.

ETHICS AS A TOOL TO PROMOTE NAZI IDEAS WITHIN THE MEDICAL CURRICULUM

The question of how best to form future physicians is not a new one. In the 1930s, even Nazi politicians and medical functionaries were concerned with this issue. Their main objective, however, was not to reform the students' curriculum for the sake of higher quality medical care or for the well-being of the patients. Instead, their intention was, first and foremost, to inculcate their ideology into an important profession (Bestvater 1939). From the viewpoint of the Nazi authorities, a new curriculum for medical students to substantiate and legitimatize the Nazi health policy was needed but still lacking. Soon, it became clear that, unlike in the humanities, it was difficult to politicize an academic discipline that was very much based on science and manual skills.

In the first years after Hitler's coming into power, a widely accepted Nazi version of specialties like Internal Medicine or Surgery—subjects that constituted the core of the curriculum—did not exist. Textbooks at that time stemmed from the pre-Nazi era, and most of the relevant lectures were given by professors who were born in the nineteenth century. Only a minority of them were willing to immediately rewrite their lectures and incorporate Nazi party ideology. While many medical professors had some sympathy for the Nazi movement, they mistrusted the enthusiasm for alternative medicine and natural healing that several high-ranking Nazis displayed, with Hitler's deputy Rudolf Hess and SS chief Heinrich Himmler leading the way. In short, the curriculum left little room for imparting the Nazi worldview to students. For Nazi propagandists, this was a serious problem since prospective medical doctors were seen as a particularly important target group. They were deemed the coming *Gesundheitsführer* (health leaders) designated to implement Nazi health and race policies in the future.

In the end, adding new subjects to the curriculum seemed to be the only choice for Nazi health activists to gain influence in academic teaching. Initially, restructuring the curriculum met resistance even from Nazi officials since further expanding the overloaded curriculum interfered with the Nazis' goal of shortening it, thereby encouraging early marriage and procreation among physicians (Ramm 1942, 33). Eventually, the addition of new subjects was accepted by Nazi authorities as a necessary evil to gain a foothold in teaching medical students. Simultaneously, in the late 1930s, the faculties had been brought into line to such an extent that their initial reluctance gave way to acceptance of the curricular changes.

So, after years of preparation and lobbying, *Reichsärzteführer* (Reich physicians' leader) Leonardo Conti together with the Ministry of Science and Education introduced a revised medical curriculum in April 1939. It included newly designed lectures in Racial Hygiene, Genetics, Military Medicine, Natural Healing, and the History of Medicine, subjects particularly suitable for promoting Nazi ideology to students (Kater 1989, 111–126). The same can be said for MLPS, another new course of obligatory lectures for students in their last semester, which was intended to provide "an understanding of both the written and unwritten laws of medical ethics" (Ramm 1942, Preface).

The nationwide introduction of compulsory ethics lectures in the medical curriculum was, on an international scale, extraordinary at that time. At the beginning of the twentieth century, medical ethics did not exist as a formal teaching subject in Germany because in Germany, as in other Western countries, medical ethical thinking was expressed primarily in medical literature and codes of conduct rather than didactic teaching (Maehle 2009; Baker and McCullough 2009). Traditionally, ethical debates had mostly revolved around professional etiquette rather than patient care or human subjects research (Dingwall and Rozelle 2011). The "guidelines for new therapy and human experimentation," issued in 1931 by the German Ministry of the Interior, were a notable exception in that they set out standards for informed consent and protection of vulnerable groups, examples of regulations that were remarkably advanced compared with international standards at that time. However, the guidelines' normative impact was limited, and they were disregarded without further ado when research on coerced concentration camp inmates began during World War II (Bruns 2014; Roelcke 2017).

Altogether, medical ethics was poorly represented in medical training until the curriculum emerged in 1939. The new MLPS course focused for the first time on physicians' moral and legal obligations to their patients as well as to their profession and the state, which was the Nazi racial state, of course. From then on, students were required to attend a set of 14 MLPS lectures during the tenth and final semester of medical studies (Bruns 2009, 102). The revised curriculum and MLPS were explicitly designed to create a new type of physician who would abandon the individualist ethical tradition of Hippocratic medicine. For example, Ehrhardt Hamann, MLPS lecturer at Halle University and member of the Nazi Party since 1929, felt the time was ripe to get rid of the Hippocrates-based medical ethics: "Every time has its own ethos, our time has the national socialist one." Instead, the new health leader would devote himself to the general welfare of the "Aryan" German people (Hamann 1940, 161–162).

The first MLPS lectures appeared in the course catalogs of German medical schools in the winter semester of 1939/40 (Course Catalogs 1939–1945). By the end of 1939, 13 out of the 28 or 46.4 percent of medical faculties in the *Grossdeutsches Reich* (Greater German Reich) offered lectures in MLPS, and in the winter semesters of 1942/43 and 1943/44, 89.3 percent of all faculties had begun MLPS training (see table 4.1).

By the winter semester of 1944/45, the last regular semester held at German universities prior to the end of the Nazi regime, the number of faculties offering lectures in MLPS had declined to 22 of 28 (78.6 percent). This decline was probably due to the war and its impact on universities' structural

Table 4.1. Lectures on MLPS at German medical faculties 1939–1945, including annexed Austria and the Danzig medical academy. Not included: Strassburg, Posen, Prague, that were temporarily annexed during war. Shown are absolute numbers; percentages are in parentheses.

	Winter Semester					
	1939/40	*1940/41*	*1941/42*	*1942/43*	*1943/44*	*1944/45*
German medical faculties	28 (100)	28 (100)	28 (100)	28 (100)	28 (100)	28 (100)
With lectures on MLPS	13 (46.4)	17 (60.7)	23 (82.1)	25 (89.3)	25 (89.3)	22 (78.6)

Created by Florian Bruns

and personnel resources. Despite these impediments, however, between 1939 and 1945, all the 28 German medical faculties offered, at least temporarily, a course on MLPS.

ARDENT NAZIS AS ETHICS LECTURERS

Who was eligible to teach ethics to medical students at that time? There were few full-time ethicists; there were only a handful of medical scholars from various specialties who pursued medical ethics besides their major occupation. Examples are Emil Abderhalden, a physiologist in Halle, Paul Diepgen, a medical historian in Berlin, and Georg Benno Gruber, a pathologist in Göttingen. Albert Moll, a Berlin psychiatrist and one of the most renowned ethicists, died in 1939 (Maehle 2012, 217–36). Even though Abderhalden, Diepgen, and Gruber were zealous to cooperate and align both themselves and their moral views with the Nazi regime, they were considered not radical enough. Diepgen, for example, a Catholic and a non-member of the Nazi Party, was deemed politically unreliable and subsequently sidelined (Bruns 2009, 72).

Therefore, starting in 1939, Reich Physicians' Leader Conti and the Ministry of Science and Education sought to appoint long-standing members of the Nazi Party as MLPS lecturers. Most of them were medical doctors not affiliated with a university but with a background as *Gauamtsleiters* (functionaries in the regional branches of the Nazi health administration) (NSDAP and Reichsärztekammer Membership Files, RÄK 9345). Conti, a member of the Nazi Party since 1927, selected mostly elderly general practitioners who desired academic honor as a reward for their longtime party loyalty (Ramm 1944). Choosing general practitioners, ideally country doctors, reflected the Nazis' belief that these physicians had a kind of "natural" attitude toward medicine and ethics that was "unspoiled" by academic scholarship. Their moral attitude, per Conti's notion, would be closer to the crude worldview of the Nazis.

In the winter semester of 1944/45, half of all MLPS lectures at German medical faculties were given by such physicians, and archival data reveals that every one of them was an early member of the Nazi Party. Most of them had signed up before 1933 and, therefore, could claim to be *Alte Kämpfer* (old fighters) of the Nazi movement; that is, they had joined the party prior to Hitler's rise to power and before party membership became popular for career advancement. All of these lecturers had their own Nazi background, either as *Gauamtsleiter*, as members of the Nazi Physicians' League (a party organization for doctors, founded in 1929), or as members of either the notorious *Sturmabteilung*, or SA (Stormtroopers) or *Schutzstaffel*, or SS (see table 4.2). As such, they were all staunch supporters of the Nazi health care policy with

Table 4.2. Medical and political backgrounds of the MLPS lecturers in Nazi Germany. Modified and revised from Bruns (2009).

Name Year of Birth	Medical Faculty	Medical Specialty	Member of the NSDAP Since	Other Nazi Organizations
Special Lecturers of Medical Ethics				
Eduard Eschbacher 1897	Freiburg	Pediatrics	1933	None reported
Ehrhardt Hamann 1900	Halle	General Medicine	1929	Nazi Physicians' League, SS, Gauamtsleiter
Rudolf Hartung 1891	Cologne	General Medicine	1930	Nazi Physicians' League, Gauamtsleiter
Wilhelm Mörchen 1891	Frankfurt, Giessen	General Medicine	1931	Nazi Physicians' League, SA, Gauamtsleiter
Rudolf Ramm 1887	Berlin	General Medicine	1930	Nazi Physicans' League, Gauamtsleiter
Heinrich Reinhardt 1894	Marburg	General Medicine	1925	Gauamtsleiter
Hans Rinne 1888	Kiel	Surgery	1931	Nazi Physicians' League, SS, Gauamtsleiter
Richard Rohde 1882	Jena	General Medicine	1930	Gauamtsleiter
Paul Schroeder 1894	Königsberg	General Medicine	1933	Nazi Physicians' League
Eugen Stähle 1890	Tübingen	Neurology	1927	Nazi Physicians' League, Gauamtsleiter
Lecturers from Other Fields Who Taught Medical Ethics				
Kurt Böhmer 1895	Düsseldorf	Forensic Pathology	Candidate from 1937	SA
Gerhard Buhtz 1896	Breslau	Forensic Pathology	1933	SS
Hans Demme 1900	Hamburg	Neurology	1933	Hereditary Health Court
Herbert Elbel 1907	Heidelberg	Forensic Pathology	1932	Nazi Physicians' League, SS

Name Year of Birth	Medical Faculty	Medical Specialty	Member of the NSDAP Since	Other Nazi Organizations
Walther Fischer 1882	Rostock	Forensic Pathology	Non-Member	None reported
Curt Goroncy 1896	Greifswald	Forensic Pathology	1933	None reported
Gottfried Jungmichel 1902	Göttingen	Forensic Pathology	1937	Nazi Physicians' League
Hermann Merkel 1873	Munich	Forensic Pathology	1937	Hereditary Health Court
Hans Molitoris 1874	Erlangen	Forensic Pathology	1933	None reported
Friedrich Pietrusky 1893	Bonn	Forensic Pathology	1937	Hereditary Health Court
Franz Riha 1876	Innsbruck	Oral Medicine and Dentistry	1940	None reported
Otto Schmidt 1898	Danzig	Forensic Pathology	Candidate from 1938	None reported
Philipp Schneider 1896	Vienna	Forensic Pathology	1933	SS
Heinrich Többen 1880	Münster	Forensic Pathology	Non-Member	SS ("passive member")
Kurt Walcher 1891	Würzburg	Forensic Pathology	1933	Nazi Physicians' League
Johannes Weicksel 1882	Leipzig	Medico- Actuarial Science	1933	Nazi Physicians' League
Anton Werkgartner 1890	Graz	Forensic Pathology	1936	Hereditary Health Court

its focus on exclusion of people who were deemed inferior: the hereditary ill, the incurable sick, the handicapped, and the Jews (Bruns 2009, 102–116).

Where it was not possible to fill the new lecturing posts with a qualified party veteran, the faculties drew on other medical professors to teach MLPS, mostly forensic pathologists experienced in medicolegal issues. The vast majority of these professors also were members of the Nazi Party, had applied for membership, or belonged to other Nazi organizations (see table 4.2). At least four of them implemented Nazi eugenic policy as judges in the *Erbgesundheitsgerichte* (Hereditary Health Courts). Beginning in 1934, these courts were established throughout Germany to adjudicate cases arising from the 1933 eugenic Sterilization Law. They were presided over by a lawyer and two physicians who passed judgments on which patients should be sterilized against their will (Proctor 1988, 95–117). All in all, only medical doctors served as MLPS lecturers. No other faculties or professions were involved. According to the lecturers' curricula vitae that can be viewed in their personnel files, none of them had any further academic qualifications in either ethics or philosophy (Ramm 1944; Proctor 1988, 95–117).

An illustrative example is the Berlin-based lecturer Rudolf Ramm. Because he taught MLPS at the prestigious Faculty of Medicine in Berlin and wrote the pertinent textbook on this subject, Ramm was probably the most influential protagonist of MLPS. Holocaust survivor Elie Wiesel has rightly named him "the eminent Nazi doctor responsible for 'ethical' questions" (Wiesel 2005, 1512). Ramm had worked as a general practitioner in the provincial town of Pirmasens where he joined the Nazi Party in 1930. Two years later he was elected deputy to the German Reichstag. From 1934 on, he served as mayor of Pirmasens, albeit not very successfully—he was removed from his post in 1937 because of financial mismanagement. In spring of 1938, the party sent him to Vienna to reorganize, under Nazi rule, the medical profession in newly annexed Austria. Ramm proved his abilities by effectively organizing the persecution and expulsion of Jewish physicians from Austria. Ramm then moved to Berlin and, in 1940, became editor-in-chief of the journal of the German Medical Association, *Deutsches Ärzteblatt* (German Medical Journal). He published several anti-Semitic articles that demanded a "complete solution to the Jewish Question in Europe" and a "radical elimination of the Jews" (Ramm 1941, 175–78). These articles in the widely read *Ärzteblatt*, written in the language of extermination and anticipating the Holocaust, suggests, at the very least, the acquiescence of large parts of the German medical profession.

With his biography and "merits," Ramm was seen as the ideal candidate to teach MLPS at Berlin University. Conti appointed him as lecturer at the Faculty of Medicine in 1940 (Ministry of Science and Education 1940). Now, Ramm was a multi-functionary who held numerous positions within the Nazi Party and the health care system. He was also in charge of organizing nationwide continuing medical education and setting up a compulsory program intended to indoctrinate doctors who were already on the job. After publishing his MLPS textbook in 1942, Ramm became the most prominent Nazi medical ethicist.

TOPICS ADDRESSED IN THE LECTURES

Because Ramm's textbook was the only one available for MLPS lecturers, it provides insight into the contents of the ethics lectures given in German medical schools during World War II. The book outlined the National Socialist version of medical ethics and the mission of doctors in the Nazi state. Ramm identified "racial miscegenation," a declining birthrate, and the "growth of inferior elements" in the German population as relevant dangers for the German people (Ramm 1942, 130). He denounced the former Weimar welfare state and democracy as weak and full of compassion for the wrong people, meaning the sick and needy. Ramm explained that in Hitler's state every person had a moral duty to keep healthy. "It is the everlasting service of the [Nazi] Party to have changed the belief in the 'right to one's own body,' derived from crass individualism, to belief in an 'obligation to stay healthy' and to have presented this as a demand arising from the National Socialism's worldview" (Ramm 1942, 148).

Without any irony, Ramm stated that it was the Nazi movement that finally brought the "reinstatement of a high level of professional ethics" to the German medical profession. According to Ramm this had been achieved, after "the profession had been extensively cleansed of politically unreliable elements foreign to our race" (Ramm 1942, 69). By this, Ramm alluded to the expulsion of approximately 8,000 German-Jewish physicians (about 2,000 of them were murdered), a process that had been almost completed by the time Ramm's book came out (Ramm 1942).

With a view to eugenics and racial hygiene, Ramm described the forced sterilization of people who were deemed hereditary ill as a "sacrifice an individual makes in the interests of the good of the *Volksgemeinschaft*" (people's community) (Ramm 1942, 134). Consequently, he praised the Sterilization Law that compelled physicians to report patients with alleged hereditary diseases to state medical authorities for sterilization.

Ramm also mentioned the "problem of euthanasia" and did not mask his point of view. He advocated "mercy killing" of the disabled: "These creatures merely vegetate and constitute a serious burden on the national community. They not only reduce the standard of living of the rest of their family members because of the expenses for their care but also need a healthy person to take care of them throughout their lives" (Ramm 1942, 103–104). The students, therefore, were taught that it was morally necessary to eliminate such patients in order to relieve their relatives and the state of the burden they posed. Such unequivocal words and, in particular, the unashamed economic justification for murdering the sick were remarkable even for Nazi standards. No Nazi author named the principles behind the killing of the mentally ill and disabled as openly as Ramm did in his book.

Ramm also addressed, without a strong Nazi ideological bias, some other medical ethical issues. He emphasized, for example, that patients should have the right to choose a doctor of their choice (Ramm 1942, 96). He also warned that billing for unnecessary procedures contradicts medical ethics. Ramm further reminded his students and colleagues of the obligation to seek collegial advice and to transfer patients in a timely manner to specialists when confronted with difficult cases (Ramm 1942, 99–100). However, Ramm clarified that these ethical principles only applied to members of the *Volksgemeinschaft*, not to those patients who were deemed "inferior."

In contrast to medical historians who strove to provide a new exegesis of the *Corpus Hippocraticum* that would fit with Nazi medicine, Ramm did not waste much thought on a reinterpretation of the Hippocratic Oath (Bruns 2009, 78–84, 117). In line with the Nazis' common metaphor of the *Volkskörper* (people's body), Ramm simply insinuated an analogy between the German people and a sick patient, so that the Hippocratic Oath seemed to fit with Nazi medical ethics: exterminating Jews or patients with hereditary diseases was morally acceptable and medically required in order to heal the organism of the German people (Ramm 1942, 130–135, 141).

Ramm's book, which was written not only for medical students but also for postgraduate physicians, received positive reviews in German medical journals, even in the popular Nazi Party newspaper *Völkischer Beobachter* (National Observer) (Bruns and Chelouche 2017, 593). The book sold out within a year. A second, slightly extended edition was published in 1943, and it was out of print by 1944 (Archive of Walter de Gruyter Publishing, Deposit 42, 213(2)). Neither the author nor his opus survived the end of the Third Reich. As a high-ranking Nazi medical functionary, Ramm was sentenced to death by a Soviet military tribunal and executed in Berlin in August 1945 (Bruns 2009, 129). His book was banned by government authorities in the same year (Bruns and Chelouche 2017, 594).

FINAL REMARKS

In contrast to the common perception, the Nazis neither ignored nor abandoned medical ethics. From 1939 onward, Nazi medical authorities inaugurated systematic teaching in medical ethics at all German medical faculties. Until then, as in other countries, medical deontology had not played a prominent role in medical training. Despite the war and its consequences, compulsory ethics lectures were swiftly established at all medical schools in Nazi Germany and annexed Austria.

The textbook of the Berlin-based MLPS lecturer Rudolf Ramm formed the basis of ethical education for medical students in Nazi Germany. In this context, *ethical education* means imparting Nazi moral values to future physicians. In his book, Ramm detailed the ethical duties of the Nazi physician that were based on the principles of racial purity, a belief in the unequal worth of human beings, the alleged supremacy of the Aryan race, and the willingness to sacrifice the individual's well-being for the good of society. He believed in the authoritarian role of the doctor as a "health leader," and openly defined the Nazi doctor's ethical obligation to rid society of certain groups:

Jews, the handicapped, and other individuals who were unable to contribute to society. This moral stance was not entirely new; rather, it drew upon values and attitudes that were already rooted in parts of German society prior to this period (Weindling 1989). The traditional Hippocratic ethos did not work as a safeguard because it turned out to be susceptible to various interpretations.

It is important to realize that ethical reasoning can be corrupted, and that teaching medical ethics is, in itself, no guarantee of the moral integrity and humanitarian quality of physicians. The professional ethos of doctors is more fragile than we might think since it depends to a large extent on sociopolitical circumstances that are, from a historical perspective, subject to change (Lerner and Caplan 2016). Getting to know and analyzing the Nazi version of medical ethics forces us to constantly reexamine our own central assumptions, our moral stances, and our personal and professional responsibilities.

BIBLIOGRAPHY

Archive of Walter de Gruyter publishing company. Deposit 42, 213(2). Located at: Berlin State Library, Berlin, Germany.

Baker, Robert B., and Laurence B. McCullough. eds. 2009. *The Cambridge World History of Medical Ethics.* Cambridge: Cambridge University Press.

Bestvater, Horst. 1939. "Gedanken und Anregungen zur Neuordnung des Medizinstudiums." *Deutsches Ärzteblatt* 69: 408–11.

Bialas, Wolfgang. 2013. "Nazi Ethics: Perpetrators with a Clear Conscience." *Dapim: Studies on the Holocaust* 27, no. 1 (August): 3–25.

Bruns, Florian. 2009. *Medizinethik im Nationalsozialismus. Entwicklungen und Protagonisten in Berlin (1939–1945).* Stuttgart: Franz Steiner.

Bruns, Florian. 2014. "Medical Ethics and Medical Research on Human Beings in National Socialism." In *Human Subjects Research after the Holocaust,* edited by Sheldon Rubenfeld and Susan Benedict, 39–50. New York: Springer.

Bruns, Florian, and Tessa Chelouche. 2017. "Lectures on Inhumanity: Teaching Medical Ethics in German Medical Schools Under Nazism." *Annals of Internal Medicine* 166, no. 8 (April): 591–95.

Caplan, Arthur L. 2010. "The Stain of Silence: Nazi Ethics and Bioethics." In *Medicine after the Holocaust: From the Master Race to the Human Genome and Beyond,* edited by Sheldon Rubenfeld, 83–92. New York: Palgrave Macmillan.

Course Catalogs. 1939–1945. Course catalogs of 28 German medical faculties between 1939 and 1945 in Berlin, Bonn, Breslau, Danzig, Düsseldorf, Erlangen, Frankfurt, Freiburg, Giessen, Göttingen, Graz, Greifswald, Halle, Hamburg, Heidelberg, Innsbruck, Jena, Kiel, Cologne, Königsberg, Leipzig, Marburg, Munich, Münster, Rostock, Tübingen, Wien, and Würzburg. Located at: Berlin State Library, Berlin, Germany.

Dingwall, Robert, and Vienna Rozelle. "The Ethical Governance of German Physicians, 1890–1939: Are There Lessons from History?" *Journal of Policy History* 23, no. 1 (January): 29–52.

Hamann, Ehrhardt. 1940. "Gedanken zum Thema: Ärztliches Ethos." *Ärzteblatt für Mitteldeutschland* 3: 161–62.

Kater, Michael H. 1989. *Doctors under Hitler*. Chapel Hill, London: University of North Carolina Press.

Lerner, Barron H., and Arthur L. Caplan. 2016. "Judging the Past: How History Should Inform Bioethics." *Annals of Internal Medicine* 164, no. 8 (April): 553–57.

Maehle, Andreas-Holger. 2009. *Doctors, Honour and the Law: Medical Ethics in Imperial Germany*. Basingstoke: Palgrave Macmillan.

Maehle, Andreas-Holger. 2012. "'God's Ethicist': Albert Moll and His Medical Ethics in Theory and Practice." *Medical History* 56, no. 2 (April): 217–36.

Ministry of Science and Education. 1940. Letter of appointment as a lecturer for Rudolf Ramm, October 11, 1940. Archival signature: UK PA, R 16, Bd. 1. Located at Archive of Humboldt University, Berlin, Germany.

NSDAP and Reichsärztekammer (Reich physicians' chamber). RÄK 9345. Membership files of E. Eschbacher, E. Hamann, R. Hartung, W. Mörchen, H. Reinhardt, R. Ramm, H. Rinne, R. Rohde, P. Schroeder, and E. Stähle. Archival signature: RÄK 9345. Located at: National Archives, Berlin, Germany.

Proctor, Robert N. 1988. *Racial Hygiene: Medicine under the Nazis*. Cambridge, MA, London: Harvard University Press.

Proctor, Robert N. 1992. "Nazi Doctors, Racial Medicine, and Human Experimentation." In *The Nazi Doctors and the Nuremberg Code. Human Rights in Human Experimentation*, edited by George J. Annas and Michael A. Grodin, 17–31. New York: Oxford University Press.

Proctor, Robert N. 2000. "Nazi Science and Medical Ethics: Some Myths and Misconceptions." *Perspectives in Biology and Medicine* 43, no. 3 (Spring): 335–46.

Ramm, Rudolf. 1941. "Die Aussiedlung der Juden als europäisches Problem." *Die Gesundheitsführung. Ziel und Weg* 11: 175–78.

Ramm, Rudolf. 1942. *Ärztliche Rechts- und Standeskunde. Der Arzt als Gesundheitserzieher*. Berlin: Walter de Gruyter.

Ramm, Rudolf. 1944. Letter to the dean of the Berlin faculty of medicine. April 23, 1944. Archival signature: UK PA, R 16, Bd. 2. Located at: Archive of Humboldt University, Berlin, Germany.

Reich, Warren T. 2001. "The Care-Based Ethic of Nazi Medicine and the Moral Importance of What We Care About." *American Journal of Bioethics* 1, no. 1 (November): 64–74.

Roelcke, Volker. 2017. "The Use and Abuse of Medical Research Ethics: The German *Richtlinien*/guidelines for Human Subject Research as an Instrument for the Protection of Research Subjects—and of Medical Science, ca. 1931–61/64." In *From Clinic to Concentration Camp. Reassessing Nazi Medical and Racial Research, 1933–1945*, edited by Paul Weindling, 33–56. London: Routledge.

Weikart, Richard. 2009. *Hitler's Ethic: The Nazi Pursuit of Evolutionary Progress*. New York: Palgrave Macmillan.

Weindling, Paul. 1989. *Health, Race and German Politics between National Unification and Nazism, 1870–1945*. Cambridge: Cambridge University Press.

Wiesel, Elie. 2005. "Without Conscience." *New England Journal of Medicine* 352 (April): 1511–13.

Chapter Five

A Protagonist's View of Euthanasia in the Netherlands Today

Eduard (A. A. E.) Verhagen

Decisions about end-of-life (EOL) treatments have been very important to the Dutch for the last 25 years. One of the interesting themes arising from many studies and surveys of death and dying during that time is that, for the Dutch, not only quality of life but also quality of death is considered important by health care providers and by the general population. In that context, it's not surprising that euthanasia, defined as death on the patient's request, was ultimately decriminalized. In this chapter, I will first describe important national developments that have resulted in legalization of euthanasia and also how medical EOL practices for adults have developed over the last decades. Next, I will focus on the developments in EOL decision-making in the pediatric population, both nationally and internationally. The last part of this chapter contains a brief summary and some thoughts about similarities and differences in how euthanasia in adults and children is regulated and organized. My final words are reflections on the potential effects that these developments might have on the position of, and support for, special-needs infants and children in current Dutch society.

HEALTH CARE ORGANIZATION IN THE NETHERLANDS

The Netherlands is a tiny and densely populated country in northwestern Europe, with a population of around 17 million inhabitants living in 16,000 square miles. The Netherlands has a universal health care system managed by the government and supplemented by private insurers. Anyone living or working in the Netherlands is entitled to basic health insurance (with or without additional coverage) from a Dutch provider. The philosophy underpinning the Dutch health care system is based on several more or less universal principles: access to care for all, solidarity through medical insurance (which is compulsory for all and available to all), and high quality health care services (Ministry of Health, Welfare and Sport 2018). To access the health care system, residents must register with a *huisarts* (general practitioner) who is the "gatekeeper" for referrals to medical specialists.

In 2017, around 150,000 adults died in the Netherlands, with cancer being the leading cause of death (31 percent) (Ministry of Health, Welfare and Sports 2018). The basic health insurance not only covers regular oncology treatments, but it also fully covers terminal and palliative care, which is provided either at home or in one of the 2,300 nursing homes, 100 hospitals, or 140 hospices. Approximately 7,900 general practitioners take care of roughly 70 percent of cancer patients dying at home. Palliative care consultation teams are available in each region to support health care providers.

Also, in 2017, approximately 1,100 children died. Most of them (51 percent) were infants between 0–12 months of age with perinatal problems and congenital malformations (Central Bureau of Statistics 2019). It is estimated that most of these infants and children died in the hospital, with a minority dying at home or in a pediatric hospice.

END-OF-LIFE DECISIONS AND EUTHANASIA
FOR ADULTS AND CHILDREN 12–15 YEARS OLD

Terminology

At the end of life, many patients need comfort-oriented care that frequently includes EOL decisions defined as medical decisions that cause or hasten death, such as withholding or withdrawing life-sustaining treatment, administering comfort-medication that may shorten life as a side-effect, and providing euthanasia. The term *euthanasia* in the Netherlands is reserved for terminating the life of a mentally competent patient at the patient's considered request. The decision to use lethal drugs to deliberately end the life of a pediatric patient who suffers unbearably is sometimes referred to as *neonatal* or *pediatric euthanasia*. However, newborns and children younger than 12 years of age are not considered competent by law in the Netherlands, so they cannot legally make that request. Therefore, some Dutch authors use the term *deliberate ending of life* of newborns/children (Willems, Verhagen, and van Wijlick 2014). In this chapter, I also choose to use the term *deliberate ending of life*, while acknowledging that the alternative terms, *neonatal* or *pediatric* euthanasia, are used in many other international publications.

Toward Legalization of Euthanasia

It is probably fair to say that during the past decades, the Dutch have been "obsessed" by death and dying, with the majority of the population in favor of euthanasia since 1966 in public opinion polls (Griffiths, Weyers, and Adams 2008). Frequent surveys among doctors in the last 30 years have consistently shown their willingness to perform euthanasia for patients with unbearable suffering. A landmark publication in the developments toward legalization of euthanasia was the 1985 report by the State Commission on Euthanasia (Staatscommissie Euthanasie), which recommended that euthanasia should be allowed under specific conditions. The government subsequently chose to investigate EOL decisions, including euthanasia, in two ways. First, by "examining and monitoring" medical EOL practice through anonymous surveys among a large group of physicians based on data from death certificates and repeating them every five years. (Data about the deaths of infants between 0–12 months of age were occasionally included.) Second, they designed a reporting and review procedure to make sure all cases of deliberate life-ending were registered.

During the Dutch debate about euthanasia in the 1980s and 1990s, several doctors were prosecuted after reporting they had, at a patient's request, ended the life of a patient who suffered unbearably. Of the many court rulings over these two decades, the 1984 Alkmaar case resulted in a landmark Supreme Court decision that, for the first time, introduced a potential legal justification for not prosecuting doctors who perform euthanasia, the concept of necessity resulting from a conflict of duties (Thomas 1984). The conflict was between the duty to alleviate the patient's hopeless suffering and the duties to obey the law and to preserve the patient's life. Governmental committees and the medical profession then successfully translated the court's criteria into practical recommendations to guide physicians, ultimately resulting in the enactment of the Dutch Termination of Life on Request and Assisted Suicide Act (*Wet toetsing levensbeëindiging op verzoek en hulp bij zelfdoding*) in 2002. Briefly, the law provides that physicians may perform euthanasia (or physician-assisted suicide) if they are convinced that: (1) the patient made a voluntary and well-considered request; (2) the patient is suffering unbearably with no prospect of improvement; (3) the situation and prognosis are both known and understood by the patient; (4) the joint conclusion by the patient and the doctor is reached that there is no reasonable alternative to relieve suffering; (5) an independent physician is consulted who must visit the patient; and (6) the physician performs the act with due care and reports the case to the regional review committee. The patient must be a legally competent adult or child 12–15 years of age to make a valid euthanasia request. (Legally, a mentally competent person who is 16 years or older is considered to have the rights and responsibilities of an adult.) Additional requirements concerning the physician's role, not in the euthanasia law but derived from case law, are that either the physician has to take control if a request is made or refer the patient to a colleague if the physician cannot or will not provide euthanasia. The physician must be resistant to (improper) pressure, keep a professional distance, and communicate with and guide other caregivers and family in the process.

Ethical and Political Justification of Legalizing Euthanasia

The ethical justification of voluntary euthanasia in adults has been widely debated in the Netherlands. In my view, the debate is summarized best by the influential Dutch ethicist Widdershoven, who states that justification originates in a combination of principles: self-determination, beneficence, responsibility, and compassion/care (2002). From a political perspective, the broad acceptance of euthanasia in the population, as demonstrated in polls and surveys, also justified legalization of euthanasia. Of course, there were political differences regarding justification and extent of the new law, but at the same time there was also a deeply rooted view among most politicians that the lawmaker should provide "freedom" for all people to live their lives in line with their norms and views. Euthanasia can be an option; it can never be an obligation.

Developments Regarding Euthanasia after Legalization

Many people wondered if and how legalization of euthanasia would change EOL practice for adults, so they read and analyzed the detailed quinquennial national surveys that are published in Dutch with a summary of the main findings in English (Onwuteaka-Philipsen et al. 2007; van der Heide et al. 2012; Onwuteaka-Philipsen et al. 2017; van der Heide, van Delden, and Onwuteaka-Philipsen 2017). Some are also published in high-impact international biomedical journals (van der Heide, van der Maas, and Kollée 1997; van der Heide et al. 1997; van der Heide et al. 2007; Onwuteaka-Philipsen et al. 2012). In addition, the regional euthanasia review committees publish annual reports with figures relating to euthanasia notifications received in the year in question. It explains how the committees review the actions of physicians who have notified them of cases of euthanasia or assisted suicide. It also describes cases that are relevant to the development of standards or are noteworthy for other reasons. Findings are published on the RTE Regional Euthanasia Review Committees' website, https://english.euthanasiecommissie.nl/the-committees/annual-reports, throughout the year under the heading "Findings & explanatory notes." A small selection is included in the committees' annual report, which is published in Dutch and English. Table 5.1 summarizes the results of the five-year surveys from 1990 to 2015, and Table 5.2 describes the relationship

Table 5.1. Frequency of medical end-of-life decisions, continuous deep sedation, and ending of life by the patient*

	2015		2010		2005		2001		1995		1990	
	No. of Cases	%	No. of Cases	%	No. of Cases	%	No. of Cases	%	No. of Cases	%	No. of Cases	%
Total number of cases studied	7,761		6,861		9,965		5,617		5,146		5,197	
Medical EOL decisions	4,397	58.1	3,685	57.8	2,580	42.5	2,899	43.8	2,604	42.6	2,361	39.4
Euthanasia	829	4.5	475	2.8	294	1.7	310	2.6	257	2.4	141	1.7
Physician-assisted suicide	22	0.1	21	0.1	17	0.1	25	0.2	25	0.2	18	0.2
Ending of life without explicit patient request	18	0.3	13	0.1	24	0.4	42	0.7	64	0.7	45	0.8
Intensified alleviation of symptoms	2,469	35.3	2,202	36.4	1,478	24.7	1,312	20.1	1,161	19.1	1,166	18.8
Forgoing of life-prolonging treatment	1,041	17.4	974	18.2	767	15.6	1,210	20.2	1,097	20.2	991	17.9
Continuous deep sedation	1,288	18.3	789	12.3	521	8.2	NA		NA		NA	
Ending of life by the patient												
Intentionally stopping eating and drinking	25	0.5	18	0.4	NA		NA		NA		NA	
Taking self-collected medication	73	0.2	47	0.2	NA		NA		NA		NA	
Other methods	403	1.2	267	1.0	NA		NA		NA		NA	

NA: not available

*Sources: Death certificate studies, summarized in van der Heide et al. 2012; Onwuteaka-Philipsen et al. 2017; van der Heide, van Delden, and Onwuteaka-Philipsen 2017

Table 5.2. Euthanasia cases reported to the regional review committees, annual reports, 2011–2016.

	2016 No. (%)	2015 No. (%)	2014 No. (%)	2013 No. (%)	2012 No. (%)	2011 No. (%)
Cancer	4,137 (68.0)	4,000 (73.0)	3,888 (73.0)	3,581 (81.0)	3,251 (77.0)	2,797 (76.0)
Dementia	141 (2.3)	109 (1.9)	81 (1.5)	97 (2.2)	42 (1.0)	49 (1.3)
Psychiatric disease	60 (1.0)	56 (1.0)	41 (0.8)	42 (1.0)	14 (0.3)	13 (0.4)
Accumulation of various old-age afflictions	244 (4.0)	183 (3.3)	257 (4.8)	251 (5.7)	NA	NA
Remaining diseases	1,509 (24.7)	1,531 (24.0)	1,039 (19.9)	457 (10.3)	881 (21.7)	836 (22.3)

Source: KNMG 2017, Euthanasia in Figures.

between euthanasia and the underlying disease for each year between 2011 and 2016. The data are based on the annual reports of the euthanasia review committees (Royal Dutch Medical Association [KNMG] 2017).

Four new issues emerged from the data in the most recent report describing practice in 2015: (1) living wills of people who have developed advanced dementia; (2) suffering in patients with refractory psychiatric symptoms such as depression; (3) approval of euthanasia for patients without a clear medical condition but with a well-considered opinion that their lives are complete, "fulfilled" lives; and (4) euthanasia in children less than 12 years old (Onwuteaka-Philipsen et al. 2017). Most or all of these emerging subjects will eventually be translated into research questions and become new studies.

THE SITUATION FOR NEWBORNS AND CHILDREN IN THE NETHERLANDS BEFORE 2005

The Acceptability of Neonatal End-of-Life Decisions

In the slipstream of the developments around EOL decisions and euthanasia for adults, a similar debate started about decision-making for severely ill newborns (Verhagen and Sauer 2005a; Dorscheidt 2006; Griffiths, Weyers, and Adams 2008). Between 1990 and 1997, influential reports by the Royal Dutch Medical Association (KNMG) and by the Dutch Pediatric Association (NVK) on the medical and ethical acceptability of EOL decisions for newborns were published, with the intention of reflecting the views of the medical profession (Nederlandse Vereniging voor Kindergeneeskunde 1992; KNMG

Commissie Aanvaardbaarheid Levensbeeindigend handelen 1997). The reports recognize two reasons for withholding or withdrawing life-sustaining treatment in newborns: treatment has no chance of success and treatment would be pointless. In the former situation, the physician would withhold and withdraw life-sustaining treatment. Regarding pointless treatment, the report's position is that both the survival of the infant and the child's quality of life are very important. The reports share the view that both life-ending decisions (withholding and/or withdrawal of care) and life-prolonging decisions must be legitimized. According to these reports, prolongation of intensive care treatment when the infant's prognosis is very grim might not always be in the best interest of the child. Quality-of-life (QOL) considerations, operationalized in the reports, must be strictly bound to medical criteria (Leenen 2000). The KNMG and NVK reports note that disagreement exists among physicians about the acceptability of deliberately ending the life of a severely ill newborn, which was a criminal offense in the Netherlands at the time of the reports. Based on the Prins and Kadijk cases in the mid-1990s, physicians could legally claim impunity on the grounds of necessity (Gerechtshof Leeuwarden 4 April 1996; Gerechtshof Amsterdam 7 November 1995, 1996). This is the same defense that was accepted for the first time for adults in the Alkmaar case described above. In order to claim necessity, the patient's suffering must be very severe, compelling the physician to choose between the duty to save a life and to do everything possible to prevent unbearable suffering. If the physician exercised the required due care formulated in the Prins and Kadijk cases, then deliberately ending a newborn's life may be justified.

Based on the 1994 reporting procedure, physicians had the legal obligation to report cases of deliberate ending of life of newborns to the Public Prosecution Service, which reviewed each case and decided whether to prosecute the doctor (Dorscheidt 2005). Not all cases, however, were reported (Verhagen et al. 2005). Fear of criminal prosecution and uncertainty about the consequences of reporting were the most important barriers to reporting (van der Wal and van der Maas 1996; van der Maas et al. 1996). In 1996, the ministers of Health and Justice appointed a consultative committee to improve the review procedure. The committee advised, among other things, the creation of a multidisciplinary review committee (consisting of physicians, a lawyer, and a medical ethicist) to review reported cases of deliberate ending of life of newborns and to advise the prosecutorial officials (Overleggroep toetsing zorgvuldig medisch handelen rond het levenseinde bij pasgeborenen 1997). This advice was strongly supported by the Dutch Pediatric Association (2005). In the meantime, a guideline about deliberate ending of life was created and accepted by Dutch pediatricians (Verhagen and Sauer 2005b). It was not until 2006, however, that a multidisciplinary advisory committee was finally installed and became operational (De Minister van Justitie en de Staatssecretaris van Volksgezondheid Welzijn en Sport 2007). Currently, the advisory committee reviews all cases of deliberate ending of life of newborns (Verhagen 2009).

Medical Practice in the Netherlands and Abroad before 2005

At the time the KNMG and NVK reports were issued, no systematic data were available about the circumstances and frequency of neonatal EOL decisions. The first nationwide surveys about newborns were in 1995 and 2001, revealing that in the Netherlands, a substantial proportion (65 percent) of newborn deaths below 12 months of age were preceded by an EOL decision (van der Heide et al. 1997; Vrakking et al. 2005). In 18 to 23 percent of cases, the decision was based on the poor prognosis of the child. Palliative care medication (analgesics and sedatives) with potentially life-shortening effect were used in around 50 percent of patients in the neonatal intensive care unit (NICU) (van der Heide et al. 2000). Administration of medication with the intention to hasten death in newborns without a preceding decision to withhold or withdraw life-sustaining therapy occurred in 1 percent of deaths (van der Wal et al. 1996; van der Heide et al. 1997; Vrakking et al. 2005). Based on these data, it was estimated that at least 15–20 cases of deliberate ending of life take place every year (van der Heide et al. 1997; Verhagen and Sauer 2005b). In the Netherlands, no national guidelines about the administration of analgesics, sedatives, and neuromuscular blockers as part of EOL care had been issued.

Studies about the EOL practice in other European countries have confirmed that withholding and withdrawing treatment became a common mode of death in most European NICUs (Costeloe et al. 2000; Cuttini et al. 2000; Roy et al. 2004; Hagen and Hansen 2004; Provoost et al. 2005; Schulz-Baldes et al. 2007; Arlettaz et al. 2005; Vanhaesebrouck et al. 2004; Larroque et al. 2004). The proportion of newborns that died with a preceding decision to withhold or withdraw life support has increased to at least 60 percent during the past 10 years in most European centers (Schulz-Baldes et al. 2007; Hagen and Hansen 2004; Arlettaz et al. 2005). QOL considerations were reported by neonatologists as reasons for these decisions in 20–50 percent of deaths (Schulz-Baldes et al. 2007; Arlettaz et al. 2005; Provoost et al. 2005). Only a few authors have reported details about what these considerations were. Provoost et al. (2005) reported that "no hope for a bearable future" was the most frequent QOL consideration used by physicians in Flanders. In 2006, Hentschel et al. reported that severe disabilities and long-term, far-reaching therapy were the considerations used by neonatologists in Freiburg, Germany.

A European survey in 1996–97 showed that the proportion of neonatologists who had ever made the decision to administer medication to hasten death varied considerably between countries (Cuttini et al. 2000). In the Netherlands and France, 75 percent and 43 percent, respectively, had done so, while in countries such as Italy and Spain, the percentages were much smaller (2 to 4 percent). Data from Flanders showed that administration of drugs was intended to hasten death in 7 percent of newborn deaths and clearly resulted in the hastening of death without the physician's explicit intention to do so in an additional 11 percent of cases (Provoost et al. 2006). A survey among European neonatologists published in 2004 by Cuttini et al. showed that opinions on the acceptability of deliberate ending of life varied widely between physicians in Europe at that time. Other publications stated that deliberate ending of life had been reported to occur in exceptional situations in Flanders and France (Provoost et al. 2005; Cuttini et al. 2000).

Most studies reporting on neonatal EOL practice in the United States before 2005 describe the situation in individual units, with the decision to withhold or withdraw treatment preceding death in 14 to 30 percent in early publications (Duff and Campbell 1973; Whitelaw 1986). Reports that were published around 2004 describe rates between 25 percent and 72 percent (Wall and Partridge 1997; Singh, Lantos, and Meadow 2004; Barton and Hodgman 2005; Abe, Catlin, and Mihara 2001; Pierucci, Kirby, and Leuthner 2001; Moseley et al. 2004). The proportion of EOL decisions based on QOL considerations was reported in only a few publications and varied between 40 to 83 percent of deaths (Singh, Lantos, and Meadow 2004; Abe, Catlin, and Mihara 2001; Wall and Partridge 1997). A more detailed description of these considerations is found only in two reports. In 1997, Wall and Partridge reported the prognosis for severe disabilities and the infant's predicted suffering as the main QOL concerns, and in 2004, Sing et al. described that treatment was limited if the burden of continuing interventions outweighed the benefits of prolonging life. Empiric data about the use of drugs as part of EOL care in the United States are not available.

Guidelines on palliative/comfort care recommend that physicians increase analgesics and sedatives at the end of life to make sure that the patient is comfortable, even if side effects of these drugs could hasten death (Liben and Lissauer 2006; Anand and Pain International Evidence-Based Group for Neonatal 2001; Carter and Bhatia 2001). The use of neuromuscular blockers as a part of EOL decision-making has not been accepted in the United States (Truog et al. 2000; Munson 2007; Davies and de Vlaming 2006). Catlin and Carter published a paper in 2002 about a newly developed neonatal palliative care protocol that stated: "If at all possible, neuromuscular blockers should be weaned from a child's system prior to any form of treatment withdrawal."

The main reasons for not giving neuromuscular blockers were: (a) Paralysis precludes the possibility of survival; (b) Paralysis may hinder the clinician's assessment of the patient's comfort; and (c) The opportunities for interaction between dying patients and their families are diminished (Truog et al. 2000). Ending a newborn's life is very controversial in the United States and, as far as I know, no American cases have been published (Catlin and Novakovich 2008; Chervenak, McCullough, and Arabin 2006; Jotkowitz and Glick 2006; Kodish 2008; Kon 2007; Lindemann and Verkerk 2008; Manninen 2006; Curlin 2005; Oakley 2005; Verhagen and Sauer 2008).

A limitation of most Dutch and international studies reporting on neonatal EOL decisions is that they describe the physician's attitude but not actual practice (Singh et al. 2007; Rebagliato et al. 2000; Saigal et al. 1999; Streiner et al. 2001; Barr 2007; Norup 1998). Publications about NICU outcomes seldom provide explicit descriptions of withholding and withdrawing care. Even when withdrawal of care is described, the distinction is rarely made between the babies who would have died despite intensive interventions (moribund babies extubated to spend their last moments in their parent's arms), and those who were extubated to die for QOL reasons (de Leeuw et al. 1996; Cuttini et al. 1997; Cook and Watchko 1996; van der Heide et al. 1997; Hagen and Hansen 2004). Moreover, studies are often very difficult to compare because authors use different definitions of patient groups and interventions. A final limitation is that most studies provide only crude data about the physician's reasons for administering potentially life-shortening medication and incomplete data on the dosages used (van der Heide et al. 2000; Provoost et al. 2006).

The Groningen Protocol for Newborn Euthanasia

Data from several studies mentioned above, as well as from reports and court cases, have confirmed that neonatal euthanasia, although rare, was consistently part of EOL care in the Netherlands. Our group developed and published in the *New England Journal of Medicine* in 2005 a protocol identifying situations in which neonatal euthanasia might be appropriate (Verhagen and Sauer 2005b). This "Groningen Protocol for Neonatal Euthanasia" (GP) has five major criteria: (1) Diagnosis and prognosis must be certain; (2) Hopeless and unbearable suffering must be present; (3) A confirming second opinion must be obtained from an independent doctor; (4) Both parents must give informed consent; and (5) The procedure must be performed carefully, in accordance with medical standards.

The GP arose from our conflict over the best care for a baby girl with the severest type of epidermolysis bullosa (Crouch 2005; Yuen et al. 2012; Verhagen 2013). The disease caused excruciating pain and suffering, her parents requested euthanasia, and a large multidisciplinary group of health care providers agreed that her suffering was intolerable and, hence, the request understandable. The doctors, fearing possible prosecution for murder, refused the request, and the patient was discharged to the care of the referring pediatrician. When the group was notified how the baby had died three months later, they developed and published the GP, which immediately generated an international controversy (Lindemann and Verkerk 2008; Chervenak, McCullough, and Arabin 2006; Kon 2007; Jotkowitz and Glick 2006; Jotkowitz, Glick, and Gesundheit 2008; Gesundheit et al. 2009; de Vries and Verhagen 2008) and prompted an analysis of the different approaches to EOL in pediatric palliative care.

It is clear that the ethical justification for neonatal euthanasia cannot be self-determination. The GP demands parental agreement, an extension of the principle of self-determination that Brouwer et al. (2018) have called *parental determination*, a bridge between self-determination and beneficence, another justifying principle. This view presumes that parents are the appropriate surrogate decision makers that give primacy to the best interests of their child.

If doctors are to behave beneficently, they must have sufficient understanding of the child's suffering. The parents—informed by their family values, intimate knowledge of their child, and their assessment of the child's quality of life—provide a specific and necessary perspective on the child's suffering. This parental determination prevents euthanasia for incompetent children from becoming an out-of-balance decision only based on beneficence.

One of the main international objections raised was that the GP is the first step down a slippery slope or erosion of norms that would lead to widely increased use of neonatal euthanasia. It was also argued that ending the life of a newborn is a violation of the doctor's obligation to preserve life and would negatively impact how the medical profession is regarded by the public (Nuffield Council on Bioethics 2006; Costeloe 2007). Proponents of the GP argued that the protocol makes doctors accountable for their decisions to all members of society and, therefore, strengthens patients' trust in their physicians (Lindemann and Verkerk 2008; Griffiths, Bood, and Weyers 1998). The key questions at the time, which I will address below, were: Would euthanasia increase or decrease after the GP? Would all cases be reported?

THE SITUATION IN THE NETHERLANDS AFTER 2005

Medical Practice in the Netherlands

Several studies were carried out to monitor the effects of the GP on EOL care. We also wondered if and how the approach toward EOL care was truly different from that of NICUs in other parts of the developed world.

In 2006, we conducted a pilot study in two large university-based NICUs to investigate how often newborn deaths were preceded by EOL decisions and to determine whether it was possible, retrospectively, to obtain accurate information about the decision-making process (Verhagen et al. 2007). We subsequently performed a nation-wide study to determine when and how physicians in the Netherlands made EOL decisions for severely ill newborns and found that EOL decisions were made in 95 percent of 359 deaths over a period of 12 months in 10 NICUs (Verhagen, Dorscheidt, et al. 2009b). In the remaining 5 percent, no decision to terminate the lives of the infants had been made, and treatment was continued until the newborn's death. Of all the newborns that died, 58 percent had been classified as having no chance of survival, and 42 percent were stabilized newborns with a poor prognosis. Withdrawal of life-sustaining treatment was the main mode of death in both groups. We found one case of deliberate termination of life.

In addition to reviewing the medical files, we interviewed the attending physicians in 147 out of 150 deaths preceded by an EOL decision based on QOL considerations. In 92 percent of deaths in the poor prognosis group, EOL decisions were based on the newborns' future QOL and future suffering and, in 44 percent of deaths, the newborns' present QOL was also considered. Consultation with colleagues on the medical team occurred in 99 percent of cases. We also found that parents had been involved in all EOL decisions and, in all cases, consensus had been reached between the parents and the team (Verhagen, de Vos, et al. 2009). Differences of opinion between parents and the medical team occurred sporadically, which led to a postponement of the EOL decision in the majority of these cases. We also studied and described in detail the types and dosages of analgesics and sedatives administered and the rationale for, and the use of, neuromuscular blockers (NMBs) (Verhagen, Dorscheidt, et al. 2009a). We reported that NMBs were administered in 16 percent of dying patients either because they already had received these agents or for the treatment or prevention of gasping. One of the striking findings was that physicians had different rationales for using NMBs in the final phase of dying: some viewed it as palliative care, while others viewed it as deliberate life-ending, which needed to be reported and reviewed.

In 2011, in response to a request from the Royal Dutch Medical Association to address the problem of health care providers using different definitions of newborn euthanasia and palliative care, a multidisciplinary group of experts was created. After a thorough analysis of medical policy statements, reports, scientific publications, ethics, and the law, it formulated general recommendations about EOL decision-making and care for very sick newborns (Willems, Verhagen, and van Wijlick 2014). In the discussion about the decision to withdraw life-supporting treatments, the group's report focused on several specific treatments, including withdrawal of respiratory support. Step by step, the report described the usual clinical course following withdrawal of a ventilator. Recommendations were made about communication with the parents and about treatment of symptoms and suffering in the dying newborn. The use of NMBs, always in addition to sedatives and analgesics, was discussed in great detail. According to the expert group, administration of NMBs is permitted if the aim is to stop prolonged gasping during ventilator withdrawal and to end a dying process presumed to take several hours or more, which only adds to the suffering of the parents. This uncommon situation may occur when even state-of-the-art palliative sedation is insufficient to relief pain and suffering and despite the medical team's careful preparation of the parents. The group ultimately concluded that administering NMBs in these circumstances should be regarded as "good medical practice," but they recommend that, in view of the ongoing debate about its legality, all cases must be reported for review to maintain full transparency and accountability. As far as I know, this is the first time that parental suffering was explicitly mentioned as a legitimate reason, under strict circumstances, to administer life-shortening medication to dying newborns. A substantial proportion of the recommendations of the multidisciplinary group corresponded with, and referred to the evidence-based Guidelines for Pediatric Palliative Care that were issued by the Dutch Pediatric Association in 2013, whose ultimate goal was to improve palliative care for children and create quality indicators to measure the quality of care. The guidelines included recommendations about palliative sedation and euthanasia in newborns and in older children, all in line with the KNMG document discussed above. Interestingly, the debate about NMB use has faded during the last two years, as indicated by our recent informal survey confirming that NMBs are no longer used in end-of-life care and that most units have removed NMBs from their EOL care protocols and palliative plans.

In 2015, the results of a study evaluating the effects of the GP were published (ten Cate and van de Vathorst 2015; ten Cate et al. 2015). The main findings were that in 2010, 63 percent of all deaths of children under one year of age were preceded by an EOL decision, mainly for withdrawal or withholding potentially life-sustaining treatments. This percentage was comparable to that found in studies before the GP. The percentage of cases in which drugs were administered with the explicit intention to hasten death was 1 percent in 2010, 9 percent in 1995 and 2001, and 8 percent in 2005 (ten Cate and van de Vathorst 2015; ten Cate et al. 2015). The overall conclusion was that there had been a considerable reduction of infant deaths that followed administration of drugs with the explicit intention to hasten death, possibly related to the introduction of routine ultrasound examination around 20 weeks of gestation with a subsequent increase in abortions of fetuses that might otherwise have been born and euthanized. In addition, the introduction of legal criteria and a review process for deliberately ending the life of a newborn may have left Dutch physicians with less room to hasten death.

Around the time these results were published, it became clear from the review committee's annual reports that in the five years following the publication of the GP, euthanasia had decreased from 15 to 2 cases over five years. The two reported cases, both babies with lethal epidermolysis bullosa, were reviewed post-hoc, considered to have been handled carefully, and no one was prosecuted (Committee Late Termination of Pregnancy and Termination of Life in Newborns 2010). For infants with spina bifida, euthanasia decreased from 15 to 0 cases. Those in favor of the GP argue that the decrease of euthanasia is the effect of more transparency and wise regulation resulting in appropriate control of EOL practice. There is increasing evidence, however, that the transformation of the health care system in 2007 when antenatal screening became a part of routine antenatal care, was probably the most important reason—increased abortions led to less euthanasia (Verhagen 2013; ten Cate et al. 2015).

COMPARING END-OF-LIFE PRACTICES IN THE NETHERLANDS, CANADA, AND THE UNITED STATES

In 2010, we also reported on the results of a comparative study of EOL decision-making in four NICUs in three culturally different countries: the United States (Chicago and Milwaukee), Canada (Montreal), and The Netherlands (Groningen) (Verhagen et al. 2010). We reviewed the medical files of all newborns older than 22 weeks of gestation who had died either in delivery rooms or in NICUs over a 12-month period. We categorized deaths using a 2-by-2 matrix and determined whether mechanical ventilation was withdrawn/withheld and whether the child was dying despite ventilation, or physiologically stable but extubated for a poor neurological prognosis. In all four NICUs, most of the unstable newborns died in their parents' arms after artificial ventilation was withdrawn. The decision to electively extubate newborns for QOL reasons was made in 19 to 35 percent of deaths in three units and never in Chicago. The proportion of newborns that died while receiving cardiopulmonary resuscitation varied between 4 to 12 percent in Wisconsin, Montreal, and Groningen and was 31 percent in Chicago. The percentage of delivery room deaths in Wisconsin, Montreal, and Groningen was 16 to 22 percent and zero in Chicago. We concluded that the deaths occurred under different conditions in the four NICUs and that distinctive EOL decisions could be categorized separately using a two-dimensional model. Cross-cultural and intra-cultural comparisons of EOL practices are feasible and important when comparing outcomes between NICUs.

We also compared the use of comfort medications in the delivery room and in the NICU before and after the decisions to withhold/withdraw life-supporting interventions (Janvier et al. 2011). We found that none of the babies who died in the delivery room received comfort medications. The use of opioids or benzodiazepines (87 percent) preceding death was similar in all NICUs. Increasing these medications around extubation occurred most often in Montreal, rarely in Milwaukee and Groningen, and never in Chicago. Comfort medications had no significant impact on the time between extubation and death. NMBs were never used around death in Chicago, once in Montreal, and more frequently in Milwaukee and Groningen. Initiation of NMBs several hours after extubation occurred in 12 out of 23 dying infants, only in Groningen, and at the explicit request of the parents to relieve agonal suffering. The team considered this "appropriate palliative care" and not euthanasia. We concluded that comfort medications were administered to almost all dying infants in each NICU. Some, but not all, centers were comfortable increasing these medications around or after extubation. In three centers, NMBs were at times present at the time of death. However, only in Holland were NMBs initiated after extubation.

WHERE ARE WE NOW?

This chapter illustrates that the practice of EOL decisions for adults and newborns in the Netherlands has been well studied for the past 25 years. The studies have provided valuable data and good insight into how, why, and when decisions to withhold/withdraw life-supporting treatment were made. The discussion about the most controversial EOL decisions, euthanasia and deliberately ending the lives of newborns, was characterized by the intention to reach full accountability and transparency. The debates about both groups of patients shared interesting similarities and resulted in regulations with considerable overlap in structure and content. Developments in medical practice in both groups are carefully and systematically monitored with detailed studies based on the outcome of surveys. Armed with these scientific data, adjustments in regulations are implemented, and the effects of each adjustment are studied in new surveys.

However, the developments regarding newborns stand out because these patients are totally dependent on surrogate decision-making, which might be seen as inevitable and acceptable by those who claim that parents are the best advocates for their children. Others might worry about potential misuse of parental authority and/or erosion of norms, leading to ending life for dubious reasons. Another well-known argument against allowing newborn euthanasia is that it sends the wrong message to society: Children suffering from severe disabilities are not welcome. Parents who care for them could feel social pressure to explain why they did not terminate their pregnancy or why they did not end the life of their child.

References are sometimes made to the developments in Germany and several other countries in the years before the Holocaust that led to the gradual dismissal and, ultimately, the death of vulnerable groups. Personally, I think these arguments are a warning for the Dutch to take precautions by monitoring and reviewing each case critically. In addition, we must ensure that disabled children and their parents feel welcome by taking steps such as providing sufficient facilities, reliable and easily accessible financial support, health care insurance, and incentives for optimal care for disabled children and families. I am convinced that the Dutch government tries to make provisions for disabled children and their families, but I also hear complaints about bureaucracy, waiting lists, and a sudden lack of support when the children become 18 years old.

As a pediatrician interested in EOL care for several decades, it strikes me that considerable energy has been put into regulation of newborn euthanasia and clarification of the indications for and implementation of withholding/withdrawing life-sustaining treatments. We, the Dutch, started by regulating and defining euthanasia, the complex endpoint of unsuccessful palliative care. We then reorganized, defined, and improved palliative care, unlike most other industrialized countries that first developed pediatric palliative care and then decided how to manage those rare cases when palliative care is insufficient. However, developments toward making high quality pediatric palliative care available in the Netherlands are accelerating. In 2013, the NVK published its national evidence-based guidelines for pediatric palliative care (Dutch Pediatric Association 2013; Knops, Kremer, and Verhagen 2015). In addition, the NVK recently launched the national knowledge center for pediatric palliative care that links practice, such as local palliative teams, regional collaboration, and consultation, to development of new knowledge and implementation by, for example, research agendas and pilot projects. Furthermore, we need to intensify and optimize pediatric palliative care for our several thousand pediatric patients with life-limiting diseases.

I want Dutch society's message to be: We feel responsible for providing optimal support of and quality of life to all children with chronic and life-limiting conditions and special needs and to their families; when children's suffering becomes refractory, we will listen to children and their parents and provide careful and tailored support in a transparent manner that ensures full accountability for all prescribed treatments, including the euthanasia of children.

BIBLIOGRAPHY

Abe, N., Anita Catlin, and D. Mihara. 2001. "End of Life in the NICU: A Study of Ventilator Withdrawal." *MCN The American Journal of Maternal/Child Nursing* 26, no. 3 (May): 141–6.

Anand, Karthika, and the International Evidence-Based Group for Neonatal Pain. 2001. "Consensus Statement for the Prevention and Management of Pain in the Newborn." *Archives of Pediatrics and Adolescent Medicine* 155, no. 2 (February): 173–80.

Arlettaz, Romaine, Dieto Mieth, Hans Ulrich Bucher, Gabriel Duc, and Jean-Claude Fauchere. 2005. "End-of-life Decisions in Delivery Room and Neonatal Intensive Care Unit." *Acta Paediatrica* 94, no. 11 (December): 1626–31.

Barr, Peter. 2007. "Relationship of Neonatologists' End-of-Life Decisions to their Personal Fear of Death." *Archives of Disease in Childhood. Fetal Neonatal Edition* 92, no. 2 (February): F104–7.

Barton, Lorayne, and Joan Hodgman. 2005. "The Contribution of Withholding or Withdrawing Care to Newborn Mortality." *Pediatrics* 116, no. 6 (December):1487–91.

Brouwer, Marije, Christopher Kaczor, Margaret Battin, Els Maeckelberghe, John Lantos, and Eduard Verhagen. 2018. "Should Pediatric Euthanasia be Legalized?" *Pediatrics* 141, no. 2 (February): doi: 10.1542/peds.2017-1343.

Carter, Brian, and Jatinda Bhatia. 2001. "Comfort/Palliative Care Guidelines for Neonatal Practice: Development and Implementation in an Academic Medical Center." *Journal of Perinatology* 21, no. 5 (August): 279–83.

Catlin, Anita, and Brian Carter. 2002. "Creation of a Neonatal End-of-Life Palliative Care Protocol." *Journal of Perinatology* 22, no. 3 (Apr–May): 184–95.

Catlin, Anita, and Renee Novakovich. 2008. "The Groningen Protocol: What Is It, How Do the Dutch Use It, and Do We Use It Here?" *Pediatric Nursing* 34, no. 3 (May–June): 247–51.

Central Bureau of Statistics. 2019. "Deaths." Accessed November 15, 2019. https://opendata.cbs.nl/statline/#/CBS/en/dataset/7052eng/table?ts=1540079787243.

Chervenak, Frank, Laurence McCullough, and Birgit Arabin. 2006. "Why the Groningen Protocol Should Be Rejected." *Hastings Center Report* 36, no. 5 (September–October): 30–3.

Committee Late Termination of Pregnancy and Termination of Life in Newborns [Commissie Late Zwangerschapsafbreking en levensbeeindiging bij pasgeborenen]. 2007. "Annual Report 2007 (Jaarverslag 2007)." Accessed November 15, 2019. http://www.lzalp.nl/documenten/publicaties/websitepublicaties/jaarverslagen/2007/jaarverslag-2007.

Committee Late Termination of Pregnancy and Termination of Life in New-borns [Commissie Late Zwangerschapsafbreking en levensbeeindiging bij pasge-borenen]. 2008. "Annual report 2008 (Jaarverslag 2008)." Accessed November 15, 2019. http://www.lzalp.nl/documenten/publicaties/websitepublicaties/jaarversla gen/2008/jaarverslag-2008.

Committee Late Termination of Pregnancy and Termination of Life in New-borns [Commissie Late Zwangerschapsafbreking en levensbeeindiging bij pasge-borenen]. 2010. "Annual Report 2009–10 (Jaarverslag 2009–10)." Accessed No-vember 15, 2019. http://www.lzalp.nl/documenten/publicaties/websitepublicaties/ jaarverslagen/2009-2010/jaarverslag-2009-2010.

Cook, Lynley A., and Jon F. Watchko. 1996. "Decision Making for the Critically Ill Neonate Near the End of Life." *Journal of Perinatology* 16, 2 Pt 1 (March–April): 133–6.

Costeloe, Kate. 2007. "Euthanasia in Neonates." *British Medical Journal* 334, no. 7600 (May 5): 912–3.

Costeloe, Kate, Enid Hennessy, Alan Gibson, Neil Marlow, and Andrew Wilkinson. 2000. "The EPICure Study: Outcomes to Discharge from Hospital for Infants Born at the Threshold of Viability." *Pediatrics* 106, no. 4 (October): 659–71.

Crouch, Gregory. 2005. "A Crusade Born of a Suffering Infant's Cry." *New York Times*, March 19, 2005.

Curlin, Farr. 2005. "Euthanasia in Severely Ill Newborns." *New England Journal of Medicine* 352, no. 22 (June): author reply 2353–5.

Cuttini, Marina, Monique Kaminski, Rodolfo Saracci, and Umberto de Vonderweid. 1997. "The EURONIC Project: A European Concerted Action on Information to Parents and Ethical Decision-Making in Neonatal Intensive Care." *Paediatric Perinatal Epidemiology* 11, no. 4 (October): 461–74.

Cuttini, Marina, M. Nadai, M. Kaminski, et al. 2000. "End-of-life Decisions in Neonatal Intensive Care: Physicians' Self-Reported Practices in Seven European Countries. EURONIC Study Group." *Lancet* 355, no. 9221 (June): 2112–8.

Davies, Dawn, and Debbie de Vlaming. 2006. "Symptom Control at the End-of-Life." In *Oxford Textbook of Palliative Care for Children*, edited by Ann Goldman, Rich-ard Hain, and Stephen Liben, 497–520. Oxford: Oxford University Press.

de Leeuw, Richard, Arnout de Beaufort, Martin de Kleine, Karin van Harrewijn, and Louis Kollée. 1996. "Foregoing Intensive Care Treatment in Newborn Infants with Extremely Poor Prognoses: A Study in Four Neonatal Intensive Care Units in The Netherlands." *Journal of Pediatrics* 129, no. 5 (November): 661–6.

De Minister van Justitie en de Staatssecretaris van Volksgezondheid Welzijn en Sport. 2007. "Regeling centrale deskundigencommissie late zwangerschapsaf-breking in een categorie 2-geval en levensbeëindiging bij pasgeborenen." Sta-atscourant (51): 8.

de Vries, Martine, and A. A. Eduard Verhagen. 2008. "A Case Against Something That Is Not the Case: The Groningen Protocol and the Moral Principle of Non-Maleficence." *American Journal of Bioethics* 8, no. 11 (December): 29–31.

Dorscheidt, Jozef. 2005. "Assessment Procedures Regarding End-of-Life Decisions in Neonatology in the Netherlands." *Medicine and Law* 24, no. 4 (December): 803–29.

Dorscheidt, Jozef. 2006. "Levensbeeindiging bij gehandicapte pasgeborenen. Strijdig met het non-discriminatie beginsel?" [Medical Termination in Disabled Newborns: Compatible with the Principle of Non-Discrimination?] (doctoral thesis). Den Haag: SDU.

Duff, Raymond, and A. G. M. Campbell. 1973. "Moral and Ethical Dilemmas in the Special-Care Nursery." *New England Journal of Medicine* 289, no. 17 (October): 890–4.

Dutch Pediatric Association (NVK). 2005. "Point of view NVK on 'Procedure Active Life-Ending Treatment of Newborns.'" Accessed October 11, 2019. https://www .nvk.nl/Nieuws/Dossiers/Levensbeeindiging-bij-pasgeborenen/Archief-berichten/ articleType/ArticleView/articleId/830/Standpunt-NVK-Procedure-actieve-levens beeindiging-pasgeborenen.

Dutch Pediatric Association (NVK). 2013. Richtlijn Paliatieve Zorg voor Kinderen [Clinical Guideline for Pediatric Palliative Care]. Accessed November 4, 2019. https://www.nvk.nl/Kwaliteit/Richtlijnen-overzicht/Details/articleType/Article View/articleId/894.

Dutch Termination of Life on Request and Assisted Suicide Act [*Wet toetsing levensbeëindiging op verzoek en hulp bij zelfdoding*]. 2002. Accessed November 29, 2019. https://www.government.nl/topics/euthanasia/euthanasia-assisted-suicide -and-non-resuscitation-on-request.

Gerechtshof Amsterdam 7 November 1995 [Amsterdam Court of Appeal]. 1996. *Tijdschrift voor Gezondheidsrecht* [Dutch Journal of Health Law] 20, no. 1 (April): 30–6.

Gerechtshof Leeuwarden 4 April 1996 [Leeuwarden Appeal Court]. 1996. *Tijdschrift voor Gezondheidsrecht* [Dutch Journal of Health Law] 20, no. 35: 284–91.

Gesundheit, Benjamin, Avraham Steinberg, Shraga Blazer, and Alan Jotkowitz. 2009. "The Groningen Protocol—The Jewish Perspective." *Neonatology* 96, no. 1 (January): 6–10.

Griffiths, John, Alex Bood, and Heleen Weyers. 1998. *Euthanasia and Law in the Netherlands*. Amsterdam: Amsterdam University Press.

Griffiths, John, Heleen Weyers, and Maurice Adams, eds. 2008. *Euthanasia and Law in Europe*. Oxford: Hart Publishing.

Hagen, Cathrin, and Thor Hansen. 2004. "Deaths in a Neonatal Intensive Care Unit: A 10-Year Perspective." *Pediatric Critical Care Medicine* 5, no. 5 (September): 463–8.

Hentschel, Roland, Katharina Lindner, Markus Krueger, and Stella Reiter-Theil. 2006. "Restriction in Ongoing Intensive Care in Neonates: A Prospective Study. *Pediatrics* 118, no. 2 (August): 563–9.

Janvier, Annie, William Meadow, Steven Leuthner, et al. 2011. "Whom Are We Comforting? An Analysis of Comfort Medications Delivered to Dying Neonates." *Journal of Pediatrics* 159, no. 2 (August): 206–10.

Jotkowitz, Alan, and Shimon Glick. 2006. "The Groningen Protocol: Another Perspective." *Journal of Medical Ethics* 32, no. 3 (March):157–8.

Jotkowitz, Alan, Shimon Glick, and B. Gesundheit. 2008. "A Case Against Justified Non-Voluntary Active Euthanasia (the Groningen Protocol)." *American Journal of Bioethics* 8, no. 11 (December): 23–6. https://doi.org/10.1080/15265160802513085.

KNMG Commissie Aanvaardbaarheid Levensbeeindigend handelen. 1997. Medisch handelen rond het levenseinde bij wilsonbekwame patiënten [Medical end-of-life pactice in incompetent patients]. Houten: Bohn Stafleu Van Loghem.

Knops, Rutger R. G., Leontien C. M. Kremer, and A. A. Eduard Verhagen. 2015. "Paediatric Palliative Care: Recommendations for Treatment of Symptoms in the Netherlands." *BMC Palliative Care* 14, no. 57 (November): 57.

Kodish, Eric. 2008. "Paediatric Ethics: A Repudiation of the Groningen Protocol." *Lancet* 371, no. 9616 (March): 892–3.

Kon, Alexander. 2007. "Neonatal Euthanasia Is Unsupportable: The Groningen Protocol Should Be Abandoned." *Theoretical Medicine and Bioethics* 28, no. 5 (October): 453–63.

Larroque, B., G. Breart, M. Kaminski, et al. 2004. "Survival of Very Preterm Infants: Epipage, a Population Based Cohort Study." *Archives of Disease in Childhood: Fetal & Neonatal Edition* 89, no. 2 (March): F139–44.

Leenen, H. J. J. 2000. "Einde van het leven" [The End of Life]. In *Handboek gezondheidsrecht. Deel 1. Rechten van mensen in de gezondheidszorg* [Handbook of Health Law. Volume 1. Individual Rights in the Context of Medical Care], edited by H. J. J. Leenen and J. K. M. Gevers, 302–78. Houten: Bohn Stafleu van Loghum.

Liben, Stephen, and Tom Lissauer. 2006. "Intensive Care Units." In *Oxford Textbook of Palliative Care for Children*, edited by Ann Goldmann, Richard Hain, and Stephen Liben, 549–56. New York: Oxford University Press.

Lindemann, Hilde, and Marian Verkerk. 2008. "Ending the Life of a Newborn: The Groningen Protocol." *Hastings Center Report* 38, No. 1 (Jan–Feb): 42–51.

Manninen, Bertha A. 2006. "A Case for Justified Non-Voluntary Active Euthanasia: Exploring the Ethics of the Groningen Protocol." *Journal of Medical Ethics* 32, no. 11 (November): 643–51.

Ministry of Health, Welfare and Sport. 2018. *Healthcare in the Netherlands*. The Hague. "Sterfte naar hoofdgroepen van doodsoorzaken [Main causes of Death]." Accessed October 20, 2018. https://www.volksgezondheidenzorg.info/onder werp/sterfte-naar-doodsoorzaak/cijfers-context/huidige-situatie#node-sterfte-naar -hoofdgroepen-van-doodsoorzaken.

Moseley, Kathryn L., Annamaria Church, Bridget Hempel, Harry Yuan, Susan Goold, and Gary Freed. 2004. "End-of-Life Choices for African-American and White Infants in a Neonatal Intensive-Care Unit: A Pilot Study." *Journal of National Medical Association* 96, no. 7 (July): 933–7.

Munson, David. 2007. "Withdrawal of Mechanical Ventilation in Pediatric and Neonatal Intensive Care Units." *Pediatric Clinics of North America* 54, no. 5 (October): 773–85.

Nederlandse Vereniging voor Kindergeneeskunde. 1992. *Doen of laten. Grenzen van het medisch handelen in de neonatologie* [To Treat or Not to Treat? Limits for Life-Sustaining Treatment in Neonatology]. Utrecht: Den Daas.

Norup, M. 1998. "Limits of Neonatal Treatment: A Survey of Attitudes in the Danish Population." *Journal of Medical Ethics* 24, no. 3 (June): 200–6.

Nuffield Council on Bioethics. 2006. "Decision Making: Ethical Issues." In *Critical Care Decisions in Fetal and Neonatal Medicine*, 7–26. London: Nuffield Council on Bioethics.

Oakley, Godfrey. 2005. "Euthanasia in Severely Ill Newborns." Letter to the editor. *New England Journal of Medicine* 352 (June): 2353–5.

Onwuteaka-Philipsen, Bregje, Arianne Brinkman-Stoppelenburg, Corine Penning, Gwen de Jong-Krul, Johannes van Delden, and Agnes van der Heide. 2012. "Trends in End-of-Life Practices before and after the Enactment of the Euthanasia Law in the Netherlands from 1990 to 2010: A Repeated Cross-Sectional Survey." *Lancet* 380, no. 9845 (September): 908–15.

Onwuteaka-Philipsen, Bregje, Johan Legemaate, Agnes van der Heide, et al. 2017. "Derde evaluatie Wet toetsing levensbeëindiging op verzoek en hulp bij zelfdoding" [Third evaluation of the Dutch Termination of Life on Request and Assisted Suicide Act]. In *Evaluatie regelgeving*. Den Haag: ZonMW.

Onwuteaka-Philipsen, Bregje, J. K. M. Gevers, Agnes van der Heide, et al. 2007. "Evaluatie Wet toetsing levensbeëindiging op verzoek en hulp bij zelfdoding" [Evaluation of the Termination of Life on Request and Assisted Suicide Act, practice, reporting and review]. Den Haag: ZonMW.

Overleggroep toetsing zorgvuldig medisch handelen rond het levenseinde bij pasgeborenen. 1997. Toetsing als spiegel van de medische praktijk [Assesment as Mirror of Medical Practice]. Rijswijk: Ministerie van Volksgezondheid Welzijn en Sport.

Pierucci, Robin, Russell Kirby, and Steven Leuthner. 2001. "End-of-life Care for Neonates and Infants: The Experience and Effects of a Palliative Care Consultation Service." *Pediatrics* 108, no. 3 (September): 653–60.

Provoost, Veerl, Filip Cools, Johan Bilsen, et al. 2006. "The Use of Drugs with a Life-Shortening Effect in End-of-Life Care in Neonates and Infants." *Intensive Care Medicine* 32, no. 1 (January): 133–9.

Provoost, Veerl, Filip Cools, Freddy Mortier, et al. 2005. "Medical End-of-Life Decisions in Neonates and Infants in Flanders." *Lancet* 365, no. 9467 (April): 1315–20.

Rebagliato, Marisa, Marina Cuttini, Lara Broggin, et al. 2000. "Neonatal End-of-Life Decision Making: Physicians' Attitudes and Relationship with Self-Reported Practices in 10 European Countries." *Journal of the American Medical Association* 284, no. 19 (November): 2451–9.

RTE Regional Euthanasia Review Committees. 2017. *Annual Report 2017*. Accessed November 16, 2019. https://english.euthanasiecommissie.nl/the-commit tees/annual-reports.

Roy, R., Narendra Aladangady, Kate Costeloe, and V. Larcher. 2004. "Decision Making and Modes of Death in a Tertiary Neonatal Unit." *Archives of Disease in Childhood: Fetal & Neonatal Edition* 89, no. 6 (November): F527–30.

Royal Dutch Medical Association (KNMG). 2017. "Euthanasia in figures april 2017." https://www.knmg.nl/web/file?uuid=6883ab97-053d-4426-a33b-bb711ab4 dd21&owner=5c945405-d6ca-4deb-aa16-7af2088aa173&contentid=63173.

Saigal, Saroj, Barbara Stoskopf, David Feeny, et al. 1999. "Differences in Preferences for Neonatal Outcomes Among Health Care Professionals, Parents, and Adolescents." *Journal of the American Medical Association* 281, no. 21 (June):1991–7.

Schulz-Baldes, A., Dieter Hüseman, A. Loui, Joachim Dudenhausen, and M. Obladen. 2007. "Neonatal End-of-Life Practice in a German Perinatal Centre." *Acta Paediatrica* 96, no. 5 (April): 681–7.

Singh, Jaideep, Jon Fanaroff, Bree Andrews, et al. 2007. "Resuscitation in the "Gray Zone" of Viability: Determining Physician Preferences and Predicting Infant Outcomes." *Pediatrics* 120, no. 3 (September): 519–26.

Singh, Jaideep, John Lantos, and William Meadow. 2004. "End-of-Life After Birth: Death and Dying in a Neonatal Intensive Care Unit." *Pediatrics* 114, no. 6 (December):1620–6.

Staatscommissie Euthanasie (State Commission on Euthanasia). 1985. Euthanasie: rapport van de Staatscommissie Euthanasie. Volume 1. Advies [Report of the State Commissien on Euthanasia]. The Hague.

Streiner, David, Saroj Saigal, Elizabeth Burrows, Barbara Stoskopf, and Peter Rosenbaum. 2001. "Attitudes of Parents and Health Care Professionals Toward Active Treatment of Extremely Premature Infants." *Pediatrics* 108, no. 1 (July): 152–7.

ten Cate, Katja, and Suzanne van de Vathorst. 2015. "Dutch Pediatricians' Views on the Use of Neuromuscular Blockers for Dying Neonates: A Qualitative Study." *Journal of Perinatology* 35, no. 7 (January): 497–502.

ten Cate, Katja, Suzanne van de Vathorst, Bregje D. Onwuteaka-Philipsen, and Agnes van der Heide. 2015. "End-of-Life Decisions for Children Under 1 Year of Age in the Netherlands: Decreased Frequency of Administration of Drugs to Deliberately Hasten Death." *Journal of Medical Ethics* 41, no. 10 (October): 795–8.

Thomas, Jo. 1984. "Dutch Court Acts on 'Right to Die.'" *New York Times*, November 28, 1984.

Truog, Robert, Jeffrey Burns, Christine Mitchell, Judy Johnson, and Walter Robinson. 2000. "Pharmacologic Paralysis and Withdrawal of Mechanical Ventilation at the End of Life." *New England Journal of Medicine* 342, no. 7 (February): 508–11.

van der Heide, Agnes, J. Legemaate, Bregje Onwuteaka-Philipsen, et al. 2012. *Tweede evaluatie Wet toetsing levensbeëindiging op verzoek en hulp bij zelfdoding* [Second Evaluation of the Dutch Termination of Life on Request and Assisted Suicide Act]. Den Haag: ZonMW.

van der Heide, Agnes, Bregje Onwuteaka-Philipsen, Mette Rurup, et al. 2007. "End-of-Life Practices in the Netherlands under the Euthanasia Act." *New England Journal of Medicine* 356, no. 19 (May): 1957–65.

van der Heide, Agnes, Johannes van Delden, and Bregje Onwuteaka-Philipsen. 2017. "End-of-Life Decisions in the Netherlands over 25 Years." *New England Journal of Medicine* 377, no. 5 (August): 492–94.

van der Heide, Agnes, Paul van der Maas, and Louis Kollée. 1997. "End-of-Life Decisions in Dutch Paediatric Practice." *Lancet* 350, no. 9092 (December): 1711.

van der Heide, Agnes, Paul van der Maas, Gerrit van der Wal, et al. 1997. "Medical End-of-Life Decisions Made for Neonates and Infants in the Netherlands." *Lancet* 350, no. 9073 (July): 251–5.

van der Heide, Agnes, Paul van der Maas, Gerrit van der Wal, Louis Kollée, and Richard de Leeuw. 2000. "Using Potentially Life-Shortening Drugs in Neonates and Infants." *Critical Care Medicine* 28, no. 7 (July): 2595–9.

van der Maas, Paul, Gerrit van der Wal, Ilinka Haverkate, et al. 1996. "Evaluation of the Notification Procedure for Physician-Assisted Death in the Netherlands." *New England Journal of Medicine* 335, no 22 (November): 1706–12.

van der Wal, Gerrit, and Paul van der Maas. 1996. "Medische beslissingen rond het levenseinde bij pasgeborenen en zuigelingen." In *Euthanasie en andere medische beslissingen rond het levenseinde: de praktijk en de meldingsprocedure*, 181–201. The Hague: SDU Uitgevers.

Vanhaesebrouck, Piet, Karel Allegaert, Jean Bottu, et al. 2004. "The EPIBEL Study: Outcomes to Discharge from Hospital for Extremely Preterm Infants in Belgium." *Pediatrics* 114, no. 3 (September): 663–75.

Verhagen, A. A. Eduard. 2009. End-of-life Decisions in Dutch Neonatal Intensive Care Units (thesis, University of Groningen). Zuthphen: Paris Legal Publishers.

Verhagen, A. A. Eduard. 2013. "The Groningen Protocol for Newborn Euthanasia; Which Way Did the Slippery Slope Tilt?" *Journal of Medical Ethics* 39, no.5 (May): 293–5.

Verhagen, A. A. Eduard, Mirjam de Vos, Jozef Dorscheidt, Bernadette Engels, Joep Hubben, and Pieter Sauer. 2009. "Conflicts about End-of-Life Decisions in NICUs in the Netherlands." *Pediatrics* 124, no. 1 (July): e112–9.

Verhagen, A. A. Eduard, Jozef Dorscheidt, Bernadette Engels, Joep Hubben, and Pieter Sauer. 2009a. "Analgesics, Sedatives and Neuromuscular Blockers As Part of End-of-Life Decisions in Dutch NICUs." *Archives of Disease in Childhood: Fetal & Neonatal Edition* 94, no. 6 (November): F434–8.

Verhagen, A. A. Eduard, Jozef Dorscheidt, Bernadette Engels, Joep Hubben, and Pieter Sauer. 2009b. "End-of-life Decisions in Dutch Neonatal Intensive Care Units." *Archives Pediatric Adolescent Medicine* 163, no. 10 (October): 895–901.

Verhagen, A. A. Eduard, Annie Janvier, Steven Leuthner, B. Andrews, J. Lagatta, Arend Bos, and William Meadow. 2010. "Categorizing Neonatal Deaths: A Cross-Cultural Study in the United States, Canada, and the Netherlands." *Journal of Pediatrics* 156, no. 1 (January): 33–7.

Verhagen, A. A. Eduard, and Pieter Sauer. 2005a. "End-of-Life Decisions in Newborns: An Approach from the Netherlands." *Pediatrics* 116, no. 3 (September): 736–9.

Verhagen, A. A. Eduard., and Pieter Sauer. 2005b. "The Groningen Protocol—Euthanasia in Severely Ill Newborns." *New England Journal of Medicine* 352, no. 10 (March): 959–62.

Verhagen, A. A. Eduard, and Pieter Sauer. 2008. "'Are Their Babies Different from Ours?' Dutch Culture and the Groningen Protocol." *Hastings Center Report* 38, no. 4 (Jul–Aug): 7; author reply 7–8.

Verhagen, A. A. Eduard, J. J. Sol, O. F. Brouwer, and Pieter J. Sauer. 2005. "Actieve levensbeeindiging bij pasgeborenen in Nederland, analyse van alle meldingen van 1997/'04. [Deliberate termination of life in newborns in The Netherlands; review of all 22 reported cases between 1997 and 2004]." *Nederlands Tijdschr voor Geneeskunde* 149, no. 4 (January): 183–8.

Verhagen, A. A. Eduard, Mark van der Hoeven, R. Corine van Meerveld, and Pieter Sauer. 2007. "Physician Medical Decision-Making at the End of Life in Newborns: Insight into Implementation at 2 Dutch Centers." *Pediatrics* 120, no. 1 (July): e20–8.

Vrakking, Astrid, Agnes van der Heide, Bregje Onwuteaka-Philipsen, Ingeborg Keij-Deerenberg, Paul van der Maas, and Gerrit van der Wal. 2005. "Medical End-of-Life

Decisions Made for Neonates and Infants in the Netherlands, 1995–2001." *Lancet* 365, no. 9467 (April): 1329–31.

Wall, Stephen, and John Partridge. 1997. "Death in the Intensive Care Nursery: Physician Practice of Withdrawing and Withholding Life Support." *Pediatrics* 99, no. 1 (January): 64–70.

Whitelaw, Andrew. 1986. "Death As an Option in Neonatal Intensive Care." *Lancet* 328, no. 8502 (August): 328–31.

Widdershoven, Guy. 2002. "Beyond Autonomy and Beneficence: The Moral Basis of Euthanasia in the Netherlands." *Ethical Perspectives* 9, no. 2–3 (2–3): 96–102.

Willems, Dick, A. A. Eduard Verhagen, and Eric van Wijlick. 2014. "Infants' Best Interests in End-of-Life Care for Newborns." *Pediatrics* 134, no. 4 (October): e1163–8.

Yuen, Wing Yan, José Duipmans, Bouwe Molenbuur, I. Herpertz, J. M. Mandema, and M. F. Jonkman. 2012. "Long-Term Follow-Up of Patients with Herlitz-Type Junctional Epidermolysis Bullosa." *British Journal of Dermatology* 167, no. 2 (April): 374–82.

Chapter Six

The Case Against Physician-Assisted Suicide and Euthanasia

Stephan Sahm

The admissibility of physician-assisted suicide (PAS) and/or euthanasia has been the subject of discussion for many years. In the Netherlands, Belgium, Luxembourg, Canada, Australia's Victoria state, nine American states, and the District of Columbia, medical acts designed to end a patient's life are immune from prosecution under certain conditions. Because of Germany's history of "euthanasia" programs during the Third Reich, these legislative decisions have inevitably led to intense debate in Germany about PAS and euthanasia.

When the president of the German *Bundestag* (Federal Parliament) instigated a public debate, there was concern that playing the "Nazi card" could inhibit or distort discussion. But, prior to the passage of relevant legislation in 2015, both advocates and opponents avoided drawing parallels with the crimes of Nazi terror. The arguments brought forward were the same as in other countries, indicating that the German debate was open and unconstrained (Oduncu and Sahm 2010).

In this chapter, I will examine the relevant regulations in Germany (Bundesaerztekammer 2011, A 346–48). My view, as a teacher of medical ethics and a physician who practices palliative care in the treatment of patients with cancer, is consistent with the ethical codes of the World Medical Association (WMA), which rejects both PAS and active euthanasia (AE) (World Medical Association 2019) or voluntary killing on demand (as opposed to "passive euthanasia" and "indirect euthanasia" that will be addressed later in the chapter).

THE FUNDAMENTAL AXIOM
UNDERPINNING LIBERAL SOCIETIES

In a free society, people have the right to decide how they live and how they die. The decision to depart from this life is an individual's inalienable right. This right is a negative right or a right of defense, not a claim right, that is, other persons and governmental institutions must not interfere without good reason—for example, when a third party is endangered or affected, or if the person claiming the right is unduly constrained when making the claim. Although psychology, sociology, and other human sciences teach us that the freedom to make decisions never actually exists without limitations, this (fictional) right of defense is an essential feature of a liberal society.

Notwithstanding this position, any humane society that operates on the principles of solidarity must acknowledge a fundamental axiom—a preference for the existence as against the non-existence of any member of the society. Human rights are based on this fundamental axiom. For example, the axiom is the rationale for organizing a health care system built on the principles of solidarity and fairness. Furthermore, the axiom includes a secular prohibition of killing and the justification for state interference in order to protect and preserve life and to protect life from interference by others. It, therefore, justifies state institutions intervening in the self-endangerment of persons if, for example, the person is in a state of diminished freedom, such as mental illness, psychological crisis, or pressure. Disregarding the fundamental axiom is tantamount to abolishing human rights.

The fundamental axiom cannot be justified on philosophical grounds alone (Spaemann 2000; 2006). In searching for the basis of the fundamental axiom—the preference for the life and existence of the members of a society—all that remains is reference to religious sources and moral intuitions. The philosophers Max Horkheimer and Theodor Adorno stated that prohibiting killing cannot be inferred by reason (Horkheimer and Adorno 1988, 127). Sources of knowledge beyond rational consideration are vital in view of the motivational aspect of ethical action, which is absolute in terms of the motivation to act on the basis of solidarity (Kolakowski 1989, 19–33). Yet, the motivation to act does not follow from the mere insight into the positive normative evaluation of an action—morality arises only when insight and the unconditioned experience of what ought to be come together.

NORMATIVE CONCEPTS OF
MEDICAL ACTS AT THE END OF LIFE

With the advent of modern medical technology like the respirator, the question of the limitations of treatment has become increasingly acute—there are few medical situations in which modern medicine does not offer life-prolonging treatment options. It follows that for many patients approaching the end of their lives, decisions are (or must be) made about the limitations of medical procedures (van der Heide et al. 2013), including palliation, the alleviation of symptoms and pain. Once an incurable disease progresses, the objective changes from curative and life-prolonging treatment to relief of symptoms. This modification includes not only withholding life-prolonging treatments, especially if the patient does not want them, but also terminating futile treatments. The obligation to sustain life does not, therefore, come without its limits. If the prolongation of life is no longer the objective, the alleviation of symptoms remains an indispensable duty (Sahm 2000; 2006).

Some have described this change in treatment objective as *passive euthanasia*, but this term is misleading (Rachels 1975; Beauchamp and Walters 1989, 248–255; Beauchamp 1997). The change involves the actual *action* of doing something: for example, when a treatment is discontinued or even when the instruction to stop treatment is given. As action is always being taken, the word *passive* causes confusion in those acting (Sahm 2000). The phrase also contains the word *euthanasia*, which suggests that the act of limiting treatment is bound up with the intention of bringing about the death of the patient. However, this view is wrong. The understanding that a treatment is no longer successful or is associated with unacceptable burdens or has been rejected by the patient cannot be equated with bringing about the death of the patient: letting a patient die is not tantamount to killing the patient (Sulmasy 1998; Sulmasy and Courtois 2019).

The same applies to the term *indirect euthanasia*, which implies that doctors and nurses indirectly bring about the death of the patient, for example, by treating pain. While some may argue that bringing about the death of the patient is a necessary component of palliative medicine, this argument is medically erroneous and ethically misleading. Properly administered pain therapy, including palliative sedation, does not necessarily shorten life (Wiffen, Wee, and Moore 2016; Wiffen et al. 2017). Furthermore, side effects of palliative pain therapy should not be assessed differently than unwanted side effects from any other medical treatment—patients die from medical interventions even when they are carried out in an expert manner with curative intention. Associating palliative therapy with acts of killing is misleading and wrong.

The terms *passive euthanasia* and *indirect euthanasia* are not used by the European working groups of palliative care physicians (Materstvedt et al. 2003), the WMA (2019), and the German Medical Association (Bundesaerztekammer, 2011). Palliative care does not differ from other medical procedures in terms of its normative structure (Sahm 2016). Treatment requires a medical indication, a positive goal (in this case, symptom relief), and the administration of the treatment in accordance with good medical practice.

THERAPEUTIC SEDATION

When discussing PAS and AE, palliative sedation—or better, therapeutic sedation—is often listed as a special case. If symptoms cannot be alleviated in any other way, long-term sedation up to loss of consciousness is a therapeutic option. Advocates of PAS and AE often claim that those who allow palliative sedation would also, for reasons of consistency, have to endorse PAS and AE and advocate their decriminalization. However, because palliative sedation is symptom-guided and indicated if symptoms cannot be relieved in any other way, their claim is unwarranted. State-of-the-art palliative sedation is reversible, variable, monitored, and the depth of sedation is carefully controlled. Patients may wake up after several hours or days, by which time the constellation of symptoms has often changed, and the patient can again communicate, enjoy company, and interact with relatives. Palliative sedation does not intend to bring about the death of the person affected. Furthermore, the frequency of unwanted side effects is not higher and might be lower than with other medical procedures (Lynn 1998). When properly carried out, palliative sedation does not differ in terms of its normative content from other medical procedures used for the benefit of patients (Curlin 2018; Sahm 2000).

On the other hand, empirical data from the Netherlands suggest that palliative sedation may be used as a pretext for practicing AE—18 percent of deaths in the Netherlands were by palliative sedation in 2017 (Royal Dutch Medical Association 2017, 20). When AE is carried out under the guise of palliative sedation, those responsible are not required to report the case and, therefore, they avoid the required assessment by a euthanasia committee. The suspicion that palliative sedation is used as a pretext for AE in the Netherlands is not easy to brush aside.

ETHICAL EVALUATION OF SUICIDAL
ACTS AND ASSISTANCE WITH SUICIDE

As stated above, people determining how they live their lives and how they die is an inalienable human right. The negative right not to be hindered in committing suicide applies only if the decision is made with unrestricted freedom from psychiatric illness, external pressure, and other factors influencing the decision, the so-called rational suicide. Only in such cases can people who wish to commit suicide claim not to be hindered in their actions. In all other cases—patients with psychiatric illness or family coercion, for example—society has a duty to prevent the suicide based on the fundamental axiom. These patients deserve psychiatric care and help in improving their living conditions. Offering support and reinforcement of a patient's intent to commit suicide is a breach of the fundamental axiom. A liberal society must also safeguard patients from outside influences that encourage suicide.

Rational suicides are a rare exception. Suicide research indicates that well over 95 percent of suicidal acts are triggered by external and mental compulsions (Fischer 2001; Schneider 2017, 616). The appropriate moral position toward expressions of suicidal ideation is, therefore, to refrain from moral judgment in the case of a (rare) rational suicide, to refrain from providing any support or encouragement for suicide, to make every effort to provide patients with other options, to reserve moral judgment, and to regret the suicide if it occurs. This moral position also applies to the increasingly frequent expressions of suicidal ideation among geriatric patients in response to various social causes (Dzeng and Pantilat 2018).

The ethical considerations presented so far provide the basis for current end-of-life legislation in Germany. The penal code does not prohibit suicidal acts. Because support for a non-criminal act is not itself a criminal offense, someone assisting with a suicide is not liable to prosecution. On the other hand, any offer to assist in a suicide is an independent risk factor for completing suicide (Jones and Paton 2015). The new law banned business-like assistance with suicide (Sahm 2016; Radbruch 2017), such as that provided by Exit and Dignitas in Switzerland, meaning that PAS is prohibited when it is performed on a repetitive basis as a professional medical activity. This view is supported by a majority of doctors in the German Medical Association, which decided that suicide assistance should not be a part of medical practice (Bundesaerztekammer 2011, A 346–48).

Therefore, when PAS is provided in the private sphere and in a spirit of profound trust, it is not criminalized in Germany. Moreover, based on my participation as an expert in parliamentary hearings, I do not think PAS performed in a setting of privacy and trust will be criminalized or subject to jurisdiction in the current political climate. Yet, the ban on business-like PAS is crucial because it rejects commercialization and broad social and medical acceptability of the procedure—the ban protects patients' lives.

An Interim Summary

I have argued that preference for life is the foundation of all human rights, a fundamental axiom, which states that the existence of members of a society is preferable to their non-existence. This axiom results in and is final justification for the prohibition of killing. The motives for accepting this axiom are as empirically diverse as there are people. However, the axiom cannot be inferred by pure rationality—it draws on resources beyond pure reason, such as religious sources, especially the Judeo-Christian revelation.

Normative assessment of end-of-life medical treatment demonstrates that treatment limitations are commonplace and indicated because, otherwise, medicine would become a hell in the face of technological progress. Palliative treatments are not different from other forms of medical treatments; they require a medical indication and they have side effects. No special associations can, therefore, be inferred between palliative medicine and intentional homicide. There is also no medical reason for ending a patient's life; palliative medicine experts maintain that almost all conditions can be treated.

The fundamental axiom also underpins the Hippocratic Oath, which proscribes killing, a ban that is accepted by the majority of medical organizations worldwide (World Medical Association 2019). Only medical associations in the Benelux countries, some US states, and Canada have abandoned this principle. In Switzerland, business-like assistance with suicide by laypersons is non-punishable by law.

FLAWS IN THE ARGUMENTS FOR PHYSICIAN-ASSISTED SUICIDE AND ACTIVE EUTHANASIA

The history of medicine in the Third Reich highlights the importance, in general, of being vigilant when life is at stake and, in particular, of examining the justifications for hastening a patient's death. While the Nazi medical crimes are not analogous to contemporary PAS and AE, Nazi physicians and ethicists did have justifications for their involuntary euthanasia programs, which are outlined elsewhere in this book. We would, therefore, be remiss if we did not carefully examine the arguments put forward by advocates of legalized PAS and euthanasia to be certain that those arguments can withstand ethical scrutiny.

In general, the reasons given by advocates of PAS and by advocates of AE do not differ. However, many of the advocates of PAS do not want to go so far as to justify the killing of patients by physicians; PAS seems to be an acceptable alternative for them. On the other hand, those who oppose PAS can rightly claim that their arguments against PAS are also applicable against AE. The legislation permitting PAS and AE in some countries has been published elsewhere (Jones, Gastmans, and Mackellar 2017; Keown 2018), and the justifications for them can be divided into two overlapping groups: basic arguments and arguments from medical practice.

Basic Arguments in Favor of Physician-Assisted Suicide and Active Euthanasia

Proponents cite the right of patients to determine their own fates, including an entitlement to seek PAS or euthanasia. A second basic argument is that some patients are tormented by untreatable and intolerable symptoms that can be relieved only by their death.

The first argument, based on self-determination, is inherently contradictory. Eligibility for PAS and AE is usually limited to patients with advanced disease near the end of life, which requires a determination by a third party; because the patient's request requires a doctor's permission, it is not self-determined. Therefore, it is not surprising that in the Netherlands, where doctors make this determination, a movement has emerged to provide support for patients whose doctors are unwilling to provide suicide assistance or assist in voluntary euthanasia. For example, the Dutch Right to Die Society has established Expertisecentrum Euthanasie, which offers PAS and AE when a patient's doctor will not give permission (2019). If self-determination provides the justification, it must always apply, but if it is subject to permission, then it is no longer autonomy. Establishing eligibility criteria for PAS and AE nullifies self-determination.

Advocates of PAS prefer that doctors endorse PAS, and patients usually follow the advice of their doctors. "The biggest thief of autonomy is sickness," wrote American bioethicist Eric Cassell (2005). However, if a physician offers assistance with a patient's suicide, either with or without a patient's request, the physician is further limiting the patient's unconditional freedom and autonomy. By not opposing PAS, either by raising the possibility of PAS or by giving the impression that PAS is ethically permissible, the physician implies social and medical acceptance of PAS, which contradicts the fundamental axiom. Therefore, withholding an endorsement of PAS and maintaining an intimate doctor-patient relationship are precisely what ensures freedom and self-determination for the patient.

The other basic argument in favor of PAS and AE is that physical suffering can be untreatable and intolerable, in which case PAS and AE are justifiable on ethical grounds and medically indicated. This claim may spring from lack of knowledge about or experience with palliative care, which can always offer symptomatic treatment, including palliative sedation as previously described. Moreover, patients seek PAS and AE because of social deprivation and the fear of loss of independence more than the presence or fear of physical ailments (Ganzini et al. 2002). In my experience, palliative care and the assurance that the limits of treatment set by the patient will be respected almost invariably cause the disappearance of death wishes. In addition, meaning-centered group psychotherapy has been demonstrated to reduce the desire for hastened death (Breitbart 2015). If physical symptoms are no longer the reason to commit suicide, restricting eligibility for PAS and AE to terminally ill patients with presumed intolerable and untreatable physical symptoms is only a rhetorical appeasement. Finally, establishing universal criteria for intolerable and unbearable suffering to shorten patients' lives would be a violation of the fundamental axiom.

If intolerable and untreatable suffering exists, then advocates should force their colleagues to offer PAS and AE; otherwise, their colleagues would be acting inhumanely. However, there are no agreed upon medical criteria to establish that patient suffering is sufficiently unbearable to justify an offer of PAS or AE. Forcing colleagues to make such judgments would be ethically monstrous.

Medical Practice Arguments in Favor of Physician-Assisted Suicide and Active Euthanasia

Proponents also put forward reasons from medical practice in favor of PAS and AE. First, they claim that the offer of suicide assistance engenders trust and strengthens the doctor-patient relationship. This assumption is mistaken. While acceding to a patient's request for assistance with suicide may avoid a difficult confrontation and appear to engender trust, the physician is actually undermining the doctor-patient relationship and the fundamental axiom by increasing the danger to the life of a vulnerable patient. For example, suicidal people, almost without exception, experience phases of dramatic ambivalence about committing suicide. In Germany, approximately 100,000 people attempt suicide each year, and 10,000 die as a result (completed suicides) (Krokauer 2017). Of the remaining 90,000, the overwhelming majority do not repeat the act in the following years. Because legalizing PAS in American states has been associated with an increased rate of total suicides relative to states that have not legalized PAS (Paton and Jones 2015), legalization appears to increase the likelihood that an ambivalent patient will become a completed suicide.

Completed suicides also encourage others to attempt suicide; they are, as it were, contagious and endanger people experiencing severe mental stress and/ or a personal crisis, as portrayed in Goethe's *Sorrows of Young Werther*, first published in 1774. At the end of the eighteenth century, some young men took their own lives after reading this novel, a phenomenon known as the "Werther effect" that has been confirmed by suicide research (Phillips 1974; Kogler and Noyon 2018). In November 2009, for example, the number of suicides and suicidal acts increased following the televised memorial service for the German goalkeeper Robert Enke, who took his own life (Cadenbach 2010). Similarly, scientists observed spikes in suicides after television programs about suicides of young students (Cheng et al. 2007; Schmidtke and Haefer 1988; Gould and Shaffer 1986).

It is also wrong to claim that offering suicide assistance quells patients' desires to take their own lives. Proponents of PAS argue, for example, that not all eligible Oregonians who are given a prescription for a lethal drug take it. The fact that some patients do not commit suicide does not necessarily lead to the conclusion that the offer of PAS quells patients' desires; rather, patients may have been ambivalent all along.

Based on data from Oregon, some proponents of PAS go further and claim that the offer of PAS has a preventive effect. However, while the incidence of PAS in Oregon is low in absolute terms, it is increasing in percentage terms at the same rate as in other countries where PAS is legal. It is also important to note that Oregon has a suicide rate higher than the American national average (Oregon Health Authority, n.d.) and 50 percent higher than that in Germany (Bronsich 2015). Furthermore, studies show that patients in Oregon with depressive disorders are not adequately diagnosed (Finlay and George 2010), and the offer of suicide assistance could increase the danger to the lives of these vulnerable, underdiagnosed patients. Also, empirical research suggests that the offer of PAS is an independent risk factor for committing suicide (Jones and Paton 2015).

Proponents of PAS sometimes state that doctors should be free to offer patients whom they have cared for many years a final service as an act of friendship. This argument contains dramatic potential but is misleading because it blinds physicians to generally accepted professional prohibitions governing breach of intimacy. For example, the prohibition against doctors having sexual relations with their patients is undisputed (World Medical Association 2006). It is justified by the asymmetry of power in the doctor-patient relationship, the concomitant danger of covert dependencies, and the risk of abuse of the role of medical authority, and applies unconditionally, regardless of the consent of the patients. It seems contradictory to declare that consensual sex with patients is an unethical act while maintaining that consensual killing of patients is an ethical act of friendship (Barilan 2003).

Finally, sociology and law teach us that ethical action requires not only ethical actors, but also strong institutional safeguards provided by traditional institutions like universities and churches as well as by professional organizations, ethical codes, the law, and such. Patients must be confident that doctors are thinking about cure and palliation rather than contemplating whether their lives are worth living. However, such contemplation is obligatory if doctors must judge the appropriateness of a request for PAS.

Empirical Data on Physician-Assisted Suicide and Euthanasia

The arguments presented in this chapter against PAS and AE are supported by empirical data from those countries where they are legal. While most proponents of PAS and AE want eligibility confined to cases of severe illness near the end of life, a few activists promote legalization without any restriction. For example, Roger Kusch, a former senator of justice in the State of Hamburg in Germany, founded a society called *Sterbehilfe Deutschland* (Euthanasia Germany) that offered assistance with suicide to all persons who want it; yet, after enactment of the new law, the society suspended activity (Widman 2019; Sterbehilfe Deutschland 2019).

Proponents also claim that legalization does not necessarily lead to liberalization of eligibility criteria and a concomitant increase in the number of cases of PAS and AE, and that procedural safeguards prevent abuse. However, the latest reports from Belgium show a steady increase in the number of patients euthanized since documentation began, including an increase of 13 percent from 2016 to 2017. Altogether, the number of cases of euthanasia in Belgium increased from 235 in 2003 to 2,309 cases in 2017 (Jones et al. 2017). In addition to demonstrating the liberalization of eligibility requirements and the unreliability of safeguards, these data demonstrated that doctors′ attitudes are changing with an increased willingness to accede to requests for euthanasia (Montero 2017).

In the beginning, only a slow increase in the number of cases of AE was observed in the Netherlands, where AE has been tolerated since 1985 and legal since 2002. Yet, from 2005 on, the numbers increased rapidly from 1,923 cases in 2005 to 6,991 in 2016 (Boer 2018). Proponents argued that the increase before 2005, three years after legalization of AE, was explained by physicians reporting previously unreported procedures, but this explanation is unconvincing for the increased numbers since 2005, especially since mortality increased by only 7.7 percent whereas the number of euthanasia cases tripled. Currently, approximately 5 percent of all deaths are caused by explicit acts of euthanasia and another 18 percent by therapeutic sedation, which may be a pretext for covert euthanasia, as noted above. Simultaneously, the eligibility criteria have changed. Initially, almost all patients had a terminal illness; now, an increasing number of patients are euthanized for dementia, psychiatric disease, old age, or other reasons (Royal Dutch Medical Association 2017; Boer 2018). And importantly, there is still a significant number of cases of involuntary euthanasia (van der Heide, van Delden, and Onwuteaka-Philipsen 2017), which proves that safeguards do not prevent abuse.

In Switzerland, where euthanasia is not permitted but assistance with suicide by lay people is legal, the number of assisted suicides has also increased approximately from 60 in 2000 to 600 in 2015 (Hurst and Mauron 2003; Sitte 2015). These data do not include the assisted suicides of persons from other countries who travel to Switzerland seeking assistance. If one projects these numbers onto Germany with a population 10 times higher than Switzerland, it would mean an estimated 6,000 extra deaths from assisted suicide per year, the equivalent of extinguishing a small town each year.

In summary, the assertion that PAS and AE can be limited to rare patients with terminal disease is an illusion, the admissibility of PAS increases the number of suicides, and permitting PAS and AE leads to an excess mortality. Furthermore, palliative medicine provides empathetic care and decreases patient suffering without intentionally hastening death (Oduncu and Sahm 2010). I, therefore, conclude that prohibiting PAS and AE is consistent with a medical profession that knows its limitations and respects and protects vulnerable patients. Limiting medical treatments has long been part of medical practice and it goes without saying that patients´ wishes to withhold life-prolonging treatment are honored.

It behooves a free society, one that respects the lives and integrity of its citizens, to criminalize PAS and AE and prohibit physicians from either assisting with patient suicides or killing their patients.

BIBLIOGRAPHY

Barilan, Y. Michael. 2003. "Of Doctor-Patient Sex and Assisted Suicide." *Israel Medical Association Journal* 5, No. 6 (June): 460–63.

Beauchamp, Tom. 1997. "A Reply to Rachels on Active and Passive Euthanasia." In *Social Ethics: Morality and Social Policy*, edited by Thomas Mappes and J. Zembaty, 67–75. New York: McGraw-Hill.

Beauchamp, Tom, and LeRoy Walters. 1989. *Contemporary Issues in Bioethics*, 3rd ed. Belmont, CA: Wadsworth Publishing.

Boer, Theo A. 2018. "Dialectics of Lead: Fifty Years of Dutch Euthanasia and its Lessons." *International Journal of Environmental Studies* 75, no. 2 (January) 239–250. https://doi.org/10.1080/00207233.2017.1415834.

Breitbart, William, Barry Rosenfeld, Hayley Pessin, Allison Applebaum, Julia Kolokowski, and Wendy Lichtenthal. 2015. "Meaning-Centered Group Psychotherapy: An Effective Intervention for Improving Psychological Well-Being in Patients with Advanced Cancer." *Journal of Clinical Oncology* 33, no. 7 (March): 749–54.

Bronsich, Thomas. 2015. "Suicide: Epidemiology." *International Encyclopedia of the Social and Behavioral Sciences*, 2nd Edition. Science Direct (website). Accessed November 9, 2019. https://www.sciencedirect.com/topics/social-sciences/suicide-rate.

Bundesaerztekammer [German Medical Association]. 2011a. "Grundsätze zur aerztlichen Sterbebegleitung" [Principles of the German Medical Association for Medical Terminal Care]. *Deutsches Aerzteblatt* 108, no. 7: A 346, B-278, C-278.

Bundesaerztekammer [German Medical Association]. 2011b. "Principles Regarding the Accompaniment of the Dying Process by Physicians." Accessed November 9, 2019. http://www.drze.de/in-focus/euthanasia/modules/german-medical-association-principles-regarding-the-accompaniment-of-the-dying-process-by-physicians?set_language=en.

Cadenbach, Christoph. 2010. Der Enke-Effekt [The Enke Effect]. https://sz-magazin
.sueddeutsche.de/gesellschaft-leben/der-enke-effekt-77033.

Cassell, Eric. 2005. "Consent or Obedience? Power and Authority in Medicine." *New England Journal of Medicine* 352, no. 4 (January): 328–30.

Cheng, Andrew, Keith Hawton, Cheng-Ting Lee, and Tony Chen. 2007. "The Influence of Media Reporting of the Suicide of a Celebrity on Suicide Rates: A Population-Based Study." *International Journal of Epidemiology* 36, no. 6 (January): 1229–34.

Curlin, Farr. 2018. "Palliative Sedation: Clinical Context and Ethical Questions." *Theoretical Medicine and Bioethics* 39, no. 3 (August): 197–209.

Dzeng, Elizabeth, and Steven Pantilat. 2018. "Social Causes of Rational Suicide in Older Adults." *Journal of the American Geriatrics Society* 66, no. 5 (May): 853–55.

Expertisecentrum Euthanasie. n.d. "Careful and Caring." Accessed November 9, 2019. https://expertisecentrumeuthanasie.nl/en/.

Finlay, Ilora, and Rob George. 2010. "Legal Physician-Assisted Suicide in Oregon and the Netherlands: Evidence Concerning the Impact on Patients in Vulnerable Groups—Another Perspective on Oregon's Data." *Journal of Medical Ethics* 37, no. 3 (March): 171–74.

Fischer, C. 2001. "Gibt es den Suizid aus freier Entscheidung?" [Is There Suicide by Choice]. In *Vom Recht zu sterben, zur Pflicht zu sterben?* [From the Right to Die to a Duty to Die?], edited by A. Schwank and R. Spöndlin, 19–28. Zürich: Edition 8.

Ganzini Linda, Theresa Harvath, Ann Jackson, Elizabeth Goy, Lois Miller, and Molly Delorit. 2002. "Experiences of Oregon Nurses and Social Workers with Hospice Patients who Requested Assistance with Suicide." *New England Journal of Medicine* 347, no. 8 (September): 582–88.

Gould, Madelyn, and David Shaffer.1986. "The Impact of Suicide in Television Movies. Evidence of Imitation." *New England Journal of Medicine* 315, no. 11 (September): 690–94.

Horkheimer, Max, and Theodor Adorno. (1947) 1988. *Dialektik der Aufklärung* [Dialectic of Enlightment]. Frankfurt: Fischer.

Hurst, Samia, and Alex Mauron. 2003. "Assisted Suicide and Euthanasia in Switzerland: Allowing a Role for Non-Physicians." *British Medical Journal* 326, no. 383 (January): 271–73. https://doi.org/10.1136/bmj.326.7383.271.

Jones, David, and David Paton. 2015. "How Does Legalization of Physician-Assisted Suicide Affect Rates of Suicide." *Southern Medical Journal* 108, no.10 (October): 599–604.

Jones, David Albert, Chris Gastmans, and Calum Mackellar. 2017. *Euthanasia and Assisted Suicide: Lessons from Belgium.* Cambridge: Cambridge University Press.

Keown, John. 2018. *Euthanasia, Ethics and Public Policy*, 2nd ed. New York: Cambridge University Press.

Kogler, Vivien, and Alexander Noyon. 2018. "The Werther Effect—About the Handling of Suicide in the Media." Open Access Government (website). November 26, 2018. Accessed November 9, 2019. https://www.openaccessgovernment.org/the-werther-effect/42915/.

Kolakowski, Leszek. 1989. *The Presence of Myth*, translated by Adam Czerniawski. Chicago: University of Chicago Press.

Krokauer, Christine. 2017. "Selbstmordrate in Deutschland erschreckend hoch. Haü-figste Ursache: Depressionen" [Suicide Rate in Germany Alarmingly High. Most Common Cause: Depression]. Psychomeda (blog). Accessed November 9, 2019. https://www.psychomeda.de/psychologie-blog/selbstmordrate-in-deutschland-er schreckend-hoch-haeufigste-u.html.

Lynn, J. L. 1998. "Terminal Sedation." *New England Journal of Medicine* 338, no. 17 (April): 1230–31.

Materstvedt, Lars Johan, David Clark, John Ellershaw, et al. 2003. "Euthanasia and Physician-Assisted Suicide: A View from an EAPC Ethics Task Force." *Palliative Medicine* 17, no. 2 (April): 97–101.

Montero, Etienne. 2017. "The Belgian Experience of Euthanasia since its Legal Implementation in 2002." In *Euthanasia and Assisted Suicide: Lessons from Belgium*, edited by David Albert Jones, Chris Gastmans, and Calum Mackellar, 26–48. Cambridge: Cambridge University Press.

Oduncu, Fuat, and Stephan Sahm. 2010. "Doctor-Cared Dying Instead of Physician-Assisted Suicide: A Perspective from Germany." *Medicine, Health Care and Philosophy* 13, no. 4 (November): 371–81.

Oregon Health Authority. n.d. "Suicide in Oregon." Accessed November 9, 2019. https://www.arcgis.com/apps/MapSeries/index.html?appid=9c59be59ef7142dfad 40d95e3b36f588.

Phillips, David P. 1974. "The Influence of Suggestion on Suicide: Substantive and Theoretical Implications of the Werther Effect." *American Sociological Review* 39, no. 3 (June): 340–54. https://www.jstor.org/stable/pdf/2094294.pdf?seq=1#page_ scan_tab_contents.

Rachels, James. 1975. "Active and Passive Euthanasia." *New England Journal of Medicine* 292, no. 2 (January): 78–80.

Radbruch, Lukas. 2017. Interview by Adelheid Müller-Lissner, translated by Jonathan Brackett. "Euthanasia: Germany Has Found a Moderate Solution." Accessed November 9, 2019. https://www.goethe.de/en/kul/ges/20927927.html.

Royal Dutch Medical Association (KNMG). 2017. "Derde Evaluatie Wet toesting levensbeeindiging op veroek en hulp bij zelfdoding." [Third Evaluation Law on Termination of Life on Request and Assistance with Suicide]. Accessed November 9, 2019. https://www.rijksoverheid.nl/documenten/rapporten/2017/05/23/derde -evaluatie-wet-toetsing-levensbeeindiging-op-verzoek-en-hulp-bij-zelfdoding.

Sahm Stephan. 2000. "Palliative Care Versus Euthanasia. The German Position: The German General Medical Council's Principles for Medical Care of the Terminally Ill." *Journal of Medicine and Philosophy* 25, no. 2 (April): 195–219.

Sahm, Stephan. 2006. *Sterbebegleitung und Patientenverfügung* [Terminal Care and Living Will]. Frankfurt: Campus Publishing.

Sahm, Stephan. 2016. "Keine Kriminalisierung der Palliativmedizin." *Zeitschrift fuer Medizinische Ethik* 3: 219–33.

Schmidtke, Armin, and H. Haefner. 1988. "The Werther Effect after Television Films: New Evidence for an Old Hypothesis." *Psychological Medicine* 18, no. 3 (August): 665–676. Published online July 9, 2009. Cambridge Core, Cambridge University Press. DOI: https://doi.org/10.1017/S0033291700008345.

Schneider Frank. 2017. *Facharztwissen Psychiatrie, Psychosomatik und Psychotherapie.* Heidelberg: Springer.

Sitte, Thomas. 2015. "Palliative Versorgung statt Beihilfe zum Suizid und Tötung auf Verlangen? Über eine mögliche Notwendigkeit lebensverkürzender Maßnahmen" [Palliative Care Instead of Aiding Suicide and Killing on Request? On a Possible Need for Life-Shortening Measures] (doctor of medicine dissertation, University of Saarland, Homburg/ Saar, 2015).

Spaemann, Robert. 2000. *Happiness and Benevolence.* Notre Dame, IN: University of Notre Dame Press.

Spaemann, Robert. 2006. *Persons: The Difference between "Someone" and "Something."* Oxford: Oxford University Press.

Sterbehilfe Deutschland. 2019. http://www.sterbehilfedeutschland.de/index.php ?site=fragen.

Sulmasy, Daniel. 1998. "Killing and Allowing to Die: Another Look." *Journal of Law, Medicine & Ethics* 26, no. 1 (June): 55–64.

Sulmasy, Daniel, and Marielle Courtois. 2019. "Why the Common-Sense Distinction between Killing and Allowing-to-Die Is So Easy to Grasp but So Hard to Explain." *Cambridge Quarterly of Healthcare Ethics* 28, no. 2 (April): 353–58.

van der Heide, Agnes, Luc Deliens, Karin Faisst, et al. 2013. "End-of-Life Decision-Making in Six European Countries." *Lancet* 362, no. 9381 (September): 345–50.

van der Heide, Agnes, van Delden J. J. M., and Bregje D. Onwuteaka-Philipsen. 2017. End-of-Life-Decisions in the Netherlands over 25 Years." *New England Journal of Medicine* 377, no. 5: (August): 492–494.

Widmann, Marc. 2019. "Sterbehilfe: Er will es zu Ende bringen" [Euthanasia: He Wants to Finish It]. *Zeit Online*, July 2, 2019. https://www.zeit.de/2019/27/roger -kusch-sterbehilfe-assistierter-suizid-verein.

Wiffen, Philip, Bee Wee, and R. Andrew Moore. 2016. "Oral Morphine for Cancer Pain." *Cochrane Systematic Review* (website), April 22. https://www.cochrane library.com/cdsr/doi/10.1002/14651858.CD003868.pub4/full.

Wiffen, Philip, Bee Wee, Sheena Derry, Rae Frances Bell, and R. Andrew Moore. 2017. "Opiods for Cancer Pain: An Overview of Cochrane Reviews. *Cochrane Systematic Review* (website), July 6. https://doi.org/10.1002/14651858.CD12592.pub2.

World Medical Association. 2006. "WMA International Code of Medical Ethics 2006." Accessed November 9, 2019. https://www.wma.net/policies-post/wma -international-code-of-medical-ethics/.

World Medical Association. 2019. "WMA Declaration on Euthanasia and Physician Assisted Suicide." Accessed November 9, 2019. https://www.wma.net/policies -post/wma-statement-on-euthanasia-and-physician-assisted-suicide/.

ADDENDUM

As this book was preparing to go to press, the German Federal Constitutional Court delivered, on February 26, 2020, a judgment on assisted suicide (but not on euthanasia) that marked a fundamental change in the law governing end-of-life decisions. Because the ruling repeals the prohibition of "business-like" assistance with suicide as described in this chapter, I have added this addendum to highlight its potential repercussions.

Because the court ruled that there is no legal obligation to provide assistance with suicide, even for physicians, the medical profession can still maintain a strong moral stance against PAS. Indeed, the German Medical Association has rejected both PAS and euthanasia (Richter-Kuhlmann 2014). Although health care policy is left to the individual German states, each state's medical association has to adopt the position expressed in the professional code of conduct of the German Medical Association. So far, they have all either banned or refused to incorporate into medical practice both PAS and euthanasia.

This ruling, however, goes far beyond prior rulings by stating that the constitutional right to make decisions about one's life and how to end it, guaranteed in Article 2 (1) of the German Constitution (Grundgesetz), now includes the right to seek assistance with suicide from others, even in the absence of disease. In taking this stance, the court violates the basic axiom as outlined above and changes the landscape of end-of-life legislation in Germany. Although the court acknowledged caveats like those presented in this chapter, it brushed them aside, emphasized autonomy over preserving life, and recognized that its judgment might lead to a dramatic increase in the number of deaths from suicide.

The court leaves open the question of legislative safeguards to prevent abuse of the right to assisted suicide, such as waiting periods, an obligation to inform persons seeking assistance of its risks and benefits, and the creation of authorization requirements. Such legislation might be ineffective in any case—in all states where assisted dying has been decriminalized, the number of persons dying by such acts has steadily increased as outlined in this chapter. In addition, Wolfgang Thierse, the former president of the German Parliament, questioned if any legal provision limiting access to suicide assistance will withstand judicial scrutiny (Thierse 2020). Nevertheless, legislators deserve support when seeking to mitigate the potential effects of this ruling.

The judgment also raises concern about maintaining the distinction in Germany between assisted suicide wherein a patient self-administers a deadly medication and active euthanasia wherein a third party injects a patient with a deadly medication. Yet, because the court attached such importance to the right to make decisions about one's life and how to end it, one may reasonably fear that these judges might overrule this distinction if an appropriate case is brought before them.

A new debate is underway in Germany about how legislators may limit the consequences of the High Court's ruling. Legislation and court rulings may change, as they have in other countries. Yet, when the lives of its patients are at stake, the medical profession should neither adopt a position of neutrality nor abandon its principled rejection of PAS and euthanasia.

ADDENDUM BIBLIOGRAPHY

Federal Constitutional Court [Bundesverfassungsgericht]. 2020. "Criminalisation of assisted suicide services unconstitutional." Press Release No. 12/2020 of 26 February 2020. Accessed March 22, 2020. https://www.bundesverfassungsgericht.de/ SharedDocs/Pressemitteilungen/EN/2020/bvg20-012.html.

Richter-Kuhlmann Eva. 2014. "Gemeinsames Bekenntnis der Kammern: Helfen, aber nicht töten." *Deutsches Ärzteblatt* 111, no. 51–52 (December): A-2247.

Thierse, Wolfgang. 2020. "Die ethischen Grundfeste erschüttert." *Frankfurter Allgemeinen Zeitung*. February 29, 2020.

Chapter Seven

Palliative Medicine and the Debate on Physician-Assisted Death in Germany

H. Christof Müller-Busch

Up until the 1970s, "quality of dying" or "medical aid for a good death" was not discussed by health care professionals in Germany. However, skepticism about the medical profession's ability to adequately address longevity, chronic illness, and artificially prolonged life catalyzed a societal debate about "dying with dignity," "a good death," and "euthanasia." The option of dying without medical help seemed inadequate for a good quality of dying. In this context, the term *physician-assisted death* means a physician actively ending a patient's life by a medical intervention. On the other hand, from a palliative care point of view, *euthanasia* is a confusing term because it covers both *passive euthanasia* (*passive Sterbehilfe*) and *active euthanasia* (*aktive Sterbehilfe*). In palliative care, passive euthanasia means withdrawal or withholding of potentially life-prolonging interventions with the intention to "let the patient die" (*Sterben lassen*) in futile medical situations or with the patient's advance consent or explicit request. Active euthanasia means the killing of a competent, terminally ill person with intolerable suffering who has made an explicit request for death by a medical intervention in defined medical situations.

Unlike other European countries like Great Britain, where both physician-assisted suicide (PAS) and euthanasia are illegal, and the Netherlands and Belgium, where both PAS and euthanasia are legal, Germany avoided the term *euthanasia*, almost certainly the result of the criminal misuse of it during the Nazi period. Instead, they used words like *Sterbebegleitung* (terminal care) or *Sterbebetreuung* (care for the dying) to mean letting death happen naturally while simultaneously providing optimal comfort care.

Furthermore, because the term *passive Sterbehilfe* was considered too active to describe medical activities in the final stages of life, ethicists suggested replacing it with the aforementioned *Sterben lassen*, which is the basis for palliative decision-making about potentially life-limiting measures. These terms must be clearly distinguished from *aktive Sterbehilfe* that covers physician-assisted dying to shorten a patient's life either by euthanasia or PAS.

In a few countries with highly developed palliative care like Belgium, the Netherlands, Luxemburg, and Canada, both PAS and euthanasia are legal. In Switzerland and in Germany, euthanasia—a doctor killing a person on his explicit request by a lethal medication or another lethal intervention—is strictly forbidden, while assisted suicide by a non-physician is, like suicide itself, not considered criminal.

DIFFERENT APPROACHES TO THE MANAGEMENT
OF DYING IN THE TWENTIETH CENTURY

Debates regarding the management of dying and the organization of a good death are philosophical themes with societal implications and concrete legal and practical consequences. These topics attracted widespread public attention in the 1960s and 70s, especially after American attorney Luis Kutner presented the first living will in 1967, which highlighted patients' rights, living wills, advance directives, and health care proxies. In 1968, the first living will legislation was proposed in Florida's state legislature, but it failed to pass (Kutner 1969). Also in 1967, the modern hospice movement began in the United Kingdom when Dame Cicely Saunders opened the St. Christopher Hospice in a residential suburb of London to provide specialist care for dying patients with incurable diseases (Clark 1998).

In 1973, Dr. Balfour Mount, a urologist, opened the first special unit for dying patients in Montreal, Canada. He coined the term *palliative care* to highlight the protection of patients living with terminal illnesses. He is considered the father of palliative care because he emphasized attention to quality of life up until the moment of death. Dr. Mount also recognized the need for humane and compassionate "whole person" care to alleviate suffering and enhance dignity for seriously ill patients and their families (Palliative Care McGill n.d.).

Also in 1973, these debates came to the Dutch public's attention when Dr. Truus Postma was prosecuted for injecting her terminally ill mother with a lethal dose of morphine (Sheldon 2007). This case launched euthanasia movements in several countries, including the Netherlands and Belgium. In 2002, they legalized PAS and euthanasia performed by physicians under defined circumstances of intolerable suffering (Rietjens et al. 2009). In the Netherlands, the number of patients dying by euthanasia as defined and regulated by the 2002 "Termination of Life on Request and Assisted Suicide (Review Procedures) Act" has increased to more than 4.5 percent of all deaths (Regional Euthanasia Review Committees 2019), even though Holland provides highly developed palliative care.

Switzerland was the first country to permit and regulate assisted suicide (*Freitodhilfe*) for persons with intolerable suffering in defined health situations. The intention was to reduce violent suicides by shooting, hanging, strangulation, suffocation, jumping, intentional traffic accidents, and other violent acts. In 1977, the canton of Zurich conducted a plebiscite, which surprisingly passed with 60 percent of the vote, proposing submission of an initiative on "euthanasia on request for people suffering from ill health" to the federal council. This led, in 1982, after an intense debate about *Freitodhilfe*, to the founding of Exit, an organization that supports self-determined suicide with assistance of non-medical persons. The legal establishment of *Freitodhilfevereine* (membership corporations to promote help for self-determined death) was based on a 1941 law permitting altruistic help for severely ill people to perform suicide. The pragmatic Swiss regulation, which was not supported by the Swiss Academy of Medical Sciences (Hurst and Mauron 2003), led to an ethical debate about PAS and the role of physicians—as citizens and not physicians—in supporting the *Freitodhilfevereine* (Griffiths, Weyers, and Adams 2008, 463–481). In hindsight, I think that the Swiss model did not achieve the intended goal of reducing violent suicides. Currently, PAS accounts for about 1.5 percent of all deaths in Switzerland, and the number of suicides committed by Swiss people has doubled since suicide assistance became tolerated and legal (Fahy 2018; Swiss Federal Statistical Office 2018).

PALLIATIVE MEDICINE AND THE DEBATE ON ASSISTED SUICIDE AND EUTHANASIA IN GERMANY

The current debates about self-determined control of dying and organization of a good death, influenced by continuously increasing requests for assisted suicide and euthanasia in countries where these practices have been legalized, has resulted in greater public acceptance of these options (Richards and Krawczyk 2019). At the same time, palliative care encourages an alternative approach to end-of-life conflicts. After a debate on euthanasia in the European Parliament, the first position paper of the European Association for Palliative Care (EAPC) rejected euthanasia and PAS (Roy, Rapin, and EAPC

Board of Directors 1994). This position was finalized in 2002 by a task force of the EAPC: "The provision of euthanasia and physician-assisted suicide should not be part of the responsibility of palliative care" (Materstvedt et al. 2003). Although this statement has been the palliative care physician's guideline for the ethical and practical approach to patients requesting a hastened death, it was considered controversial by some palliative care specialists because (1) the wish to die is not an uncommon phenomenon in palliative care, and (2) Switzerland does not criminalize suicide assistance. Nevertheless, the EAPC position was adopted by the German Medical Association (*Bundesärztekammer*) in the most recent version (2011) of the *Grundsätze zur ärztlichen Sterbebegleitung* (Principles of Medical Aid in Dying), which outlines the obligations of physicians caring for severely ill and dying patients.

In contrast to Switzerland, where non-physician-assisted suicide has been facilitated by membership organizations like Exit and Dignitas, Germany changed section 217 of the criminal code to explicitly forbid organizations offering assisted suicide (Melching 2017), which has provoked a debate among palliative care physicians about the appropriate response to a patient's request for assisted suicide. While the change in the criminal code, which explicitly forbids commercial, or business-like, assisted suicide appears to have allayed some concerns, doctors continue to worry (Hauptmeier 2019) about their legal exposure if they assist in a patient's suicide.

Suicide and assisted suicide occur very rarely in German palliative care. A retrospective survey of physicians on causes of death in 17,772 patients treated with specialized palliative care revealed only 17 cases of suicide (0.1 percent) (Sitte, Gronwald, and Gottschling 2016). The debate over assisted death in Germany arose not because of the number of suicides but because of the term *business-like* in the 2015 law. Although the Federal Constitutional Court has received constitutional complaints and petitions to lift the ban on suicide assistance, a final decision on the legality of assisted suicide has not yet been made. On the other hand, in 2017, the Federal Administrative Court decided that patients have the right to get a sufficient dose of lethal medication to commit suicide in exceptional cases. So, while the legal situation in Germany is complex, assisted suicide or euthanasia in palliative settings remains extremely rare.

Comprehensive care for the severely ill and the dying has become one of the great challenges in palliative care, including enabling a good death (Smith 2000). Core principles in the debate about what is a good death include optimal medical care, relief of suffering, recognition of patients' perspectives and rights, and respect for autonomy. The palliative care physician must consider not only the subjective views of the patient but also the subjective views of those who live on after their loved one's death, especially when the patient has made a request to hasten death (Hendry et al. 2013). Although there is no general definition of a good death in palliative care, it could be defined as a process of dying, not just the final moment of life, that is consistent with inherent dignity and tolerated and accepted by all involved. Quality in end-of-life care and in death is a dynamic process that is negotiated and renegotiated between patients, families, and health care professionals.

REQUESTS FOR HASTENED DEATH IN PALLIATIVE CARE

Patients and their families confronting life-limiting disease or old age need respectful help from physicians and multiple professional care teams, acknowledging that each participant may have different views on hastened death by assisted suicide and euthanasia. Currently, physicians in favor of life-shortening medical interventions are constrained by the government's and the German Medical Association's statements that active euthanasia is illegal. But opinion surveys in Germany, as in most industrialized countries, are clearly in favor of a legal option to terminate life by euthanasia or assisted suicide (Statista 2017; Roesinger et al. 2018). In addition, German doctors' views about end-of-life options are influenced by reflections on Nazi euthanasia programs and the Nuremberg Medical Trial (Spitshuis 2018). Nonetheless, one must admit that the general debate on euthanasia today is insufficiently influenced by what we can and need to learn from medicine during the Third Reich.

While patients with progressive terminal diseases receiving palliative care make explicit requests for assisted suicide and euthanasia, these requests are rare. The prevalence of wishes for hastened death from all palliative care patients ranges between 1.5 and 40 percent. The great variability is likely due to disparities in the definition and scope of practices encompassed by the phrase "hastened death," as well as the characteristics of the patient samples studied, the assessment instruments used, and the kind and quality of care (Bellido-Pérez et al. 2017; Ferrand et al. 2012; Oregon Health Authority 2018). In this context, it is important to differentiate between the wish to die and the wish to hasten death either by the discontinuation of life-prolonging treatment, by an explicit request for a deadly medication for self-administration, or by a deadly medical intervention (Ohnsorge, Gudat, and Rehmann-Sutter 2014).

My personal experience of over 25 years in palliative care supports the idea that only a small percentage of patients receiving quality palliative care find their suffering so intolerable that they request either assisted suicide or euthanasia. When these requests are made, they raise the question of an appropriate moral response, which will define the available options for a hastened death.

In 2015, before the German parliament voted for the new regulation, the German Association for Palliative Medicine surveyed its members about their attitudes toward end-of-life practices including PAS. The response rate was 36.9 percent for the 5,152 members invited to participate in the survey: Physicians accounted for nearly 50 percent of the respondents, nurses 17.8 percent, other professionals 14.3 percent, and about 20 percent did not have socio-demographic information. More than 90 percent agreed that "wishes for physician-assisted suicide may be ambivalent" and "are rather a wish to end an unbearable situation." Of the 833 participating physicians, 74.2 percent had been asked to perform PAS, and 3 percent actually performed it. More than 60 percent of all professionals agreed that PAS is not part of palliative care (Jansky, Jaspers, Radbruch, and Nauck 2016). The results of this study essentially confirmed a similar study that was conducted ten years earlier (Müller-Busch et al. 2005).

WHAT TO DO WHEN THE PATIENT ASKS

The encounter with a palliative care patient asking for hastened death is an ethical as well as a medical challenge, which might be seen as provocative but also as a chance to reflect on personal values. In 2017, in order to clarify the complex legal situation, the board of the German Medical Association published a position paper on hastened death that expanded upon its 2011 Principles of Medical Aid in Dying, which had outlined the obligations of physicians caring for severely ill and dying patients. The paper provided information and recommendations for dealing with patients' dying wishes and requests for PAS, including various case scenarios that illustrated the relevant legal and moral obligations. In 2018, recommendations for the assessment, evaluation, and management of wishes for hastened death were formulated in guidelines for palliative care physicians caring for cancer patients. They were published in 2019 (Leitlinienprogramm Onkologie 2019).

These guidelines encourage physicians to acknowledge patients' requests for PAS or euthanasia with respect and in a sensitive manner—the inclusion of somebody else in the planned ending of one's own life is a sign of great trust and confidence. And, because the physician's response to such a request depends on the stage of the patient's illness and prognosis, these issues should be addressed in an empathic way with the patient and the family when indicated.

In most patients with advanced and terminal illnesses, the focus of palliative care physicians is ensuring that optimal medication regimens keep patients as comfortable and unstressed as possible, including palliative or terminal sedation to reduce or temporarily eliminate consciousness for patients with intolerable somatic, psychological, or even existential suffering. While palliative sedation therapy is an acknowledged therapeutic option for patients with intolerable suffering and refractory symptoms, the palliative care physician must carefully review with the patient (and family, if indicated) the medical and ethical aspects of this form of treatment (Müller-Busch, Andres, and Jehser 2003). The reason is that using sedation in end-of-life care as a substitute for euthanasia represents "an unacceptable, and often illegal, deviation from normative ethical clinical practice" according to the EAPC Task Force position paper and other guidelines that can help identify the appropriate place of sedation in end-of-life care and diminish misuse by adequate consideration of moral and ethical concerns (Cherny and Radbruch 2009).

In earlier stages of the patient's illness, the psychosocial and existential catalysts of the patient's wish for assisted suicide or euthanasia should be investigated and addressed sensitively, and other options should be explored. In my experience, the conflicts underlying the patient's request can be identified and sufficiently resolved so that the patient no longer requests a hastened death. It is sometimes helpful to point out that there is no death that burdens survivors with as much dismay, shame, and guilt as a suicide. Also, in palliative and hospice care, no other type of patient death professionally and personally affects clinicians and staff as much as a suicide (Fairman et al. 2008).

Occasionally, despite the best efforts of the palliative care team, patients choose suicide. The ethical challenge of continuing to care, in a palliative setting, for a patient who wants to die by suicide requires a deliberative patient-physician relationship that empowers the patient "not simply to follow unexamined preferences, but to consider, through dialogue, alternative health-related values, their worthiness and their implications for treatment" (Emanuel, E. and Emanuel, L. 1992). Such a relationship cannot be regulated by rules of professional conduct alone—it also depends on the physician's personal values, beliefs, and responsibility.

One of the controversial issues in this context is the management of patients who choose to hasten death by Voluntary Stopping Eating and Drinking, also known as VSED (Jox et al. 2017), a method increasingly sought to end intolerable situations in nursing homes and home care settings. Caring for these patients is a medical and an emotional challenge that requires multidisciplinary palliative care (Radbruch, Münch, and Maier 2019).

Palliative care cannot solve all health problems and conflicts, and it is important to recognize that the prevention of suicide is an important goal in palliative care. In the rehabilitative and the preterminal stages of palliative care, when explicit requests for assisted suicide and euthanasia are most often made, it is important to create a problem-based deliberative patient-physician relationship that respects both the patient's and the physician's ethical viewpoint. In most cases, it is possible to identify the patient's motivations for a suicide plan and discuss the impact of suicide on survivors. While some have argued that palliative care and legalization of euthanasia are nonantagonistic (Bernheim et al. 2008), I view the concept of integrating euthanasia and assisted suicide into palliative care as misleading, not least from an epistemological perspective. The benefit of death as a therapeutic goal cannot be justified on a normative basis or assumed by empirical experience or scientific results. The therapeutic goals in palliative care are always about life, even when death is accepted and respected as an inevitable fact but not as a therapeutic goal (Müller-Busch 2016).

BIBLIOGRAPHY

Bellido-Pérez, Mercedes, Cristina Royo, Joaquin Tomás-Sábado, Josep Porta-Sales, and Albert Balaguer. 2017. "Assessment of the Wish to Hasten Death in Patients with Advanced Disease: A Systematic Review of Measurement Instruments." *Palliative Medicine* 31, no. 66 (June): 510–525.

Bernheim, Jan L., Reginald Deschepper, Wim Distelmans, et al. 2008. "Development of Palliative Care and Legalisation of Euthanasia: Antagonism or Synergy?" *British Medical Journal* 336, no. 7649 (April): 864–867.

Cherny, Nathan I., Lukas Radbruch, and Board of the European Association for Palliative Care. 2009. "European Association for Palliative Care (EAPC) Recommended Framework for the Use of Sedation in Palliative Care." *Palliative Medicine* 23, no. 7 (October): 581–593.

Clark, David. 1998. "Originating a Movement: Cicely Saunders and the Development of St. Christopher's Hospice, 1957–1967." *Mortality* 3, no. 1 (January): 43–63.

Emanuel, Ezekiel J., and Linda L. Emanuel. 1992. "Four Models of the Physician-Patient Relationship. *Journal of the American Medical Association*, 267, no. 16 (April), 2221–2226.

Fahy, Jo. 2018. "A Way Out: Growing Number of People Sign Up for Assisted Suicide." Swiss News/Swissinfo.ch (website), February 14, 2018. https://www .swissinfo.ch/eng/a-way-out_growing-number-of-people-sign-up-for-assisted-sui cide/43899702.

Fairman, Nathan, Lori P. Montross Thomas, Stephanie Whitmore, Emily Meier, and Scott A. Irwin. 2014. "What Did I Miss? A Qualitative Assessment of the Impact of Patient Suicide on Hospice Clinical Staff." *Journal of Palliative Medicine* 17, no. 7 (July): 832–836.

Federal Administrative Court [Bundesverwaltungsgericht]. 2017. "Urteil vom 02.03.2017-BVerwG 3 C 19.15." Accessed November 25, 2019. https://www .bverwg.de/020317U3C19.15.0.

Ferrand, Edouard, Jean-Francois Dreyfus, Mélanie Chastrusse, et al. 2012. "Évolution des demandes de mort anticipées exprimées auprès des équipes de soins palliatifs en France. L'enquête multicentrique Demande." *Médecine Palliative: Soins de Support-Accompagnement-Éthique* 11, no. 33 (June): 121–132.

German Medical Association. 2011. "Principles of Medical Aid in Dying." [Bundesärztekammer *Grundsätze der Bundesärztekammer zur ärztlichen Sterbebegleitung*]. Deutsches Ärzteblatt 108, no. 7: A346–A348.

German Medical Association. 2017. "Principles of Medical Aid in Dying." Bundesärztekammer Bekanntmachungen. *Deutsches Ärzteblatt* 114, no. 7: A334-A336. Accessed November 26, 2019. https://www.aerzteblatt.de/archiv/186360/Verbot-der-geschaeftsmaessigen-Foerderung-der-Selbsttoetung-(-217-StGB)-Hinweise-und-Erlaeuterungen-fuer-die-aerztliche-Praxis.

Griffiths, John, Heleen Weyers, and Maurice Adams. 2008. *Euthanasia and Law in Europe*. Portland, OR: Hart Publishing.

Hauptmeier, Carsten. 2019. "Germany Reopens Painful Debate on Assisted Suicide." *Mail & Guardian*, April 16, 2019. https://mg.co.za/article/2019-04-16-germany-reopens-painful-debate-on-assisted-suicide.

Hendry, Maggie, Diana Pasterfield, Ruth Lewis, et al. 2013. "Why Do We Want the Right to Die? A Systematic Review of the International Literature on the Views of Patients, Carers and the Public on Assisted Dying." *Palliative Medicine* 27, no. 1 (November): 13–26.

Hurst, Samia A., and Alex Mauron. 2003. "Assisted Suicide and Euthanasia in Switzerland: Allowing a Role for Non-Physicians." *British Medical Journal* 326, no. 7383 (February): 271–273. doi:10.1136/bmj.326.7383.271.

Jansky, Maximiliane, Birgit Jaspers, Luke Radbruch, and Friedemann Nauck. 2016. "Einstellungen zu und Erfahrungen mit ärztlich assistiertem Suizid." *Bundesgesundheitsblatt-Gesundheitsforschung-Gesundheitsschutz* 60, no. 1 (November): 89–98.

Jox, Ralf J., Isra Black, Gian Domenico Borasio, and Johanna Anneser. 2017. "Voluntary Stopping of Eating and Drinking: Is Medical Support Ethically Justified?" *BMC Medicine* 15, no. 186 (October). https://doi.org/10.1186/s12916-017-0950-1.

Kutner, Luis. 1969. "Due Process of Euthanasia: The Living Will, A Proposal." *Indiana Law Journal* 44, no. 4 (Summer): 539–554.

Leitlinienprogramm Onkologie. 2019. *Erweiterte S3-Leitlinie Palliativmedizin für Patienten mit einer nicht-heilbaren Krebserkrankung*. Langversion 2.0–August 2019 AWMF-Registernummer: 128/001-OL. Accessed November 26, 2019. https://www.leitlinienprogramm-onkologie.de/fileadmin/user_upload/Downloads/Leitlinien/Palliativmedizin/Version_2/LL_Palliativmedizin_2.0_Langversion.pdf.

Materstvedt, Lars Johan, David Clark, John Ellershaw, et al. 2003. "Euthanasia and Physician-Assisted Suicide: A View from an EAPC Ethics Task Force." *Palliative Medicine* 17, no. 2 (March): 97–101; discussion 102–179.

Melching, Heiner. 2017. "Neue gesetzliche Regelungen für die Palliativversorgung und ihre Implikationen für Politik und Praxis." *Bundesgesundheitsblatt-Gesundheitsforschung-Gesundheitsschutz* 60, no. 1: 4–10.

Müller-Busch, H. Christof. 2016. "Entscheidungen am Lebensende und Respekt vor Autonomie–Möglichkeiten und Grenzen der Palliativmedizin." In *Entscheidungen am Lebensende*, edited by Johann Pltzer and Franziska Brosschåadl,17–30. Baden Baden, Germany: Nomos.

Müller-Busch, H. Christof, Inge Andres, and Thomas Jehser. 2003. "Sedation in Palliative Care—A Critical Analysis of 7 Years Experience." *BMC Palliative Care* 2, no. 2 (May): 2.

Müller-Busch, H. Christof, Fuat Oduncu, S. Woskanjan, and E. Klaschik. 2005. "Attitudes on Euthanasia, Physician-Assisted Suicide and Terminal Sedation—A Survey of the Members of the German Association for Palliative Medicine." *Medicine, Health Care and Philosophy* 7, no. 3 (January): 333–339.

Ohnsorge, Kathrin, Heike Gudat, and Christoph Rehmann-Sutter. 2014. "Intentions in Wishes to Die: Analysis and a Typology–A Report of 30 Qualitative Case Studies of Terminally Ill Cancer Patients in Palliative Care." *Psycho-Oncology* 23, no. 9 (September): 1021–1026.

Oregon Health Authority: Public Health Division. 2018. *The Oregon Death with Dignity Act Annual Reports*, September 2, 2018. https://www.oregon.gov/oha/PH/PROVIDERPARTNERRESOURCES/EVALUATIONRESEARCH/DEATHWITHDIGNITYACT/Documents/year20.pdf.

Palliative Care McGill. n.d. "History." Accessed November 25, 2019. https://www.mcgill.ca/palliativecare/about-us/history.

Radbruch, Lukas, Urs Münch, and Bernd-Oliver Maier. 2019. "Palliativmedizin: Umgang mit Sterbewünschen." *Deutsches Arzteblatt* 116, no. 41: A-1828 / B-1508 / C-1481.

Regional Euthanasia Review Committees. 2019. "Annual Report 2018." Accessed November 25, 2019. https://english.euthanasiecommissie.nl/the-committees/documents/publications/annual-reports/2002/annual-reports/annual-reports.

Richards, Naomi, and Marian Krawczyk. 2019. "What Is the Cultural Value of Dying in an Era of Assisted Dying?" *Medical Humanities* (July 26): medhum-2018-011621. doi: 10.1136/medhum-2018-011621.

Rietjens, Judith A. C., Paul van der Maas, Bregje Onwuteaka-Philipsen, Johannes van Delden, and Agnes van der Heide. 2009. "Two Decades of Research on Euthanasia from the Netherlands. What Have We Learnt and What Questions Remain?" *Journal of Bioethical Inquiry* 6, no. 3 (September): 271–283.

Roesinger, Mathias, Laura Prudlik, Sara Pauli. et al. 2018. "Factors which influence the position toward euthanasia. Results of a representative survey among older people in Germany." *Zeitschrift für Gerontologie und Geriatrie* 51, no. 2 (February): 222–230.

Roy, David J., Charles-Henri Rapin, and the EAPC Board of Directors. 1994. "Regarding Euthanasia." *European Journal of Palliative Care* 1, no.1 (Spring): 57–59.

Sheldon, Tony. 2007 "Andries Postma." *British Medical Journal* 334, no. 7588 (February): 320. doi: 10.1136/bmj.39111.520486.FA.

Sitte, Thomas, Benjamin Gronwald, and Sven Gottschling. 2016. "Palliative Versorgung statt Beihilfe zum Suizid und Tötung auf Verlangen?" *Schmerzmedizin* 32, no. 3 (August): 25–33.

Smith, Richard. 2000. "A Good Death." *British Medical Journal* 320: 129–130.

Spitshuis, G. A. H. 2018. "'Euthanasie'noch immer ein Tabu? Einfluss der Erinnerungskultur auf die Einstellungen bezüglich der aktiven Sterbehilfe in Deutschland im Vergleich zu den Niederlanden." Bachelor's thesis, Radboud Universiteit, June 14, 2018.

Statista. (2017). "Umfrage zur aktiven Sterbehilfe." https://de.statista.com/statistik/daten/studie/318894/umfrage/aktive-sterbehilfe-meinungen-nach-soziodemografischen-merkmalen/.

Swiss Federal Statistical Office. 2018. "Statistique des causes e décès 2016: Le nombre de décès par démence a reculé pour la première fois en 2016." Press release, December 17, 2018. https://www.bfs.admin.ch/bfs/en/home/news/whats-new.assetdetail.6728285.html.

Part II

PHYSICIAN-ASSISTED SUICIDE AND EUTHANASIA AFTER THE HOLOCAUST

Chapter Eight

Helping the Few

Historical Perspectives on Aid in Dying

Barron H. Lerner

Physician aid in dying (PAD) has become a very important topic in American medicine. As of now, PAD is legal in nine states and the District of Columbia, and other state legislatures are considering bills to permit the practice. PAD is the latest chapter of a much longer standing debate as to whether physicians should ever expedite the deaths of their patients.

Not surprisingly, a very substantial literature exists by writers, including Resier (1992), Emanuel (1994), Snyder and Sulmasy (2001), and Gorsuch (2006), that explores the philosophical arguments both for and against speeding death—as well as historical explorations of past efforts to do so.

I am choosing a different way to explore this history. First, I will create a hypothesis: *Physician aid in dying is a useful and appropriate intervention for a very small percentage of the population but raises substantial moral and logistical issues that make it highly problematic.* Next, I will look at a series of other past medical interventions in which a similar calculus existed. In each instance, I will explore what we can learn from these earlier efforts to help a small percentage of patients with a morally problematic intervention. Although none of the other examples is a perfect fit, they do raise similar historical concerns to those raised by PAD: healing, harming, suffering, morality, and patient autonomy.

HISTORY OF EUTHANASIA

Among the earliest mentions of the topic of euthanasia is in the Hippocratic Oath, which dates from Greece in 300–400 BCE. Physicians who adhered to the Oath vowed never to "administer a poison to anyone," that is, to not participate in euthanasia. Most Western physicians have generally honored this admonition.

The next major chapter in the history of euthanasia took place in Nazi Germany from 1939 to 1941. As part of a global movement to promote eugenics, the theory that societies should promote the propagation of "good" genes and discourage the propagation of "bad" genes, the Nazis initiated the notorious *Aktion* T4 program, discussed throughout this book. In this program, Nazi physicians euthanized "unfit" Germans with mental illnesses and intellectual deficiencies.

Not surprisingly, perhaps, enthusiasm for having doctors speed death waned after the revelations about Nazi Germany. But two concurrent movements emerged beginning in the 1980s. First, Holland, in a series of court cases, articulated circumstances in which euthanasia would not be prosecuted (de Haan 2002). In subsequent decades, several other European countries passed laws that either legalized or tolerated actual euthanasia. And recently, in some of these countries, growing numbers of individuals with mental illnesses or who are "tired of life" are finding physicians who will end their lives (Lane 2018).

Second, in the United States, activists began pushing for laws that would legalize some type of PAD. Two cases eventually made it to the U.S. Supreme Court, which, in 1997, ruled that there was no constitutional right to PAD (Vacco v. Quill, 521 U.S. 793, 1997; Washington v. Glucksberg, 521 U.S. 702, 1996). But the court allowed individual states to enact their own laws legalizing the process. Also in 1997, the nation's first such law, Oregon's Death with Dignity Act, went into effect. In this program, physicians merely supply the medications that patients may or may not eventually use (Oregon Health Authority 2019). PAD is now legal in the District of Columbia as well as Washington, Vermont, Montana, California, Hawaii, Colorado, New Jersey, and Maine.

PREMISE

Those debating a controversial practice such as PAD generally argue that it is either right or wrong. But what if it was sometimes right, and usually wrong? This chapter takes this notion as its premise. Specifically, what if a very small percentage of dying individuals will not be adequately served by palliative care, hospice, or other interventions designed to limit pain and suffering? To benefit them, are we willing to countenance, legalize, and/or operationalize a procedure—PAD—that goes against thousands of years of admonitions that doctors should not speed death? Moreover, are we willing to approve a procedure closely related to one that was thoroughly abused by supposedly "ethical" physicians in Nazi Germany and is perhaps being misused by modern-day clinicians in Europe?

To explore this premise further, it is useful to revisit the case of Brittany Maynard (Span 2014). In January 2014, at age 29, she was diagnosed with glioblastoma, a terminal brain cancer. She underwent standard treatment but eventually was told by her physicians that there were no additional beneficial therapies. By this point, Maynard had moved from California to Oregon, where she could take advantage of the Death with Dignity Law.

Maynard became a vocal spokesperson for PAD, appearing on multiple media outlets. Specifically, she argued that the short time she had remaining would be full of symptoms that would cause suffering: nausea, vomiting, seizures, blindness, paralysis, and drug-resistant pain. Why, she asked, if she was going to die anyway, did she have to suffer through such discomfort beforehand?

Maynard was a perfect ambassador for PAD. Young, attractive, educated—and with a fully supportive husband—she made a compelling case. Maynard eventually took the pills and died in November 2014.

In the wake of Maynard's death, enthusiasm for PAD continues, as demonstrated by several new state laws. Polls regularly indicate public support of roughly 70 percent (Dugan 2015). And although one study from Switzerland found post-traumatic stress disorder among family and friends who witnessed assisted suicide (Wagner, Muller, and Maercker 2012), others have not. For example, research by Oregon physicians showed that over 90 percent of surviving family members were "at peace" with their relative's choice (Ganzini et al. 2009).

There are valid criticisms of Maynard's and similar cases, as discussed elsewhere in this book. But for argument's sake, what if Maynard indeed took charge of her medical care in a terrible situation, used the system properly, did not violate the safeguards put in place, and, in so doing, spared herself suffering and died on her own terms? If so, is this the sort of opportunity that everyone in Maynard's situation should have access to?

It turns out that PAD is only one of many medical procedures that have raised a similar calculus. In related ways, abortion, lobotomy, sterilization, organ transplantation, and experimental therapies have also had the potential to benefit small numbers of people while raising moral questions as to whether such procedures should be performed at all.

ABORTION

Abortion may be the most logical procedure to compare to PAD. It is inherently controversial, involving, according to some, the "taking of a life." In this manner, it resembles PAD, only at the opposite end of existence. Notably, it was also forbidden in the Hippocratic Oath. As with PAD, Hippocratic and religious admonitions against abortion generally made it both illegal and largely secret for centuries.

But in the 1970s, the histories of abortion and PAD dramatically diverged. In 1973, the U.S. Supreme Court, in *Roe v. Wade*, ruled that pregnant women had the right to an abortion during the first trimester of pregnancy. Justice Harry Blackmun, writing for the 7–2 majority, argued that a woman's right to privacy, based on the due process clause of the Fourteenth Amendment, should entitle her to a legal abortion (Roe v. Wade 410 U.S. 113, 1973).

But the court's ruling was far from an obvious conclusion. In writing his decision, Blackmun downplayed standard legal precedents and instead emphasized historical examples of legal abortion. "It perhaps is not generally appreciated," he wrote, "that the restrictive criminal abortion laws in effect in a majority of States today are of relatively recent vintage."

Some scholars have argued that Blackmun's opinion was highly irregular, having less to do with the law than the social climate in which the case was argued and decided. Nineteen seventy-three was the height of second-wave feminism, which claimed that women had been long treated as second class citizens, deprived of equal rights. The *Roe* decision, therefore, was a mechanism for the Supreme Court to rectify this—judicial activism, according to critics.

Twenty years later, when the Court leaned further to the right, abortion survived a major challenge in the case of *Planned Parenthood v. Casey* (505 U.S. 833, 1992). Writing for a 5–4 majority, Justice Anthony Kennedy rejected a Pennsylvania law seeking to restrict abortion by once again focusing on women's rights. In a famous passage from the decision, he wrote that "At the heart of liberty is the right to define one's own concept of existence, of meaning, of the universe, and of the mystery of human life."

This language created an opportunity for a new legal approach to the right to die. And indeed, in the 1990s, both the second and ninth judicial circuits ruled that state laws attempting to criminalize PAD were unconstitutional (Gorsuch 2006, 8–13). In contrast to *Roe* and *Casey*, however, the U.S. Supreme Court disagreed, ruling in *Vacco v. Quill* and *Washington v. Glucksberg* that state laws prohibiting PAD were not illegal—in other words, Americans did not have the right to have physicians speed their deaths (Vacco v. Quill, 521 U.S. 793, 1997; Washington v. Glucksberg, 521 U.S. 702, 1996). Although physicians could allow patients to die of their disease, the justices argued, PAD represented intent to kill, something the Court had no intention of protecting.

The parallel stories of abortion and PAD remind us of the historical contingency of interventions that fit the premise advanced in this chapter—potentially valuable for a small population but morally problematic. It was not that the issue of abortion was satisfactorily resolved in one direction and PAD in the other direction. Rather, the longstanding debate over abortion came to a head at a historical moment that promoted its legalization. Yet when PAD advocates later made similar arguments about rights and liberty, the Supreme Count soundly rejected them. At the end of the day, physicians, philosophers, and bioethicists may argue about what is right and wrong, but society decides what is or is not legally permitted.

LOBOTOMY

In the early to mid-twentieth century, mental hospitals teemed with chronic psychiatric patients too sick to be discharged. Many had schizophrenia, which caused delusions, confusion, and violence. Doctors tried many aggressive treatments but had little success. In 1935, Portuguese neurologist Enad Moniz proposed a radical therapy: lobotomy, in which a physician deliberately damaged brain tissue to relieve a patient's symptoms. The theory was that mental illness resulted from faulty neurological connections that gradually became fixed within the brain. Disrupting the neuronal circuits could potentially help—or even cure—patients. Between the 1940s and 1960s, roughly 40,000 lobotomies were performed. In 1949, Moniz received the Nobel Prize (Pressman 1998, 147).

Despite the popularity of lobotomy, there were many contemporaneous critics who decried the operation. It was hard to deny that it usually caused dramatic personality changes, rendering patients docile, apathetic, and dependent. Some critics went further, terming it barbaric or monstrous. For decades, this assessment persisted, both in the historical literature and in cultural renderings, such as the novel and film *One Flew Over the Cuckoo's Nest*.

But in 1998, this history was revised. In his book *Last Resort*, historian Jack Pressman convincingly argued that lobotomy had represented the "best science" of the day and was a reasonable last resort for miserable patients with no prospect of improvement or of ever being discharged (Pressman 1998). Docility and loss of personality, while objectionable and perhaps outrageous to the outside observer, might be reasonable for a small percentage of suffering patients. In this sense, lobotomy is another example of something that was highly problematic but seems to have been "indicated" in extreme circumstances.

So what light does this history throw on the issue of PAD? To answer this, it is instructive to look at the work of another historian, Joel Braslow. In his 1997 book *Mental Ills and Bodily Cures*, Braslow showed that lobotomy, while supposedly a last-ditch treatment for incurable psychiatric illness, often represented something quite different: a strategy for maintaining order in chaotic, overcrowded, underfunded institutions.

In this sense, the history of lobotomy provides a cautionary tale for morally problematic interventions that promise hope to a small number of individuals. Such people, and, by association, society more broadly, are entitled to an especially accurate account of why such procedures are justifiable and what they are supposed to achieve. This conclusion could not be more relevant for PAD. As more data about its use accumulate, it is clear that most people requesting it are not having unrelenting pain or suffering—the common assumption created by cases like that of Brittany Maynard—but rather fear future dependence and loss of control (Hedberg and New 2017). To the degree that lobotomy or PAD are being performed for what we might term "unadvertised" reasons, the argument for permitting such procedures becomes less compelling.

SEXUAL STERILIZATION

Few medical interventions in American history have a more negative legacy than sexual sterilization. Between the two world wars, building on a surge of interest in eugenics, doctors performed roughly 60,000 sterilizations—mostly of women. Proponents believed that so-called unfit individuals, such as those with mental illness and low intelligence, would transmit these conditions to their offspring. This would not only cause more disease in future generations, but also more economic dependence on the state. Sterilizations predominated among the poor and minorities—groups less able to object (Hansen and King 2013).

Sadly and ironically, American eugenics laws served as the basis for a similar program of sterilization in Nazi Germany. During the 1930s, German doctors sterilized approximately 400,000 people with many of the same characteristics as the American patients. In Germany, of course, the sterilization program progressed to euthanasia and, eventually, the extermination of unfit and "non-human" populations (Proctor 1988). In the United States, there was no such slippery slope, and Nazi atrocities led to a backlash against sterilization after World War II.

But the procedure did not disappear. In Puerto Rico and other locations during the 1960s and 1970s, government officials promulgated programs that mandated the sterilization of poor Latina women—at times as a *quid pro quo* for obtaining Medicaid (Krase 2014). Once again, there was a fierce backlash and mandatory sterilization declined.

Just because sterilization was being misused, however, did not mean it was never indicated. What if there were women with mental limitations who were at risk of being impregnated without their consent? Couldn't a case be made that these relatively small number of women were reasonable candidates for a procedure otherwise deemed morally reprehensible?

In the 1990s, I encountered just such a case in my primary care clinic. I was caring for a mother and daughter, in their late forties and early twenties, respectively. The daughter had undergone formal neuropsychiatric testing and had a very low IQ. Her mother, arguing that her daughter could neither understand the concept of raising a child nor likely resist men who wanted to have sex with her, asked me if it was possible that she be sterilized.

As a historian of medicine and a bioethicist, I found the question to be jarring. I immediately thought back to the noxious history of sterilization and could not see myself participating. But, I realized, New York in the 1990s was neither North Carolina in the 1930s nor Puerto Rico in the 1970s. So a colleague and I did some research.

We discovered that it was extremely difficult anywhere in the United States to sterilize either minors or those deemed mentally incompetent—a direct legacy of the past abuses. In New York, where I worked, a city administrative code strictly forbade this. Court decisions similarly discouraged sterilization, instructing physicians to use less restrictive measures such as long-acting hormonal agents to prevent pregnancy (Pham and Lerner 2001).

So I told the mother that the answer was "no," sterilization was not legally possible. I also discussed this issue with the daughter, who did not want to be sterilized but agreed to take hormones.

Fast forward ten years. The daughter eventually got pregnant twice, most likely due to nonadherence with the medication. She was unable to participate meaningfully in the rearing of either child, which is just what her mother had predicted when originally proposing the sterilization. The children were raised by the mother and the daughter's boyfriend's parents (they never married).

Without assessing whether the ultimate outcome was the "right" one, it is possible to conclude that what the mother proposed was a reasonable option—an intervention that would usually be reflexively rejected but might make sense in a small number of instances. But in this case, history "won." The past uses of sterilization were simply too objectionable to allow for it to return in a different historical era.

SOLID ORGAN TRANSPLANTATION

As of the early 1960s, surgeons were aggressively studying transplantation of livers and hearts. Replacing an organ with one obtained from a corpse was a disturbing concept at this time and the media avidly covered both the medical and ethical aspects of the procedure (Rothman 1991, 152–156). Barriers to transplantation generally fell into two categories. First, some critics believed that putting another person's organ into someone's body was simply wrong, bespeaking a hubris on the part of the medical profession reminiscent of Victor Frankenstein.

A second objection was more logistical. In which cases was it appropriate to try a transplant? How did one obtain proper informed consent for such a procedure? Were there adequate medications available to prevent rejection of the transplanted organ? These questions were all part of the larger one explored in this chapter: even if transplantation was a reasonable option for a small number of persons, was it appropriate to forge ahead with such controversial and complicated operations?

The answer, initially, was yes. Starting with a three-year-old boy dying of biliary atresia, doctors in 1963 performed nearly a dozen liver transplants. In all these cases, the patients survived only briefly. This glaring lack of success led the surgeons to declare an informal moratorium on liver transplants until more could be learned (Starzl 1992, 96–105).

Five years later in 1968, in the wake of Christiaan Barnard's historic first heart transplantation, surgeons performed nearly 100 cardiac transplants. As of August 1969, only nine of these patients were alive. This similar disturbing mortality rate led the heart surgeons, too, to temporarily stop doing transplants (Rothman 1991, 165–166).

But, as we know, transplantation of livers and hearts has become wildly successful. This triumph can be attributed in part to the development of better antirejection medicines. But the story of transplantation is also historically contingent. Transplantation was part of a larger post–World War II period in which aggressive surgical procedures using new technologies were celebrated. Researchers pushing the boundaries in trying to save lives, had the "courage to fail" (Fox and Swazey 1974). Which is what they did, of course, until they succeeded.

The transplant surgeons also benefitted from lax research guidelines. Despite the Nuremberg Code and other attempts to ensure informed consent, investigators at this time did pretty much what they wanted. In this setting, the acceptability of using dangerous and objectionable procedures to potentially save lives increased.

So, in the 1960s, substantial concerns were raised about the mortality and efficacy of organ transplants, but surgeons just went ahead anyway. They believed that the ultimate benefits would justify early mishaps, and this strategy ultimately won the day. Interestingly, PAD advocates might argue that a similar consequentialist mindset has also proven successful in the case of Oregon's Death with Dignity law. That is, moral objections to PAD were initially considered but ultimately rejected. And, despite early fears, there has been no slippery slope in which the law is being abused; nor has Oregon become a destination for people looking for assisted death.

RISE OF PATIENT AUTONOMY

By the 1980s and 1990s, another factor was at play when evaluating aggressive procedures that might potentially be helpful: patient autonomy. Prior to 1970, paternalism—the notion that "Doctor knows best"—dominated the doctor-patient relationship.

Historians have convincingly situated the rise of patients' rights within larger changes in American society, including the civil rights movement, opposition to the Vietnam War, and most importantly, second-wave feminism. These movements, all of which promoted rights among the previously disempowered, took hold in medicine as patients began questioning their physicians. Autonomy was also propelled by examples of unethical behavior by certain physician-researchers who had victimized disadvantaged populations. The historical literature contains dozens of examples of patients rejecting paternalism and effecting positive change within medicine (Lerner 2001).

More recently, the ethics of patient autonomy have arisen over what is called "expanded access" or "compassionate use." These are programs that potentially permit the use of an unapproved drug by people with life-threatening conditions who do not meet the enrollment criteria for clinical trials. But critics argue that such "n of 1" treatments—a clinical trial in which a single patient is the entire trial—prevent gathering of meaningful data, are highly unlikely to have a positive impact on the disease in question and may cause substantial harm (Bateman-House et al. 2015). Moreover, they reflect what Edmund Pellegrino termed the "absolutization of autonomy" (Pellegrino 1994): the false sense that people who advocate for themselves are necessarily making the best choices.

So what does the history of patient autonomy teach us about PAD? Patients who push for experimental or nonstandard treatments are by no means always "right." But they have been sometimes. From this perspective, genuine consideration of these requests—if reasonable—seems appropriate. It's hard to argue that motivated people don't deserve a chance. The same argument might be made by advocates of PAD. Yes, there are risks and serious moral concerns. But shouldn't we consider opportunities that might truly benefit needy patients—even if only a very small number of them?

CONCLUSION

This chapter has presented several instances in which controversial interventions designed for a small percentage of patients have been pursued—with variable results. It might be argued, however, that such experimentation is not mandatory. That is, there are ethically dubious medical acts that should never be performed regardless of the availability and demand. In the United States, with the exception of Jack Kevorkian's "death machine" in the 1990s (Nicol and Wylie 2006), such a moratorium has been in place for euthanasia. It is reasonable to argue that such prohibitions are appropriate for euthanasia, other morally problematic acts such as human germ line editing, and, some would say, for PAD.

But for the most part, in a country that prizes both technology and patient autonomy, such interventions eventually occur. This chapter has asked how the history of earlier efforts can inform the growing use of PAD.

As with all the other historical examples in this chapter, PAD is historically contingent. At first blush, speeding death by physicians may seem to be a timeless issue. For centuries, philosophers and, more recently, bioethicists, have argued as to whether it is right or wrong, and sought to influence clinical and policy decisions. But ultimate choices are most often determined by society—based on cultural, political, and economic factors at play in different historical eras.

We should also take patients' stories seriously. Those who request a procedure like PAD in a state where it is illegal, as with my patient in New York who wondered about sterilization of her daughter, should not simply be told that this is simply something that doctors should never do. Documents like the Hippocratic Oath, while foundational, are not necessarily binding. We should be comfortable with the idea that certain of the oath's admonitions have evolved over time, while others have not.

But having said this, when autonomous requests appear suspect or misguided, physicians should not merely accede to them. Lobotomy had a narrow indication for otherwise incurable psychiatric patients, but to the degree it was being done for custodial purposes, its rationale became dubious. So, too, we need to reexamine PAD in light of the fact that patients' reasons for requesting it have little to do with *actual* pain and suffering but more to do with *fears* that such conditions may emerge and lead to loss of control for patients. Slippery slopes can be real.

Finally, perhaps it might be helpful for clinicians involved in end-of-life care to discuss the premise of this chapter with their patients. Such a talk would indicate that PAD may be a reasonable option for a limited group of individuals but not necessarily something that they would recommend. And for those who are considering PAD, physicians might mention other past procedures that seemed to offer patients a "solution" to a vexing challenge but proved misguided and at times harmful. Such a discussion should be accompanied by a thorough delineation of what palliative care can do to ease dying, despite the recent legislative push for PAD. There will always be limits to what clinicians can promise their patients.

BIBLIOGRAPHY

Bateman-House, Alison, Laura Kimberly, Barbara Redman, Nancy Dubler, and Arthur Caplan. 2015. "Right-to-Try Laws: Hope, Hype and Unintended Consequences." *Annals of Internal Medicine* 163, no. 10 (November): 796–97.

Braslow, Joel D. 1997. *Mental Ills and Bodily Cures: Psychiatric Treatment in the First Half of the Twentieth Century.* Berkeley: University of California Press.

De Haan, Jurriaan. 2002. "The New Dutch Law on Euthanasia." *Medical Law Review* 10, no. 1 (January): 57–75.

Dugan, Andrew. 2015. "In U.S., Support Up for Doctor-Assisted Suicide." Gallup, May 27, 2015. http://www.gallup.com/poll/183425/support-doctor-assisted-suicide.aspx.

Emanuel, Ezekiel J. 1994. "Euthanasia: Historical, Ethical and Empiric Perspectives." *Archives of Internal Medicine* 154, no. 17 (September): 1890–1901.

Fox, Renee, and Judith P. Swazey. 1974. *The Courage to Fail: A Social View of Organ Transplants and Dialysis.* Chicago: University of Chicago Press.

Ganzini, Linda, Elizabeth R. Goy, Steven K. Dobscha, and Holly Prigerson. 2009. "Mental Health Outcomes of Family Members of Oregonians Who Request Physician Aid in Dying." *Journal of Pain and Symptom Management* 38 (December): 807–15.

Gorsuch, Neil M. 2006. *The Future of Assisted Suicide and Euthanasia.* Princeton: Princeton University Press.

Hansen, Randall, and Desmond King. 2013. *Sterilized by the State: Eugenics, Race, and the Population Scare in Twentieth-Century North America.* New York: Cambridge University Press.

Hedberg, Katrina, and Craig New. 2017. "Oregon's Death with Dignity Act: 20 Years of Experience to Inform the Debate." *Annals of Internal Medicine* 167, no. 8 (October): 579–83.

Krase, Kathryn. 2014. "History of Forced Sterilization and Current U.S. Abuses." Our Bodies Ourselves website, October 1, 2014. https://www.ourbodiesourselves.org/book-excerpts/health-article/forced-sterilization.

Lane, Charles. 2018. "How Many Botched Cases Would It Take to End Euthanasia of the Vulnerable?" *Washington Post*, January 24, 2018.

Lerner, Barron H. 2001. *The Breast Cancer Wars.* New York: Oxford University Press.

Nicol, Neal, and Harry Wylie. 2006. *Between the Dying and the Dead: Dr. Jack Kevorkian's Life and the Battle to Legalize Euthanasia.* Madison: University of Wisconsin Press.

Oregon Health Authority. 2019. *Oregon Death with Dignity Act: Annual Report 2018.* February 25, 2019. https://www.deathwithdignity.org/oregon-death-with-dignity-act-annual-reports.

Pellegrino, Edmund D. 1994. "Patient Autonomy and the Physician's Ethics." *Annals of the Royal College of Physicians and Surgeons of Canada* 27, no. 3 (April): 171–73.

Pham, Hoangmai, and Barron H. Lerner. 2001. "In the Patient's Best Interest? Revisiting Sexual Autonomy and Sterilization of the Developmentally Disabled." *Western Journal of Medicine* 175, no. 4 (October): 280–83.

Pressman, Jack D. 1998. *Last Resort: Psychosurgery and the Limits of Medicine.* Cambridge: Cambridge University Press.

Proctor, Robert N. (1988). *Racial Hygiene: Medicine under the Nazis.* Cambridge, MA: Harvard University Press.

Reiser, Stanley J. 1992. "Physician-Assisted Dying: Historical Perspective." *Trends in Health Care, Law & Ethics* 7, no. 2 (Winter): 11–14.

Rothman, David J. 1991. *Strangers at the Bedside: A History of How Law and Bioethics Transformed Medical Decision Making.* New York: Basic Books.

Snyder, Lois, and Daniel J. Sulmasy. 2001. "Physician-Assisted Suicide." *Annals of Internal Medicine* 135, no. 3 (August): 209–16.

Span, Paula. 2014. "A New Face on the End-of-Life Debate." *New York Times,* November 5, 2014. https://newoldage.blogs.nytimes.com/2014/11/05/a-new-face-on-the-end-of-life-debate.

Starzl, Thomas. 1992. *The Puzzle People: Memoirs of a Transplant Surgeon.* Pittsburgh: University of Pittsburgh Press.

Wagner, Brigit, J. Muller, and Andreas Maercker. 2011. "Death by Request in Switzerland: Posttraumatic Stress Disorder and Complicated Grief after Witnessing Assisted Suicide." *European Psychiatry* 27, no. 1 (October): 542–46.

Chapter Nine

Palliative Care, Hospice, and Last-Resort Options

Timothy E. Quill

PREFACE

Because I know much more about palliative care and hospice in the context of the potential and limits of modern medicine than I do about the Holocaust, I got a very sobering education in the Berlin and Houston conferences. Simply put, the Nazi adult "euthanasia" program, or *Aktion* T4, was neither euthanasia nor voluntary—it was murder and execution, initially of disabled persons and then of "undesirable" persons for the perceived good of society. There was no compassion for the targets of this program, nor was there any blurring with acceptable boundaries of medical practice. Once these first steps were taken, it became easier to understand how medical experimentation would also lose its moral grounding, with high-risk, often cruel experiments on non-consenting patients to answer research questions posed by Nazi physicians and scientists.

How did medicine become so profoundly perverted? Putting the perceived needs of society above the individual seems to have been a pivotal first step toward subsequent compromises, which then seemed to "make sense." The level to which medicine in Germany went off the rails is a reality that must be explicitly addressed lest we run the risk of not learning from and, thereby, not honoring and possibly repeating this history.

The distortion of the ethical values guiding medical experimentation was not limited to Germany—the researchers conducting the Tuskegee syphilis experiments in the United States used a similar logic (Jones 1981). The greater good of a segment of society was presumed to outweigh the good of the individual, especially a devalued individual. Does this mean that all medical experimentation cannot be trusted under any circumstances, or can trust be assured by critical safeguards, fully informed consent, and open practices? The field of medical ethics emerged in part from these experiments, and there are now widely agreed upon guidelines for consent to medical experimentation that include institutional review boards and oversight committees. Whether such protections are sufficient remains uncertain, but they are genuine attempts to protect vulnerable patients in response to this history.

Because weak and vulnerable patients were killed without consent for the perceived greater good of German society, does that mean that contemporary medicine should limit its death-hastening options for patients with severe suffering who are pleading for assistance at the end of life? If possible and if the patient agrees, the initial response to unacceptable suffering must always be to redouble our efforts to treat the underlying disease while simultaneously trying to relieve the suffering. But how should clinicians respond if unacceptable suffering persists despite our unrestrained efforts to palliate, especially when the patient expresses a clear desire for assistance in finding an escape through death *right now*?

In this chapter, I will offer guidance for how to conduct a program of care at the end of life that always begins with excellent palliative care but also includes "assisted suicide" if and when unacceptable suffering persists and if the patient is requesting it. Just as ethical guidelines potentially offer a path for socially acceptable medical research, so too might guidelines and safeguards potentially offer a path for acceptable physician-assisted suicide (PAS) or voluntary active euthanasia as a last resort. The chapter will be divided into four sections: (1) hospice and palliative care as the standards of care for seriously ill patients; (2) evaluating requests for assisted death; (3) exploring all options including last resorts for responding to unacceptable suffering; and (4) comparing an aboveboard practice of last-resort options that include safeguards with absolute prohibition. Each section will end with some reflection on how my thinking changed after these two conferences.

HOSPICE AND PALLIATIVE CARE

How should a *healer* approach a patient with a serious, potentially terminal illness? If we conceptualize healing exclusively in terms of curing or restoring health, then death might be viewed as a medical failure to be fought off by all means possible. This view may lead to invasive, end-of-life treatments with poor odds of success and additional patient suffering.

Clearly, a broader model of healing is needed as patients become sicker and approach the end of their lives, a model that does not preclude a vigorous fight against disease but is informed by realistic discussion of options and odds. It should always address the associated suffering, including attention to the physical, psychosocial, and spiritual dimensions. Every effort should be made to maintain the integrity of the patient as a person, including confirmation of his or her understanding of, and agreement with, the proposed treatment. In addition, patients should be encouraged to discuss the meaning and significance of their treatment, one of their last and most important choices, in the context of their entire life.

Hospice care has taught me that vital opportunities for personal growth and interpersonal closure persist even when the underlying disease is no longer responsive to treatment. Medical providers should not only explore all reasonable options for disease-directed therapy, but also manage symptoms and open the door to a more expansive inquiry. The commitment to face this final unknown with patients and to not abandon them, no matter how dire the medical situation, is among the most vital roles of health care providers (Quill and Cassel 1995).

Many of the best health care systems in the United States, Canada, and Western Europe are designed to deliver this broader approach. The labels vary, but the overall concept is that palliative care should be provided to all seriously ill patients. Palliative care includes the biological, psychological, social, and spiritual care of persons with serious illnesses. The goal of palliative care is to provide the best possible quality of life for the patient and their family. Palliative care can be provided alongside the most aggressive of disease-directed treatments if that, too, will benefit the patient. Palliative care allows patients to both "hope for the best" by considering all medical options and "prepare for the worst" if such treatment proves ineffective (Back, Arnold, and Quill 2003).

Hospice in the United States is an insurance-based program to provide palliative care to terminally ill patients and their families who accept that they will no longer benefit from disease-directed treatments. Once patients are enrolled in hospice care, all palliative treatments and supplies are paid for, as well as a few hours of professional home care each day to supplement the family's care of the patient (Quill et al. 2014).

I am very enthusiastic about hospice care, but the transition to hospice can be very challenging as it requires a classic "bad news" discussion about disease-directed treatment no longer working and the patient is most likely dying (Casarett and Quill 2007). Furthermore, to be admitted to hospice, the patient has to forgo additional disease-directed therapy and hospitalization. The desire for contemporaneous, even "long-shot," medical treatments often precludes timely hospice admission. On the other hand, most patients who eventually choose hospice are very satisfied if and when they make the transition.

My commitment to palliative care and hospice has increased since these two conferences about PAS and euthanasia after the Holocaust. I have learned that the transition to hospice, while always somewhat difficult, may be especially challenging for patients whose family members have had experiences with the Holocaust because "giving up" on active treatment and accepting the inevitability of death may have special meaning for them (Weiss 2017). I still have some difficulty accepting some patients' decisions to continue ineffective treatments that add substantial suffering toward the end of life, but my understanding of the historical significance of the Holocaust has helped me better comprehend the complexity of such considerations when one has been touched by this horrific history.

EVALUATING REQUESTS FOR ASSISTED DEATH

Many seriously ill patients consider this question: what are my options if my suffering becomes unacceptable to me? In Oregon, one in six terminally ill patients talks to their family about PAS, one in fifty talks to their doctors, but it accounts for only one in three hundred deaths (Tolle et al. 2004). Knowing which options are available, and knowing that one's physician has an open mind, will reassure some patients and their families. Most patients who consider PAS will never actually use it if they receive adequate palliative care. On the other hand, patients who lack access to health care or have historical knowledge of abuses in these domains may be frightened by even the existence of such options (see chapter 10 in this book).

How can we best balance responsiveness to difficult suffering with protection against abuse and bias in the modern environment? The first step is always to ensure access and adequacy of health care, including palliative care and, when appropriate, hospice care. Then, if a patient requests direct assistance in dying, all efforts to palliate should be reviewed and redoubled, as most of the time adequate palliative answers can still be found.

Some patients who raise this question are asking more about the future rather than the present (Quill 1993). Perhaps they have witnessed difficult suffering in their own families or friends. Part of the clinician's job is to ask questions about the patient's hopes and fears about the end of life (for example, "What are you most afraid of?" or "What kinds of experiences have you had in your family around death?"), and to clarify how the clinician would respond if the patient's fears become a reality. Most of the time, all that will be needed is standard palliative care and hospice, but if the clinician has made a commitment to be as responsive as possible no matter how the last phase of the illness unfolds, he or she must find common ground with the patient if unacceptable suffering emerges.

If a patient requests assistance in dying *now*, the committed physician should first fully explore the "why now" for the request, hoping to uncover treatable root causes of the patient's suffering (Quill 1993). If the patient is experiencing unacceptable, intolerable suffering that cannot be adequately relieved, then the physician must search for mutually acceptable ways of responding.

It is critical that physicians create an environment where patients can openly express their concerns and fears about severe suffering toward the end of life, as well as the specifics of any requested death-hastening interventions. Physicians must also be aware of their own views, values, and biases in this regard and assure each patient that his or her personal values and experiences will guide the treatment process. If physicians are aware that their boundaries are being tested, then discussing their struggles with trusted and experienced colleagues before acting is essential. If a death-hastening intervention is being contemplated, then formal palliative care consultation is critical to ensure that the request is fully evaluated and that all reasonable alternatives are considered. When and if the moral boundaries are still unclear, a formal ethics consultation along with an extensive discussion with the entire interprofessional palliative care team should also be obtained. The more these processes are out in the open and documented, the better for all concerned.

PALLIATIVE OPTIONS TO ADDRESS SEVERE SUFFERING TOWARD THE VERY END OF LIFE

Clinicians who care for patients nearing the end of life need to be aware of all available palliative options for addressing severe suffering, including potential last-resort options—and consider, preferably in advance, which ones they could or could not support (Quill, Lo, and Brock 1997; Quill, Lee, and Nunn 2000).

Proportionately Accelerating Opioids for Severe Pain or Dyspnea

When a patient nearing the end of life experiences severe pain or dyspnea, administration of opioids in proportion to the severity of the symptoms is a mainstay of treatment. The risks of tolerance and overuse are relatively small in this circumstance, and the risks of over-sedation, respiratory depression, and hastening death are minimal with usual pain management. The doctrine of double effect, which clearly applies in most of these cases, has four main elements: (1) The clinician's intent is to relieve pain; (2) Side effects, such as accelerating death, can be foreseen but they are not intended; (3) The need for pain relief must be proportionate to the risk of hastening death; and (4) Death cannot be intentionally hastened to relieve the patient's suffering. This doctrine comes from the Catholic moral tradition, but it has wide secular applicability when applied to aggressive symptom management toward the end of life. Opioid treatment has become much more complicated with the recent epidemic of opioid abuse and opioid-related deaths, but opioid use toward the very end of life still has strong clinical support—we can promise patients that they will not die in pain that could have been medically relieved (Schenker, Merlin, and Quill 2018).

Withholding or Withdrawing Life-Sustaining Therapies

Potentially life-sustaining therapies can be withheld or withdrawn if the patient's goals or clinical situation changes. Decisionally capable patients, or their surrogates if the patient is incapacitated, can make these choices. Justification for such actions that intentionally hasten death derives from the right to bodily integrity—we need patients' permission to invade their bodies with medical treatment, and they can take away that permission if their circumstances change. A few religious groups make firm distinctions between not starting (permissible) and stopping once started (impermissible), but secular laws in the Western world clearly permit both actions.

Withholding and withdrawing life-sustaining therapies are relatively commonplace and uncontroversial in most palliative care circles. The following four possibilities, presented in order of decreasing societal consensus about acceptability, should generally be considered last-resort options (Quill, Lo, and Brock 1997; Quill, Lee, and Nunn 2000).

Palliative Sedation (Potentially to Unconsciousness)

Two kinds of sedation are relevant here: (1) proportionate palliative sedation is the progressive increasing of doses of sedating medications to the lowest dose needed to relieve the patient's suffering. This practice usually does not expose the patient to the risk of a hastened death unless doses need to be repeatedly accelerated because of acute, otherwise intractable suffering; and (2) palliative sedation to unconsciousness is the rapid sedation of a patient to unconsciousness to relieve severe, intractable, acute suffering, such as a patient with neck cancer rapidly exsanguinating from a ruptured carotid artery (Quill, Lo, et al. 2009). Some patients may request sedation to unconsciousness in the absence of severe, acute physical suffering to achieve a wished-for death in environments where more explicit assistance is not permitted. While the doctrine of double effect may provide justification for most cases of proportionate palliative sedation, requests to intentionally hasten death with palliative sedation to unconsciousness cannot be similarly justified as death would be clearly intended, and (arguably) the response would be disproportionate if the immediate suffering was not severe and otherwise intractable (Quill, Dresser, and Brock 1997). Under such circumstances, other last-resort options could be explored depending on the patient's clinical situation and personal values.

Voluntarily Stopping Eating and Drinking

Voluntarily stopping eating and drinking, also known as VSED, is not the predictable loss of appetite and thirst that comes at the very end of the "natural" dying process. Rather, it is an active decision to hasten death made by a patient who is capable of eating and drinking—not drinking is especially important to achieve a timely death (Quill, Ganzini, Troug, and Pope 2018; Wax, Kosier, and Quill 2018; Horowitz, Sussman, and Quill 2016). When a patient voluntarily stops eating and drinking, it generally takes from 10 to 14 days to die, provided the patient assiduously avoids drinking even small amounts. This practice theoretically does not require direct physician involvement, but physicians should participate in the initial assessment and help manage symptoms, especially dry mouth and confusion, as the process unfolds. Voluntarily stopping eating and drinking is an option for patients with considerable resolve and full decision-making capacity and, because it takes too long, it is inappropriate for patients with severe, acute physical suffering.

Physician-Assisted Suicide/Physician-Assisted Death

In physician-assisted suicide (PAS), also known as physician-assisted death (PAD), the physician provides the medical means, usually a potentially lethal prescription of barbiturates, to intentionally hasten the death of a decisionally capable patient who must both request the prescription and carry out the final act himself. Even though the patient must ultimately take the medication, the physician is morally responsible as an accomplice. In the United States, PAD is legal in eight states (Oregon, Washington, Colorado, Vermont, Hawaii, California, Maine, New Jersey) and the District of Columbia. The Montana law remains in dispute. There is debate about what to call this practice. Opponents and some philosophers prefer the term *physician-assisted suicide* because it is "accurate" (Singer and Siegler 1990). Public support goes down when this language is used, so proponents prefer more general terminology like *physician-assisted death* because it is not conflated with suicide caused by mental illness (Quill and Battin 2004). Other languages have different terms for *mental-illness-related suicide*, *heroic suicide* (jumping on a bomb to save one's squad in battle), and *rational suicide* (action that makes sense given one's medical circumstance and personal values) (Battin 1996).

Voluntary Active Euthanasia

With voluntary active euthanasia (VAE), the physician provides the means to achieve a wished-for death at the patient's request and also carries out the final act, which includes both sedation to unconsciousness and then the provision of a lethal injection. VAE can respond to a wider range of clinical circumstances than PAD, but also puts more responsibility on the physician as both accomplice and final actor. In the United States, the legal prohibition against VAE is much clearer than is the prohibition against PAD—for example, Dr. Jack Kevorkian flaunted the legal prohibition against PAD, but was incarcerated after conviction in a case of VAE (Nicol and Wylie 2006, 231). In 2016, the Canadian Supreme Court determined a "fundamental right" to choose either PAD or VAE provided the patient has a "grievous and irremediable medical condition" that "causes enduring suffering that is intolerable to the individual" in situations where death is "reasonably foreseeable." In addition, several Western European countries have legalized PAD and VAE with varying stipulations. In jurisdictions such as Canada and The Netherlands, where both PAD and VAE are legally permitted, the vast majority of patients choose VAE (Health Canada 2019; RTE 2018).

While a variety of considerations go into the choice of an end-of-life option, the patient's clinical situation and personal values are clearly at the core, as are the law in the patient's jurisdiction and the clinician's values if assistance involves his or her direct participation. The requirements for legal practice of PAD and VAE are clearly spelled out in jurisdictions where they are permitted. On the other hand, there is an underground practice of PAD within the United States in states where it is prohibited (Meier et al. 1998).

In most jurisdictions where these practices are legally permitted, opt-out clauses exist for clinicians who believe they are morally wrong. The requirement to think through what one can and cannot offer under such circumstances needs to be considered for the other last-resort options as well—just because they are legal does not mean that they are morally acceptable to all clinicians. Clinicians need to decide what they would potentially do in response to unacceptable suffering as well as what they would not do. While patients' values and preferences count the most in these circumstances, physicians' values also count if the option involves their direct participation.

If these decisions are first and foremost driven by the voluntary and capable choices of patients who are otherwise receiving excellent medical care, and not by their clinicians or by overarching societal issues, then contemporary PAD and VAE can potentially be differentiated from medical practice and policies of the Holocaust.

OPEN PRACTICE WITH SAFEGUARDS VS. PROHIBITION

Wherever society chooses to draw a line demarcating the permissibility of the six palliative options to address unacceptable suffering toward the very end of life, it must also provide access to good medical care, including palliative care. When unacceptable suffering persists despite such provision, it is challenging to safeguard vulnerable patients from error, abuse, or coercion while simultaneously ensuring availability of agreed-upon last-resort options.

Categories of safeguards for last-resort options are generally agreed upon. (1) Both disease-directed and palliative treatments need to be accessible, ineffective, and/or unwanted. (2) Rigorous informed consent is required including clarity about the underlying disease and its prognosis, as well as patient understanding of the benefits and burdens of the available treatment options. (3) Independent second opinions should be available to ensure that all disease-directed therapies and palliative alternatives are fully understood, especially for the last four last-resort options. (4) The consent process should be carefully documented in the patient's medical record.

The consent process can be challenging. Clinicians might be vague about what they are offering because they fear getting into legal or professional trouble, potentially saying things like "Don't take too much of this or it will kill you," which may leave the patient wondering if the doctor is providing a genuine warning or a covert suggestion. Decision-making in this realm requires honesty to be sure that physician and patient fully understand each other. If a physician writes flexible sedation orders for proportionate palliative sedation, the orders for increasing the medication should be very clear. Secrecy and intentional ambiguity have no place in these critical discussions. The risks of a misunderstanding that results in undertreatment or overtreatment of suffering are far too great.

There are also potential risks of being explicit about these end-of-life options. Routinely informing all seriously ill patients and families about all potential last-resort choices may impair the doctor-patient relationship. For example, unsolicited disclosure may frighten some patients and families, deprive others of opportunities to benefit from improbable but possibly effective disease-directed treatments, and cause still others to lose hope or feel abandoned. Patients who have been medically discriminated against in the past, including those with personal or family Holocaust experiences, may have a particularly unfavorable reaction to unsolicited, explicit disclosures about potential methods for hastening death.

Safeguards should always be considered before initiating any end-of-life discussion that might ultimately lead to a hastened death. The first consideration is the patient's capacity for major medical decision-making. The last-resort options for fully capacitated patients might include any of the six options outlined above, whereas only three of the options might be available to patients who have lost capacity (aggressive symptom management, cessation of life supports, and proportionate palliative sedation). The second consideration is the adequacy of palliative care. Although all good doctors should be able to do basic palliative care (Quill and Abernethy 2013), if any of the six last-resort options are being considered, consultation with a board-certified, palliative care physician should be obtained if at all possible. The third consideration is the physician's level of understanding of the patient's unacceptable suffering and the patient's awareness of all available alternatives. Finally, the physician should request a formal psychiatric evaluation if the patient has a history of mental illness that might alter decision-making ability or if the patient's current capacity to make major life and death decisions is uncertain.

If safeguards are inadequate, then the patient may end his life prematurely. A relatively large number of patients think about options for hastening death, but relatively few go through with them even where they are legally permitted (Quill 1993). Patients should not be permitted to choose death based on transient feelings or impulses—evaluations must be thorough, and standards of informed consent should be uniformly applied. On the other hand, if safeguards are too burdensome, they may add to rather than alleviate suffering.

Safeguards for legal last-resort practices are also essential to prevent secret, underground, unregulated practices that are fraught with hazards, even if motivated by clinician compassion. If PAD or VAE are permitted, the entire process should be transparent and clearly documented, confirming that each requesting patient had decision-making capacity assessments and comprehensive palliative care before a decision was made about how to respond. If society, the law, and/or the medical profession choose to prohibit PAD or VAE, they need to be forthright about how clinicians should respond to patients who find themselves suffering unacceptably despite receiving the best possible palliative care.

Unacceptable suffering may primarily mean physical symptoms for some patients, while, for others, unacceptable suffering may primarily mean complex psychosocial symptoms such as dependence, loneliness, and lack of control. Clinicians must work together with patients and families to ameliorate all such suffering, but they must also listen carefully to what the patient is saying about their limits in terms of acceptability. Even if society, the law, and/or the medical profession are committed to addressing patient suffering, some patients will still choose PAD or VAE if it is legally available. Others who live in jurisdictions where PAD and VAE are prohibited may seek out underground options for hastening death to relieve their symptoms despite the inherently hazardous nature of secret practices. At the very least, the Holocaust teaches us that covert medical practices are easily abused.

PHYSICIANS RESPONSES TO UNACCEPTABLE SUFFERING IN LIGHT OF THE HOLOCAUST

Proponents of access to last-resort options put forth three main arguments: patient autonomy, beneficence, and nonabandonment (Quill and Battin 2004). (1) The suffering patient's autonomous wishes, preferences, and values count the most, although the values of the assisting clinician also count. Opt-out clauses for clinicians who cannot comply with a patient's request for a permitted option based on their own moral values are also needed. (2) Allowing and even assisting a suffering patient to achieve a wished-for death could be a beneficent act, especially if all other avenues to address their unacceptable suffering had been exhausted. (3) Clinicians must not abandon suffering patients at this time of great need (Quill and Cassel 1995). Suffering patients do not have a choice about going through this final process, but clinicians also have a responsibility to care for and respond to patients no matter where the disease takes them. Without violating their fundamental values, clinicians need to be as responsive and creative as possible in addressing patients' dilemmas.

There are also three main arguments against at least some last-resort options (Foley and Hendin 2002). (1) The immorality of "killing" absolutely prohibits clinicians from intentionally hastening death. Physicians are healers, not killers. (2) The "slippery slope" argument suggests that the inherent difficulty of determining eligibility for last-resort options inevitably leads to hastening the death of patients with lesser degrees of suffering and more ambiguous levels of consent. (3) Intentionally ending life, even at the request of a suffering patient, would be a fundamental violation of a doctor's professional integrity, stated most clearly in the prohibition "doctors must not kill" (Pellegrino 1992).

How one weighs these competing arguments will largely determine how physicians respond to inquiries about and requests for an assisted death.

However, all doctors, regardless of their position on PAD or VAE, need to address patients' ongoing medical and palliative care needs, to suggest alternative approaches, and to assess patients' capacity to make major decisions. Physicians opposed to PAD or VAE may ultimately choose to withdraw from ongoing care if patients ultimately pursue an assisted death.

While individual participation in assisted suicide is currently not illegal in Germany, a new law passed in 2015 makes it illegal to offer assistance in suicide in any systematic, or organized fashion and the German National Medical Association recommends against physician participation (Emanuel et al. 2016). In my opinion, if doctors are to participate in PAS or VAE, they should ideally be personally and directly involved in all aspects of the process unless the genuine legal risks are too prohibitive.

It is painfully clear from the German experience in the 1930s and 1940s that any of these last-resort options can be used malevolently, either without the patient's explicit consent and/or without regard to the individual patient's benefit or burden. Disregard of explicit consent can lead to utilization of last-resort options against the wishes of the individual patient, eventually bringing about killing that overrides explicit patient dissent and refusal, and even "mercy killing" of disabled children for eugenic and economic reasons based solely on perceived benefit to society. While we in the United States would like to believe we learned this historical lesson, experience suggests that one generation of medical professionals has difficulty learning the hard lessons from previous generations. For example, consider the Tuskegee experiments on the "natural history" of untreated syphilis in African American men—despite the availability of penicillin since the 1940s—under the auspices of the US Public Health Service from 1932 until newspaper articles publicized its existence in 1972 (Heller 1972). Despite the passage of 25 years since the Nuremberg Medical Trial and the Nuremberg Code, the continuation of this and other unethical human subjects research (Beecher 1966; Fairchild and Bayer 1999) in the United States undermines the belief in our ability to consistently learn from history.

How do we avoid repeating the shameful German and American medical histories while simultaneously respecting individual patient autonomy and responding to patients experiencing unacceptable suffering toward the end of life? If last-resort options are to be used benevolently with maximal protection from abuse, they must be firmly anchored in individual patient autonomy and consent and be available only to those patients who have access to palliative and hospice care. If physicians receive a request for any last-resort option from a patient who does not have access to palliative and hospice care, I recommend that they request a second opinion, preferably in person, from an experienced, board-certified palliative medicine clinician to ensure that all reasonable palliative approaches have been considered, if not tried, before exercising any of these options.

But when patients continue to suffer despite unrestrained efforts to palliate and when they ask physicians about options to escape their suffering, I continue to believe that we need to decide which last-resort options should be openly available, and then explain how we could use these options to address the patient's particular situation. Severe unrelieved suffering prior to death adversely impacts everyone involved, including the patient, family, friends, and staff at all levels. An impending bad death should be considered a medical emergency (Quill and Brody 1995) that physicians should thoroughly evaluate and openly respond to. While local laws set boundaries on legally available last-resort options, they do not free us from our continuing responsibility to care for our patients in their time of extreme need and vulnerability. We must do as much as possible to relieve the various dimensions of our patients' suffering without violating fundamental personal values of any of the direct participants.

FINAL THOUGHTS

Learning about unethical medical practices, including active killing, in Germany and elsewhere has been both sobering and enlightening, and it has helped me better understand the great hesitancy that many have about PAD and VAE. Reconciling that history with my advocacy for last-resort options is not simple. In an ideal world, we would ensure access to the best possible disease-directed treatment for all seriously ill patients and to palliative and hospice care for all dying patients, and then collectively struggle to agree upon which last-resort options should be made available to patients with unrelieved suffering at the end of life. In the real world, we must be as creative as possible to provide access to palliative care consultation in order to ensure that all reasonable palliative treatments are being considered, if not tried, before considering any last-resort options.

In my opinion, all legally available end-of-life options to address severe suffering, including the four last-resort options, should be subject to well thought-out and publicized safeguards. As a society, we may choose to prohibit some last-resort options, but we must be clear about which options *are* available and under what circumstances. More clarity and openness about these processes would potentially reassure patients who fear a bad death, increase the medical profession's responsiveness to extremes of suffering, lead to greater success in addressing unique circumstances, and provide more accountability when suffering persists.

ACKNOWLEDGMENTS

I would like to thank my good friend and colleague Dr. Bernie Sussman, who is a lifelong student of the Holocaust and also attended the conference in Berlin, for working with me to better understand the profound historical and personal issues underlying these considerations. Bernie worked diligently with me to deepen this essay, but the positions, viewpoints, and limitations are my own. I also want to thank Shelly Rubenfeld and the Center for Medicine after the Holocaust for conceiving and then implementing this experience and other related projects to help educate us all about how the Holocaust is critically relevant to medical ethics and medical practice in today's world. I may not have altered my opinions as much as Shelly would have liked, but I am seeing these questions in a much more sobering historical context than I was, and for that I am very grateful to him and the conference participants.

BIBLIOGRAPHY

Back, Anthony, Robert Arnold, and Timothy Quill. 2003. "Hope for the Best, and Prepare for the Worst." *Annals of Internal Medicine* 138, no. 5 (March): 439–43.

Battin, Margaret. 1996. *The Least Worst Death: Essays in Bioethics on the End of Life*. New York: Oxford University Press.

Beecher, Henry K. 1966. "Ethics and Clinical Research." *New England Journal of Medicine* 274, no. 24 (June): 1354–60. doi:10.1056/NEJM196606162742405.

Casarett, David, and Timothy Quill. 2007. "I'm Not Ready for Hospice: Strategies for Timely and Effective Hospice Discussions." *Annals of Internal Medicine* 146, no. 6 (April): 443–49.

Emanuel, Ezekiel, Bregje Onwuteaka-Philipsen, John Urwin, and Joachim Cohen. 2016. "Attitudes and Practices of Euthanasia and Physician-Assisted Suicide in the United States, Canada, and Europe." *Journal of the American Medical Association* 316, no. 1 (July): 79–90. doi:10.1001/jama.2016.8499.

Fairchild, Amy L., and Ronald Bayer. 1999. "Uses and Abuses of Tuskegee." *Science* 284, no. 5416 (May): 919–21.

Foley, Kathleen, and Herbert Hendin, eds. 2002. *The Case Against Assisted Suicide: For the Right to End of Life Care*. Baltimore, MD: Johns Hopkins University Press.

Health Canada. 2019. *Fourth Interim Report on Medical Assistance in Dying in Canada*. Accessed March 14, 2020. https://www.canada.ca/en/health-canada/services/publications/health-system-services/medical-assistance-dying-interim-report-april-2019.html.

Heller, Jean. 1972. "Participating Doctor Says Syphilitics Not Told of Experiment." *Birmingham News*, July 27, 1972.

Horowitz, Robert, Bernard Sussman, and Timothy Quill. 2016. "VSED Narratives: Exploring Complexity." *Narrative Inquiry in Bioethics* 6, no. 2 (Summer): 115–20.

Jones, James H. 1981. *Bad Blood: The Tuskegee Syphilis Experiment*. New York: Free Press.

Meier, Diane, Carol-Ann Emmons, Sylvan Wallenstein, Timothy Quill, R. Sean Morrison, and Christine Cassel. 1998. "A National Survey of Physician-Assisted Suicide and Euthanasia in the United States." *New England Journal of Medicine* 338, no. 17 (May): 1193–201.

Nicol, Neal, and Harry Wylie. 2006. *Between the Dying and the Dead: Dr. Jack Kevorkian's Life and the Battle to Legalize Euthanasia*. Madison: University of Wisconsin Press.

Pellegrino, Edmund. 1992. "Doctors Must Not Kill." *Journal of Clinical Ethics* 3, no. 2 (Summer): 95–102.

Quill, Timothy. 1993. "Doctor, I Want to Die. Will You Help Me?" *Journal of the American Medical Association* 270, no. 7 (August): 870–73.

Quill, Timothy, and Amy Abernethy. 2013. "Generalist Plus Specialist Palliative Care—Creating a More Sustainable Model." *New England Journal of Medicine* 368, no. 13 (March): 1173–75.

Quill, Timothy, and Margaret P. Battin, eds. 2004. *Physician-Assisted Dying: The Case for Palliative Care and Patient Choice*. Baltimore, MD: Johns Hopkins University Press.

Quill, Timothy, Kimberly Bower, Robert Holloway, et al. 2014. *Primer of Palliative Care*, 6th Edition. Chicago: American Academy of Hospice and Palliative Medicine.

Quill, Timothy, and Robert Brody. 1995. "'You Promised Me I Wouldn't Die Like This!' A Bad Death as a Medical Emergency." *Archives of Internal Medicine* 155, no.12 (June): 1250–54.

Quill, Timothy, and Christine Cassel. 1995. "Nonabandonment: A Central Obligation for Physicians." *Annals of Internal Medicine* 122, no. 5 (March): 368–74.

Quill, Timothy, Rebecca Dresser, and Dan Brock. 1997. "The Rule of Double Effect—A Critique of Its Role in End-of-Life Decision Making." *New England Journal of Medicine* 337, no. 24 (December): 1768–71.

Quill, Timothy, Linda Ganzini, Robert Troug, and Thaddeus Pope. 2018. "Voluntarily Stopping Eating and Drinking among Patients with Serious Advanced Illness: Clinical, Ethical, and Legal Aspects." *Journal of the American Medical Association* 178, no.1 (November): 123–27.

Quill, Timothy, Barbara C. Lee, and Sally Nunn. 2000. "Palliative Treatments of Last Resort: Choosing the Least Harmful Alternative." *Annals of Internal Medicine* 132, no. 6 (March): 488–93.

Quill, Timothy, Bernard Lo, and Dan Brock. 1997. "Palliative Options of Last Resort: A Comparison of Voluntarily Stopping Eating and Drinking, Terminal Sedation, Physician-Assisted Suicide, and Voluntary Active Euthanasia." *Journal of the American Medical Association* 278, no. 23 (December): 2099–104.

Quill, Timothy, Bernard Lo, Dan Brock, and Alan Meisel. 2009. "Last-Resort Options for Palliative Sedation." *Annals of Internal Medicine* 151, no. 6 (September): 421–24.

RTE (Dutch Regional Euthanasia Review Committees). 2018. *Annual Report 2018*. Accessed March 14, 2020. https://english.euthanasiecommissie.nl.

Schenker, Yael, Jessica Merlin, and Timothy Quill. 2018. "Use of Palliative Care Earlier in the Disease Course in the Context of the Opioid Epidemic." *Journal of the American Medical Association* 320, no. 9 (September): 871–72.

Singer, Peter, and Mark Siegler. 1990. "Euthanasia—A Critique." *New England Journal of Medicine* 322, no. 26 (June): 1881–83.

Tolle, Susan, Virginia P. Tilden, Linda Drach, et al. 2004. "Characteristics and Proportion of Dying Oregonians who Personally Consider Physician-Assisted Suicide." *Journal of Clinical Ethics* 15, no. 2 (February): 111–18.

Wax, John, Amy An, Nicole Kosier, and Timothy Quill. 2018. "Voluntary Stopping Eating and Drinking." *Journal of the American Geriatrics Society* 66, no. 3 (March): 441–45.

Weiss, Toby. 2017. "Caring for Holocaust Survivors with Sensitivity at the End of Life." National Hospice and Palliative Care Organization online course. https://www.nhpco.org/online_course/caring-for-holocaust-survivors-with-sensitivity-at-the-end-of-life/.

Chapter Ten

Race and Physician-Assisted Death

Do Black Lives Matter?

Alan Elbaum and LaVera Crawley

Race and racism are critical but neglected lenses of analysis in the current debate on physician-assisted death (PAD) in the United States. This chapter is an inquiry into how the stakes of the debate are clarified by consideration of health inequities and end-of-life decision-making patterns among African Americans.[1] The legalization of PAD in the United States is rapidly gathering momentum. Since Oregon passed the first "Death with Dignity Act" in 1997, eight more jurisdictions have enacted similar laws, the majority of these since 2016 (Death with Dignity n.d.).[2] Opponents of such laws frequently invoke a slippery slope moral argument, fearing that marginalized groups will be pressured to accept PAD in lieu of continued medical treatments.

The starting point of this chapter is the fact that the number of African Americans who have availed themselves of PAD is close to zero. Some commentators have taken this fact to mean that there is no slippery slope (Emanuel et al. 2016). We argue, however, that this statistic ought to spur inquiry into the historical and sociological factors that have produced aversion to PAD in the African American community. When such an analysis is done, the statistic does not reassure so much as it destabilizes abstract convictions about the ethics of PAD.

This chapter, emerging from the 2018 Physician-Assisted Suicide and Euthanasia after the Holocaust (PASEATH) working group, evaluates the legacies of eugenics and euthanasia in Nazi Germany and the United States and highlights the bioethical implications of both historical injustice and persistent racial health disparities. Legalized PAD in the United States is gaining ground in the very same era as the Black Lives Matter movement, when there is a new and widespread recognition that certain lives are ascribed intrinsic value while others must struggle for the right to exist. The present political moment is, therefore, a turning point in which there is an opportunity to shape the future of PAD as well as the boundaries of palliative care. In these projects, we ignore the lessons from the histories of racism in the Third Reich and in the United States at our peril.

Participants in the PASEATH working group studied the complicity of the medical profession in the policies of Nazi Germany, including the forced sterilization of "genetically diseased" individuals in the pre-war years, followed by the involuntary euthanasia of tens of thousands of disabled and psychiatrically ill individuals during World War II (Proctor 1988, 95–117, 177–222). The working group discussed the ethical ramifications of PAD in the post-Holocaust era, asking: Are there political and philosophical continuities between the contemporary situation and Nazi Germany? Do present-day commitments to patient autonomy and informed consent mark such a profound difference between now and then as to make the comparison valueless? Ultimately, how does mid-twentieth-century German history inform present-day debates on PAD and euthanasia?

In the first section of this chapter, we explore the continuities between practices of eugenics and racial purification in Nazi Germany and in the present-day United States. We clarify the distinction between race as a social phenomenon and race as a biological trait, a distinction that continues to elude influential policy makers. In our discussion of the complex relationship between race and the unequal distribution of wealth, we draw on Henry Giroux's analysis of Hurricane Katrina as the event that conclusively revealed the American biopolitics in which certain lives hold value and others are disposable (Giroux 2006).

In the second section, we evaluate the contemporary status of patient autonomy and voluntary consent in light of the actions of physicians and nurses at Memorial Hospital in New Orleans during Hurricane Katrina who chose to euthanize at least eight bedbound, mostly African American patients rather than evacuate them (Fink 2013). The safeguard of voluntary consent—established after the Holocaust with regard to human subjects research and now firmly integrated into medical decision-making—was suspended by the very professionals charged with protecting it. We offer an answer to the question of how involuntary euthanasia became imaginable once again in the twenty-first century in the United States and note that the "slippery slope" that is evoked in the debate on PAD is not an abstract proposition but a recent precedent.

In the third and final section, we argue that previous findings on African Americans' ambivalent reception of palliative care also illuminate their attitudes toward PAD. In particular, LaVera Crawley's ethnographic study of African Americans making medical decisions in the face of serious illness revealed a key explanatory model—the patients regarded death as a challenge to be overcome, one that was analogous to the racism and disenfranchisement they and their ancestors had struggled to overcome. In the context of the health and health care disparities that have produced an epidemic of premature African American death, the patients in the study described their tendency to resist medical interventions that would hasten death still further. These insights from Crawley's study suggest why including the lessons of twentieth-century eugenics and euthanasia and of Hurricane Katrina is essential to the PAD debate.

Our overall argument follows the model of philosopher Susan Neiman in her recent book, *Learning from the Germans: Race and the Memory of Evil.* Neiman makes a compelling case for the usefulness of comparing the ways in which America and Germany have reckoned with the respective national crimes of slavery and the Holocaust. The goal of such a comparison, she argues, is not to equate one form of evil to another, but to engage in a process of comparative redemption: "Can we compare the processes that are meant to heal the wounds of such different historical events?" (Neiman 2019, 32). At a minimum, redemption from racism requires giving due place to its memory and to its current manifestations in the ethical debates of our time.

PAD is now gathering momentum in a society where black lives appear to be disposable, in which physicians routinely undertreat African American patients and, in recent memory, actively euthanized them against their will. The notion of licensing physicians to assist in death calls first for a reckoning with the question, "Do Black Lives Matter?"

RACE AND EUGENICS IN THE
UNITED STATES AND NAZI GERMANY

In laying the groundwork for evaluating the ethics of PAD, the PASEATH working group examined the question of whether there are political and philosophical continuities between Nazi Germany and the present-day United States: our answer is "yes." Certain racial ideologies and eugenic policies were common to both Germany and the United States in the early twentieth century. In this section, we argue that aspects of present-day American racial politics remain fundamentally eugenic.

From its origins in the heyday of scientific racism and social Darwinism in nineteenth-century Europe, the concept of race has been fraught with ideologies of domination. The thinkers who first attempted to categorize human variation under the umbrella of distinct and pure races were guided by the belief that they were identifying immutably biological categories, and they used their findings to justify the supremacy of white Europeans. Such theories of scientific racism led directly to policies for the promotion of "racial hygiene" in pre-World War II Germany and America (Proctor 1988, 10–45). Yet we now know that race is not biological. Advances in human genome research have given credence to what social scientists had already observed, that is, that "race is an ideology and for this reason . . . should be more accurately described as a social construct and not a biological one" (NIH National Human Genome Research Institute n.d.).

Modern science notwithstanding, antiquated and essentialized notions of race continue to be widely held. The downstream effects of the social construction of race, such as discriminatory practices against particular races, often come to be regarded as fundamental characteristics of the group in question. Senator Lindsey Graham of South Carolina, for example, in his 2009 speech on the floor of the US Senate, argued against the Affordable Care Act on the grounds that it would expand eligibility for Medicaid—the federal system of health insurance for those requiring financial assistance that is administered by the states—and his state would, therefore, have to pay more to cover the poor. "My State is on its knees," he said, "I have a 31 percent African American population in South Carolina" (Congressional Record 2009). In other words, Graham conflated the "racial" location of being an African American with the social location of being poor. In fact, fewer than a third (28.7 percent) of African Americans in South Carolina live below the poverty line (Macartney, Bishaw, and Fontenot 2013). The irony of this example is that while African Americans have been systematically impoverished by social determinants from slavery onward, the persistent attachment to race as a biological category led Graham to see poverty as an innately African American characteristic and to attack precisely the kind of social program that could help rectify the disparity.

Graham objected to the use of government funds for the benefit of a group at the confluence of multiple axes of marginalization: the poor, the sick, and the non-white. His and others' similar rhetoric on the Affordable Care Act partake of a long American tradition of antipathy for the welfare state and its beneficiaries. In the first decades of the twentieth century, such antipathy was a driving force in the eugenics movement, which sought to improve future generations by eliminating the socially, medically, and racially unfit from the gene pool. At the 1914 First National Conference on Race Betterment, held in Battle Creek, Michigan, University of Wisconsin biologist Leon Cole delivered a speech on "The Relationship of Philanthropy and Medicine to Race Betterment," arguing that charity and social policies for the advancement of the poor were incompatible with the ultimate aim of philanthropy, namely, the improvement of the "human stock" through a process of "rational"—

rather than natural—selection. Cole drew an analogy between the social body and the physical body: "Death is the normal process of elimination in the social organism, and we might carry the figure a step further and say that in prolonging the lives of defectives we are tampering with the functioning of the social kidneys!" (Cole 1914, 503). American philanthropists and legislators took heed. The Carnegie Foundation, among others, sponsored the work of the Eugenics Records Office from 1910 until 1939, which, in turn, provided the research to back up policies being implemented by states' Boards of Eugenics. By 1939, 29 states had involuntarily sterilized over 30,000 individuals deemed "mentally ill and criminally insane," a practice the United States Supreme Court nearly unanimously upheld in 1927 in *Buck v. Bell* (Proctor 1988, 97). Such sterilization policies did not need to invoke race to achieve the eugenic goal of excluding African Americans from the gene pool of the "fit"; anti-miscegenation laws effectively accomplished the same goal.

German racial hygienists openly admired the American precedent in coercive sterilization for the betterment of the race. When the Nazis came to power in 1933, one of their first acts was the passage of the "Law for the Prevention of Offspring with Hereditary Diseases" in July 1933 (German History in Documents and Images n.d.). This law required doctors to report patients with specified diagnoses, especially "feebleminded" patients, to genetic health courts, which ultimately resulted in approximately 400,000 involuntary sterilizations during the Third Reich. As in the United States, there was no explicit provision for sterilizing people on the basis of race, yet this did not prevent the Nazis from applying the same logic to a racial group whose propagation they feared, the approximately 500 children born to German women and black French soldiers during the post–World War I occupation, also known as the "Rhineland bastards." In this case, the Gestapo bypassed the stipulations of the law and simply seized the children and extracted "consent" for the sterilizations from their parents in a secret operation in 1937 (Proctor 1988, 95–117).

By the summer of 1939, the sterilization of the "genetically diseased" was supplanted by the idea of involuntary euthanasia of the incurably sick and the mentally ill. Karl Binding, professor of law, and Alfred Hoche, professor of medicine, provided the ethical justification for voluntary and involuntary euthanasia in their 1920 book, *Permitting the Destruction of Unworthy Life: Its Extent and Form.* They wrote, "Is there human life which has so utterly forfeited its claim to worth that its continuation has forever lost all value both for the bearer of that life and for society? Initially, this question is in every case to be answered with certainty: Yes" (Binding and Hoche 1920, loc. 1016 of 1997). As historian Robert Proctor notes, these scholars were asserting that the destruction of such lives is not only tolerable but humane

(1988, 178). Since 1933, the Nazi government had been preoccupied with the "value" of the disabled and the economic burden they imposed on the taxpayer, and accordingly, the Nazis made drastic cuts to expenditures for medical services (1988, 184–185). During World War II, they pursued a more definitive solution: From January 1940 until August 1941, some 5,000 infants with physical disabilities and 70,273 adults with mental illness were secretly murdered. The adult euthanasia program was known as *Aktion* T4 (named for *Tiergartenstrasse* 4, headquarters of the Committee for the Scientific Treatment of Severe, Genetically Determined Illness) (Proctor 1988, 185–192; see chapter 3 in this book). In chapter 2 in this book, Volker Roelcke describes how *Aktion* T4 emerged from the combination of two distinct ethical justifications for euthanasia: that of providing "mercy" to the supposedly suffering patient and that of alleviating the economic "burden" that the patient imposed on society.

Two features of *Aktion* T4 are of special relevance for the upcoming discussion of the events at Memorial Hospital, race, and PAD in the contemporary American context. The first feature is that "physicians were never *ordered* to murder psychiatric patients and handicapped children. They were *empowered* to do so, and fulfilled their task without protest, often on their own initiative" (Proctor 1988, 192–193). Hospitals continued to euthanize their mentally ill patients well past the official end of *Aktion* T4 in August 1941, and in some cases even past the end of the war and into the American occupation (Proctor 1988, 192–193). The second feature is that medically-based euthanasia paved the way for the Final Solution of the Jewish Question. In December 1941, the same physicians who diagnosed patients as mentally unfit under *Aktion* T4 were newly tasked with identifying the "antisocials" in German hospitals and concentration camps—including Jews, Sinti and Roma, communists, and homosexuals—and culling them for extermination (Ley and Hinz-Wessels 2012). One of these physicians, Friedrich Mennecke, was questioned at the Nuremberg Medical Trial, "So, you had two kinds of cases: the mentally ill, which had to be evaluated according to medical criteria, and those which had to be evaluated according to political and racial criteria?" Mennecke responded, "One simply cannot distinguish the two, Herr Attorney. The two cases were simply not divided and clearly separated from one another" (Proctor 1988, 208–209).

Following World War II and the revelation of the Nazis' atrocities, the American eugenics movement would forever be tainted by association (Black 2012, 418). The number of sterilizations declined until the last American eugenic sterilization was done in Oregon in 1981 (State Library of Oregon n.d.). While eugenicists in the early part of the twentieth century did not disproportionately or explicitly target African Americans—Jim Crow and anti-miscegenation laws made eugenic policies extraneous—sterilization patterns changed in the 1960s and increasingly affected poor black women (Kluchin 2011, 202–215). In some cases, existing eugenic sterilization laws were repurposed for this new target demographic. In North Carolina, through the 1930s and 1940s, African Americans only represented approximately 25 percent both of the state's population and of the sterilized. By 1966, African Americans comprised no less than 64 percent of those sterilized by the Eugenics Board of North Carolina (Kluchin 2011, 91). African Americans and people of color also became subject to involuntary sterilization as a corollary of their representation in the ranks of welfare recipients, although it is exceedingly difficult to untangle the elements of consent and coercion in the statistics of poor women sterilized by federal family planning programs in this era (Kluchin 2011, 91). Not until 1974 did the issue come to national attention, in *Relf v. Weinberger*, a case of two African American minors who were forcibly sterilized in Alabama when their clinicians judged they would not be "disciplined enough" to take birth control pills (Ladd-Taylor 2020, 213). Judge Gerhard Gesell found that "an indefinite number of poor people have been improperly coerced into accepting a sterilization operation under the threat that various federally supported welfare benefits would be withdrawn unless they submitted to irreversible sterilization," concluding, "The dividing line between family planning and eugenics is murky" (Relf v. Weinberger, 372 F. Supp. 1196 1974).

Sterilization provides a striking example of both the continuity and the evolution of eugenic thinking throughout the twentieth century, but sterilization is only one of many forces that have impinged on the ability of African Americans to survive as individuals and as a group; reduction of the fertility of recipients of welfare benefits was another. After African American welfare advocates finally overcame the obstacles that had blocked their access to welfare, political scientist Virginia Eubanks noted, "News coverage of poverty became increasingly critical. . . . Stories about welfare fraud and abuse were most likely to contain images of Black faces. . . . [T]he percentage of African Americans represented in news magazine stories about poverty jumped from 27 to 72 percent between 1964 and 1967" (Eubanks 2017, 31). Ronald Reagan rose to the presidency on a platform that included cutting welfare expenditures, popularizing the caricature that racialized "welfare queens" were stealing the money of honest, white laborers, inviting a comparison to Nazi-era propaganda depicting the economic burden that "useless eaters" imposed on the tax-paying public (Cammett 2014). To the present day, factions that favor dismantling the social safety net for the poor, sick, elderly, and other marginalized groups are thereby eliminating resources that enable those groups' continued existence.

The response to Hurricane Katrina may have demonstrated the consequences of such policies. According to the analysis of Henry Giroux, professor of media studies at McMaster University, the images of predominantly black victims that flooded the media at that time evoked images of lynching victims from previous eras:

> The bodies of the Katrina victims . . . reveal[ed] and shatter[ed] the conservative fictions that we live in a color blind society . . . and revealed the emergence of a new kind of politics, one in which entire populations are now considered disposable, an unnecessary burden on state coffers, and consigned to fend for themselves." (Giroux 2006, 174)

Racial bias structured the media coverage of the disaster as well: images of desperate people wading through the water with supplies taken from abandoned stores were captioned as "looters" if black and, if white, simply as victims or survivors who had found the groceries (Spence 2005; Ortega 2009).

A Pew poll shortly after Katrina revealed a wide gulf between black and white Americans' willingness to recognize racism as contributing to the disaster. While 66 percent of African Americans said that "the government's response to the situation would have been faster if most of the victims had been white," only 17 percent of whites agreed, and 77 percent of whites said the race of the victims would not have made any difference (Doherty 2015). Journalist Jamelle Bouie traces the origin of Black Lives Matter to the dismissal, post-Katrina, of "the idea that black Americans had a legitimate grievance. The result was a collapse in black racial optimism . . . a deep sense that America is indifferent to their lives and livelihoods" (2015).

This section has argued that the conflation of racial and social characteristics, and the continuities between eugenic policies in Nazi Germany and in the United States, continue to reverberate in the twenty-first century. They provide the basis for understanding the euthanasia that occurred at Memorial Hospital in New Orleans in the midst of Hurricane Katrina as well as the tendency by African Americans to resist PAD.

EUTHANASIA AT MEMORIAL HOSPITAL

The second question that the PASEATH working group took up is whether present-day commitments to patient autonomy and informed consent are so strong that there can be no true analogy between euthanasia in contemporary society and in Nazi Germany. The danger of a fallacious analogy is most pronounced when one cites the Nazi precedent merely as a rhetorical flourish, usually to attack a group of people or a policy. Our intention in this section is instead to compare the circumstances of euthanasia under the Nazis to those that led to involuntary euthanasia at Memorial Hospital during Hurricane Katrina. We argue that the present-day commitment to patient autonomy and informed consent has proven to be violable, and that the Nazi analogy actually helps illuminate specific risks of PAD.

It is worth reviewing the perspectives of bioethicists and Holocaust historians regarding the relevance of Nazi euthanasia to contemporary debates. A representative range of such views can be found in the proceedings of a seminal 1976 conference entitled Biomedical Ethics and the Shadow of Nazism: A Conference on the Proper Use of the Nazi Analogy in Ethical Debate (Callahan et al. 1976). The discussion in this conference revolved around one of the starkest expressions of the slippery slope argument: Leo Alexander's claim (published in his 1949 article, "Medical Science under Dictatorship") that the Nazis' crimes originated in the concept, central to all forms of euthanasia, that there is such a thing as a life not worthy to be lived: "The infinitely small wedged-in lever from which [the Nazis'] entire trend of mind received its impetus was the attitude toward the nonrehabilitable sick" (Alexander 1949). If one holds this view, there is grave danger even in PAD administered voluntarily to a patient requesting "death with dignity." Against Alexander, Holocaust historian Lucy Dawidowicz maintained that the Nazi euthanasia program was so exceptional as to be inapplicable to contemporary debates. She argued that the word *euthanasia* in the setting of the Holocaust was simply a euphemism for the murder of "racially valueless" individuals, and that the Nazi preoccupation with the incurably sick was negligible beside their obsession with racial purification (Callahan et al. 1976, 4).

Implicit in Dawidowicz's rejection of the Nazi analogy, however, is the assumption that contemporary societies do not have pernicious racial ideologies. In the words of one of her respondents in the 1976 conference, "What got German society on the slippery slope, indeed what characterized the slope, was the racist attitudes already in place. It is a reasonable defense and distinguishes our case from theirs for us to say that we [in the United States] don't have those attitudes" (Callahan et al. 1976, 15). The assumption that there are no racist attitudes in the United States is a serious omission. In this section, we suggest a middle ground between the view of Alexander and that of Dawidowicz. In Nazi Germany, racial ideology and negative attitudes toward the incurably sick converged in a program of mass euthanasia. In the United States, implicit racism and similarly negative attitudes toward the incurably sick resulted in euthanasia in Memorial Hospital in the aftermath of Hurricane Katrina.

When Hurricane Katrina made landfall on August 29, 2005, it devastated the city of New Orleans, revealing its inadequate infrastructure and disaster preparedness, especially in poor and minority neighborhoods. The events at Memorial Hospital have been exhaustively covered by physician and journalist Sheri Fink, and our account in this chapter relies entirely on her reportage. The storm hit Memorial Hospital especially hard, and the doctors, nurses, and hospital staff who stayed behind continued to care for patients in intolerable conditions for four days. The auxiliary generators failed, leaving the hospital without power, and temperatures rose to 110°F. With meager assistance from the government and from the company that owned the hospital, and without working power or communication systems, the staff heroically managed to evacuate almost all the patients by the morning of September 1.

The disaster response leaders made the unusual decision to reverse the customary order of triage: the sickest patients were to be evacuated last. Patients with "Do Not Resuscitate" (DNR) orders, which technically means only that cardiopulmonary resuscitation (CPR) should not be performed in case of death, were also triaged to last place. On the final morning, nine patients remained on a floor leased by LifeCare Hospitals of New Orleans, L.L.C. ("LifeCare"), an outside hospital system providing long-term acute care and rehabilitation for patients with limited—but not terminal—prognoses. Several were elderly, several were on mechanical ventilators, and most were black or African American.[3] When the doctors and nurses who took charge in the crisis fell under the shared (and retrospectively mistaken) impression that it would be impossible to evacuate these patients, it appears that they took drastic measures—all nine patients were dead by that afternoon. The autopsies pointed to excess levels of morphine and midazolam in their bloodstreams as the cause of death, but these medications had previously been prescribed for only one of the nine patients as part of her care plan (Fink 2013, 356–361).

There followed the opposite of a public outcry. In the aftermath of the hurricane, state prosecutors gathered evidence to arrest Dr. Anna Pou and nurses Cheri Landry and Lori Budo, and the county coroner determined that at least four of the patients were unquestionably victims of homicide. A grand jury was convened in 2007 to determine whether Pou, Landry, and Budo would be prosecuted, but the jurors declined to hear the state's evidence or summon the witnesses. Public opinion was squarely behind the health care providers. A poll by Pou's lawyer's office found that 76 percent of people in Orleans Parish favored exoneration and only 8 percent supported indictment (Fink 2013, 412). The grand jury chose not to indict Pou on any charges. Following this episode, Pou became an advocate for "alternate standards of care" and immunity for health care providers in future disasters (Fink 2009). Lachlan Forrow, a bioethicist and palliative care physician, offers an opposing view: "Rather than thinking about exceptional moral rules for exceptional moral situations, we should almost always see exceptional moral situations as opportunities for us to show exceptionally deep commitment to our deepest moral values" (Fink 2013, 469).

How is it possible that health care providers administered involuntary euthanasia in the United States in the twenty-first century? Some of the Life-Care patients were alert, oriented, and able to engage in the process of informed consent, but the requirement for consent was waived. None, as far as can be known, asked for death. The extreme conditions in such a disaster zone reveal how care is rationed and how real or perceived exigencies can lead dedicated providers to violate the most basic of human rights. It is instructive to think back to the two salient features of *Aktion* T4 that were flagged above: first, that physicians were empowered—not ordered—to end the lives of patients deemed incurable, and second, as Mennecke testified, that there was no simple distinction between the medical and the racial inputs when assessing whether a patient could be cured or ought to be euthanized.

In the case of Katrina, providers at Memorial Hospital felt abandoned by the government and the hospital administration and were left with absolute power over their patients. Onlookers cited a (mistaken) belief that New Orleans was already under martial law when explaining why they did not challenge the physicians. There was little chance of a future reckoning—medicines were dispensed without prescriptions, and patients' charts went missing. Other factors included acute time pressure as well as a perception that these patients were suffering. Apart from the factors of sheer exhaustion and unlivable conditions, everyone in the hospital had been commanded to vacate by the evening of September 1 (Fink 2009). These conditions created an opening for snap judgments and biases to direct behavior, in the same way that high-pressure circumstances magnify police officers' well-documented tendency to see a black man carrying a gun when there is no gun (Payne 2006).

In her book *Five Days at Memorial*, Sheri Fink documents numerous implicit and explicit biases of the physicians directing the hurricane response. Most striking are the judgments, not always evidence-based, about who could survive and who could not.[4] Terence Stahelin, a LifeCare respiratory therapist appalled at the failure to evacuate his patients, suggested, "These were the 'expendable' patients. The ones who someone decided that [they] had no quality of life" (Fink 2013, 312).[5] One doctor who described to Fink his role in hastening the death of a patient also expressed a fear that "the people firing guns into the chaos of New Orleans—'the animals,' he called them—would storm the hospital, looking for drugs after everyone else was gone. 'I figured, What would they do, these crazy black people who think they've been oppressed for all these years by white people?'" (Fink 2009). Did racism have a role in the decision to euthanize the LifeCare patients? It cannot be proven, and it could not have been the sole factor, as some of the victims were white. But could it be that implicit racism was part of the white providers' emergent calculation of which lives were worth living—and saving?

In the 1976 conference proceedings cited at the beginning of this section, medical ethicist Robert Veatch proposed a careful use of the Nazi analogy in the discussion of euthanasia:

> One might resist the permitting of killing for mercy, not because logically it would lead to the principle that it is acceptable to kill for social purposes like saving the race, but because once the behavior is available it will tap already existing moral principles . . . or introduce consideration of slightly more questionable princi- ples. . . . [T]he relevant question is whether that was what happened in Germany, and if so, whether a similar historical condition of available double motivation— mercy and social interest—exists in this country. (Callahan et al. 1976)

This is the sense in which the euthanasia at Memorial Hospital is analogous to the actions of physicians under *Aktion* T4. The beleaguered providers at Memorial Hospital did not have any explicit desire to "save the race." Karen Wynn, the chair of the hospital ethics committee, drew an analogy to routine palliative care practices, suggesting that deaths may have been hastened by the administration of morphine and midazolam but that the sole intention was to offer comfort, peace, and dignity. She said, "We did the best we could do. It was the right thing to do under the circumstances" (Fink 2009). These providers acted for the "available" purpose of mercy, but in so doing, they violated the safeguard of consent and killed their most vulnerable patients. The potential danger that Veatch outlined—which is exactly what occurred at Memorial Hospital—lies at the heart of why PAD legislation evokes skepti- cism and even fear among African Americans.

AFRICAN AMERICANS, PALLIATIVE CARE, AND PHYSICIAN-ASSISTED DEATH

The third question that the PASEATH working group discussed was how mid-twentieth-century German history ultimately informs present-day de- bates on PAD. In this final section, we draw on the histories of racism and euthanasia described in the previous two sections in order to contextualize contemporary African American views of PAD. We find that these views are best understood as instances of the tendency to resist palliative care interventions in general.

When focusing on one subpopulation, in this case African Americans, it is crucial to avoid basing assumptions on stereotypes and essentializing characteristics of the group. Any general statement about blacks in the United States, for example, would have to be true across a diverse range of social locations, including socioeconomic status, immigration status, education level, geography, religion, and age. Statements that apply across such diversity likely reference the impact of racism on black bodies, and even that would apply differentially based on racial visibility.[6] As a result, any statement about African Americans as a population is merely a hypothesis when applied to individuals. That said, there are distinct and prevalent patterns of responses among many African Americans toward end-of-life issues. Specifically, there is a tendency to underutilize hospice and other palliative care interventions, such as advance directives, and African Americans are more likely than whites to opt for aggressive medical treatments and to be kept alive on life support (Sanders, Robinson, and Block 2016; Mebane et al. 1999).

Crawley observed these patterns in an ethnographic study at the Stanford University Center for Biomedical Ethics in which she followed ten African American patients with serious illness and their families over two years (Koenig and Crawley 1999). From these patients' point of entry into the hospital through their process of dying and the post-death journey, including funeral, autopsy, and the families' bereavement, Crawley focused on the complex decision-making processes that came up at each stage: receiving the terminal diagnosis, struggling with chronically debilitating disease, and preparing for death when it seemed imminent. She observed several distinct patterns in how these African American patients conceived of and confronted their mortality, two of which are most relevant to the debate on PAD.

In the first pattern, death was seen as a welcomed friend, a transition from an earthly life of pain and suffering to a joyous reunion with God in heaven (Crawley et al. 2000). This perspective is beautifully conveyed in James Weldon Johnson's 1920s poem, "Go Down Death," written in a style that mimics the sonorous, booming voice of a black preacher. The poem addresses the surviving family of an elderly matriarch, "Weep not, weep not, / She is not dead; / She's resting in the bosom of Jesus" (Johnson 2008, 27–29). Obviously, patients and families who demonstrated this pattern were religious and held strong beliefs in the afterlife.[7] In the second pattern, terminal illness and death were seen as struggles to be overcome. To understand this stance, one must consider that the entire saga of blacks on the American continent has been a continuous struggle for their individual and collective existence. From the brutal legacy of slavery, abuses in medical experimentation (most famously but by no means limited to the United States Public Health Service's Tuskegee Study of Untreated Syphilis in the Negro Male) (Washington 2006, 157–185), and eugenic sterilizations, through economic injustices and the denial of basic human and civil rights, through voter suppression, mass incarceration, and police killings—these are just a few of the examples of the historical and contemporary traumas that make life as a black person in the United States a struggle for the right to exist. Even those African Americans with economic, educational, or class privilege are subject to discrimination: recall the incident when the esteemed Harvard professor, Henry Louis Gates, was arrested while entering his own house in Harvard's faculty housing (Goodnough 2009). African Americans live with and have lived with such aggressions and existential threats for centuries.

The American medical system itself bears part of the responsibility for the fact that black deaths are often unjustly premature. Life expectancy has been persistently lower for African Americans than for whites since official estimates have been recorded (Olshansky et al. 2012). A 2002 Institute of Medicine (IOM) report on racial and ethnic health disparities reviewed a large and consistent body of research demonstrating inequities in medical care and health outcomes by race, even when insurance status, income, age, and severity of conditions are comparable (Smedley, Stith, and Nelson 2003). The IOM report highlights that African Americans die at higher rates from cardiovascular disease, cancer, and HIV/AIDS than any other US racial or ethnic group (Smedley, Stith, and Nelson 2003, 29). Black women die in or after childbirth at a rate three times higher than white women, and half of those deaths are considered preventable (Nelson, Moniz, and Davis 2018, 1007). The reasons for these findings are multifactorial and include socioeconomic and educational disparities, environmental degradation, direct and indirect consequences of discrimination, and differences in access to health care and insurance. Yet even at equivalent levels of access to care, "racial and ethnic minorities experience a lower quality of health services and are less likely to receive even routine medical procedures than white Americans" (Smedley, Stith, and Nelson 2003, 29). In the IOM report, the list of services that African Americans are less likely to receive spans pages and encompasses virtually all health conditions. These health care disparities are associated with increased mortality (Smedley, Stith, and Nelson 2003, 422–439).

The IOM report posits three levels of influences that account for the injustice of inadequate health care for certain populations: health systems-level (such as legal and regulatory systems in health care institutions), provider-level (such as conscious and unconscious bias or insufficient cultural competence), and patient-level (including individual or culture-bound preferences) (Smedley, Stith, and Nelson 2003, 125–179). This framework of analysis may also be fruitfully applied to the euthanasia of the vulnerable group of LifeCare patients at Memorial Hospital. In that example, the systems-level influence was the abandonment of the population of New Orleans by the federal and state governments and the consequent failure to provide sufficient or timely aid for evacuating the patients of Memorial Hospital. Provider-level factors included conditions of extreme duress, rationalizations that euthanasia was the only way to relieve suffering, and implicit, negative attitudes that physicians felt toward the incurably sick and toward African Americans. Seen from this perspective, while the events at Memorial Hospital were exceptional in terms of the chaos created by the hurricane and the lack of provider accountability, these events occurred within larger structures of racism and oppression and fell into predictable patterns.

With regard to the third level of influence, patient-level preferences, much has been written about the role of mistrust in African American engagement with health care, but as Crawley has previously published, this misrepresents the crux of the issue. Speaking of decontextualized "mistrust" suggests that this is a dispositional trait of African Americans and, further, that the onus is on black patients to place greater trust in their providers. Mistrust is more appropriately seen as dynamic and situational: certain behaviors of providers toward patients constitute *breaches* of trust and thereby reduce the chance that those patients will go on to place unearned trust in future providers (Crawley et al. 2000). For example, in Crawley's study of perceived discrimination in medical settings, African American participants were less likely than white patients to receive cancer screening if, within the clinical setting, they felt discrimination or mistreatment based on their race or ethnicity (Crawley, Ahn, and Winkleby 2008). The euthanasia at Memorial Hospital is an especially grave—but by no means isolated—instance of such a breach of trust.

The themes discussed in this section—the struggle of African Americans for the right to exist, the injustice of premature black deaths, and the experience of health systems-level and provider-level discrimination—underlie the perspective that death is a struggle to be overcome. While not every African American patient has had these experiences or holds these perspectives, the inequities are, nevertheless, part of the cultural narrative within the African American community. Stories about mistreatment at the hands of medical professionals abound within families and neighborhoods and in films, music, literature, and news coverage; as a result, the credibility of the health care system is limited.[8] This may account for the findings in palliative care studies that African Americans are less likely than other groups to enroll in hospice, less likely to participate in advance care planning, and more likely to prefer aggressive medical interventions even if such interventions have a low chance of success (Sanders, Robinson, and Block 2016; Mebane et al. 1999).

In Crawley's conversations about DNR orders or transitioning into hospice with the participants in her ethnographic study, she repeatedly heard statements like, "She is not going to go down without a fight." Such statements reflect two historically founded fears: that physicians may not do everything within their power to prolong the lives of their black patients, and that the mere acceptance of palliative interventions may further increase this risk and, thereby, constitute a threat to life or a surrender in the struggle against death (Sanders, Robinson, and Block 1999, 220–223). Sociologist Roi Livne suggests an important reason underlying the disjuncture between the values of palliative care and the values of many African American patients like those in Crawley's ethnography, namely, that it was white, middle- and upper-class advocates whose experiences originally shaped the growth of palliative care. He writes, "People of color, immigrants, and people of lower socioeconomic status are consequently more likely to find themselves at odds with a medical profession that pressures them to economize dying, then judges them negatively if they resist" (Livne 2019, 146).

In advance care planning conversations, physicians counsel their patients that a DNR order means one thing and one thing only: if the patient's heart or lungs cease working, she will not receive CPR. A patient with a DNR order may live in perfect health for decades and may receive aggressive medical interventions. However, the story of Memorial Hospital once again demonstrates how the meaning of DNR can creep beyond its literal, legal sense. One of the leaders of the hurricane response team told Fink that he believed patients with DNR orders had terminal or irreversible conditions. He thought they had the "least to lose" and thus should be evacuated last (Fink 2009). When Angela McManus learned that her mother Wilda McManus would not be evacuated because of this policy, she insisted that her mother's DNR order be rescinded. She was told that this could not be done as no physicians were present, and police escorted her away from her mother and out of the building. Wilda McManus became one of the victims of euthanasia (Fink 2013, 145). In an interview after Hurricane Katrina, Angela McManus echoed a sentiment that Crawley observed in her own ethnographic study: "DNR means do not resuscitate. It does not mean do not rescue, do not take care of" (Kahn 2006). In the case of Memorial Hospital, "DNR" in fact became "Do Not Rescue."

In the same way that African Americans tend to access palliative care less than other groups, they have also, for the most part, not participated in PAD. According to the data from Oregon, only one black person has taken advantage of the Death with Dignity process since 1998 (Oregon Health Authority 2018). Six of the 840 patients (0.7 percent) accessing PAD in California since 2016 have been black (California Department of Public Health 2018). Other states, such as Washington and Colorado, only report race as "white" or "non-white," making it impossible to know the race of the 2 to 5 percent non-white patients who access PAD each year in each state (Washington State Department of Health 2018; Colorado Department of Public Health and

Environment 2018). In one sense, these statistics are reassuring: they show that African Americans have not been coerced into accepting PAD as an alternative to proper medical treatment. But instead of taking this as reassurance and ending the discussion, we ought to ask, "Why is this the case?" The fact raises more questions than it answers.

There is a world of difference between palliative care and PAD in their means and their ends; however, they both stand apart from other branches of medicine in that physicians practicing palliative care and PAD do not aim to prolong the patient's life. The fear that leads African Americans to underutilize palliative care—an important health care disparity in its own right—is that the boundary between palliative care and PAD is not as solid as we would like. Undertreatment and withholding of care from African American patients by medical providers contribute to the epidemic of premature black death (Cunningham et al. 2017; Smedley, Stith, and Nelson 2003). If death is a struggle to be overcome, so too are the health care practices that either discriminate against African Americans or suggest that doctors will do less than everything in their power to prolong the lives of their patients. The legalization of PAD, the safeguard of voluntary consent notwithstanding, raises the specter that the boundary between palliative care and PAD might yet become still more porous.

CONCLUSION

Are there political and philosophical continuities between the contemporary situation and Nazi Germany? The first section of this chapter traced the parallel histories of eugenics in the United States and Nazi Germany, culminating in the mass euthanasia of children with congenital disease and adults with mental illness in Germany's *Aktion* T4. Although eugenics was formally discredited in the United States after the Holocaust, the social forces that created the conditions for eugenics persist to the present day. One can see manifestations of these forces in ongoing attacks on social welfare programs such as Medicaid that are lifelines for marginalized communities as well as in the government's inadequate response to Hurricane Katrina, which demonstrated the disposability of black lives. Legalized PAD is a rollback of protections and taboos that have prevailed since the medical abuses under the Nazi regime. In the persistence of the structural racism that contributed to American and Nazi eugenics, it is essential to determine if there are sufficient safeguards in place to protect marginalized communities.

Do present-day commitments to patient autonomy and informed consent mark such a profound difference between now and then as to make the comparison valueless? The euthanasia that occurred at Memorial Hospital demonstrates that the safeguard of voluntary consent, even now, is not absolute. In conditions of exhaustion and duress, physicians' implicit and explicit biases about which lives were worth living obscured for them the possibility of evacuating the LifeCare patients and led them to administer involuntary euthanasia. Ethicist Robert Veatch has proposed a useful criterion to consider when comparing Nazi euthanasia to present conditions: the question is "whether a similar historical condition of available double motivation— mercy and social interest—exists in this country" (Callahan et al. 1976, 17). The killings at Memorial Hospital were surely motivated by a misplaced sense of mercy, but this calculation was inextricable from providers' implicit racism and attitudes toward the incurably sick.

The final section of this chapter contextualized the view among many African Americans that death is a struggle to be overcome and reviewed the health care disparities that endanger and shorten black lives. The fear that medical providers already do not provide adequate treatment to black patients partially explains why African Americans tend to underutilize palliative care and why they have hardly used PAD at all. The experiences of African Americans and marginalized social groups have not sufficiently informed the development of either palliative care or PAD.

Ultimately, how does mid-twentieth-century German history inform the present-day debate on PAD and euthanasia? Our goal in this chapter is not to argue against the legalization of PAD. Instead, we are insisting that everyone interested in the ethics of PAD must also grapple with America's legacies of eugenics and racism. PAD is becoming legal in ever more diverse settings across the United States at the same time that the Black Lives Matter movement is increasing consciousness of how African Americans have to struggle for the right to exist. As our society negotiates the future of PAD and the boundaries of palliative care, policymakers, health systems, and health care workers must strive to eliminate racial health disparities and to continually strengthen safeguards of voluntary consent. Only then will we have learned the appropriate lessons both from the Nazi experience and from America's past and present racism.

NOTES

1. The term *African American* is more accurately a reference to ethnicity than race, as it refers to diasporic Africans whose ethnic and cultural influences reflect the American experience. The term *black* is more inclusive of the wider population of persons of African descent and is also a reference to racial visibility, which may be the more relevant term when referring to persons or groups subject to structural racism based on skin color.

2. The year 2016 also marked the first time PAD became legal in jurisdictions with substantial African American populations: California at first, followed by Washington, DC, and New Jersey.

3. Not every victim is named or identified by race in Sheri Fink's account, *Five Days at Memorial*. The statement that "most were black or African American" applies to those victims who are identified.

4. These are two examples drawn from the stories of patients who were not euthanized but who were allowed to die: "The doctor said the hospital didn't have any more oxygen and couldn't get any. 'You have to let him go.' It was not true that there was no oxygen in the hospital, but Isbell was not in a position to know this" (Fink 2013, 127); "A doctor came and peered at the lady's chart. 'She has lung cancer,' he said quietly. He turned to Green and closed the woman's chart. 'She's not going anywhere.' He looked at the oxygen tank and shook his head no. 'That's it,' he said, and chopped the air with his hand. There would be no more respiratory treatments" (Fink 2013, 162–163).

5. Dr. Horace Baltz, president of the Memorial Hospital medical staff, previously characterized his colleagues' opinions on the LifeCare patients as, "We spend too much on these turkeys. We ought to let them go" (Fink, 2013, 46).

6. For example, Anatole Broyard, an African American and the former editor of the New York Times Book Review, passed as white in order to avoid racial discrimination.

7. This correlates with a recently published study on the association between afterlife beliefs and attitudes toward PAD. Using data from the Baylor Religion Survey, the investigator found that beliefs in either heaven or hell were, separately and together, predictive of having a negative attitude toward physician aid in dying. Interestingly, they found that the belief in hell had a stronger impact than the belief in heaven on attitudes toward PAD. This may be explained by the negative perception of medical aid in dying as a form of suicide, which to some is an act punishable by being condemned to hell (Sharp 2018,1–12).

8. For example, former first lady Michelle Obama writes in her memoir, *Becoming*, about her grandfather's death from advanced lung cancer, noting his "long-held view that doctors were untrustworthy having kept him from any sort of timely intervention" (Obama 2018, 92). For a comprehensive treatment of this complex phenomenon, David Bradley's award-winning 1981 novel, *The Chaneysville Incident*, provides an excellent picture of historical and contemporary encounters with death and dying, discrimination against African Americans, and how these stories get passed through generations.

BIBLIOGRAPHY

Alexander, Leo. 1949. "Medical Science under Dictatorship." *New England Journal of Medicine* 241, no. 2 (July 14): 39–47. https://doi.org/10.1056/NEJM1949 07142410201.

Binding, Karl, and Alfred Hoche. (1920) 2012. *Permitting the Destruction of Life Unworthy of Life.* Translated by Cristina Modak. Ebook. Greenwood, WI: Suzeteo Enterprises. Kindle.

Black, Edwin. 2012. *War Against the Weak: Eugenics and America's Campaign to Create a Master Race.* Washington, DC: Dialog Press.

Bouie, Jamelle. 2019. "Where Black Lives Matter Began." *Slate,* August 23, 2015. www.slate.com/articles/news_and_politics/politics/2015/08/hurricane_ katrina_10th_anniversary_how_the_black_lives_matter_movement_was.html.

Bradley, David. 1981. *The Chaneysville Incident.* New York: Harper & Row.

California Department of Public Health. "End of Life Option Act." June 2018. Accessed January 9, 2019. https://www.cdph.ca.gov/Programs/CHSI/Pages/End-of-Life-Option-Act-.aspx.

Callahan, Daniel, Arthur Caplan, Harold Edgar, et al. 1976. "Special Supplement: Biomedical Ethics and the Shadow of Nazism." *Hastings Center Report* 6, no. 4 (August): 1–19.

Cammett, Ann. 2014. "Deadbeat Dads & Welfare Queens: How Metaphor Shapes Poverty Law." *Boston College Journal of Law and Social Justice* 34, no. 2 (June): 233–265. http://lawdigitalcommons.bc.edu/jlsj/vol34/iss2/3.

Cole, Leon. 1914. "The Relationship of Philanthropy and Medicine to Race Betterment." In *Proceedings of the first National Conference on Race Betterment, January 8, 9, 10, 11, 12, 1914,* edited by Emily Robbins. Battle Creek, MI: Race Betterment Foundation.

Colorado Department of Public Health and Environment. 2018. "Colorado End-of-Life Options Act, Year One: 2017 Data Summary." Accessed January 9, 2019. https://www.deathwithdignity.org/wp-content/uploads/2015/10/2017-CO -End-of-Life-Options-Act-Annual-Report.pdf.

Congressional Record 155, no. 196. (2009). "Proceedings and Debate of the 111th Congress, First Session," S13564 (December 20). Accessed August 14, 2020. https://www.congress.gov/111/crec/2009/12/20/CREC-2009-12-20.pdf.

Crawley, LaVera, David Ahn, and Marilyn Winkleby. 2008. "Perceived Medical Discrimination and Cancer Screening Behaviors of Racial and Ethnic Minority Adults." *Cancer Epidemiology Biomarkers & Prevention.* 17, no. 8 (August): 1937–1944.

Crawley, LaVera, Richard Payne, James Bolden, et al. 2000. "Palliative and End-of-Life Care in the African American Community." *Journal of the American Medical Association* 284, no. 19 (November): 2518–2521.

Cunningham, Timothy J., Janet B. Croft, Yong Liu, Hua Lu, Paul I. Eke, and Wayne H. Giles. 2017. "Vital Signs: Racial Disparities in Age-Specific Mortality among Blacks or African Americans—United States, 1999–2015." *Morbidity and Mortality Weekly Report* 66, no. 17 (May): 444–456.

Death with Dignity. n.d. "Death with Dignity Acts." Accessed July 8, 2019. https:// www.deathwithdignity.org/learn/death-with-dignity-acts/.

Doherty, Caroll. 2015. "Remembering Katrina: Wide Racial Divide over Government's Response." Pew Research Center. August 27, 2015. https://www.pewre search.org/fact-tank/2015/08/27/remembering-katrina-wide-racial-divide-over -governments-response/.

Emanuel, Ezekiel J., Bregje D. Onwuteaka-Philipsen, John W. Urwin, and Joachim Cohen. 2016. "Attitudes and Practices of Euthanasia and Physician-Assisted Suicide in the United States, Canada, and Europe." *Journal of the American Medical Association* 316, no. 1 (July): 79–90. https://doi.org/10.1001/jama.2016.8499.

Eubanks, Virginia. 2017. *Automating Inequality: How High-Tech Tools Profile, Police, and Punish the Poor.* New York: Picador.

Fink, Sheri. "The Deadly Choices at Memorial." *New York Times*, August 25, 2009. https://www.nytimes.com/2009/08/30/magazine/30doctors.html.

Fink, Sheri. 2013. *Five Days at Memorial: Life and Death in a Storm-Ravaged Hospital.* New York: Crown Publishers.

German History in Documents and Images. n.d. "Law for the Prevention of Offspring with Hereditary Diseases, July 14, 1933." Volume 7. Nazi Germany, 1933–1945. Accessed December 6, 2019. http://germanhistorydocs.ghi-dc.org/pdf/eng/English30.pdf.

Giroux, Henry. 2006. "Reading Hurricane Katrina: Race, Class and the Biopolitics of Disposability." *College Literature* 33, no. 3 (Summer): 171–196.

Goodnough, Abby. "Harvard Professor Jailed; Officer is Accused of Bias." *New York Times*, July 20, 2009. https://www.nytimes.com/2009/07/21/us/21gates.html.

Johnson, James Weldon. 2008. *God's Trombones: Seven Negro Sermons in Verse*, edited by Henry Louis Gates. New York: Penguin Books.

Kahn, Carrie. 2006. "New Orleans Hospital Staff Discussed Mercy Killings." *NPR.* February 16, 2006. https://www.npr.org/templates/story/story.php?storyId=5219917.

Kluchin, Rebecca M. 2011. *Fit to be Tied: Sterilization and Reproductive Rights in America, 1950–1980.* New Brunswick: Rutgers University Press.

Koenig, Barbara, and LaVera Crawley. 1999. *Final Report: Dying in an African American Community.* New York: Project on Death in America, Open Society Institute.

Ladd-Taylor, Molly. 2020. *Fixing the Poor: Eugenic Sterilization and Child Welfare in the Twentieth Century.* Baltimore: Johns Hopkins University Press.

Ley, Astrid, and Annette Hinz-Wessels. 2012. *The "Euthanasia Institution" of Brandenburg an der Havel.* Berlin: Metropol.

Livne, Roi. 2019. *Values at the End of Life: The Logic of Palliative Care.* Cambridge, MA: Harvard University Press.

Macartney, Suzanne, Alemayehu Bishaw, and Kayla Fontenot. 2013. "Poverty Rates for Selected Detailed Race and Hispanic Groups by State and Place: 2007–2011." United States Census Bureau. Accessed July 8, 2019. https://www.census.gov/library/publications/2013/acs/acsbr11-17.html.

Mebane, Eric W., Roy F. Oman, Leo T. Kroonen, and Mary K. Goldstein. 1999. "The Influence of Physician Race, Age, and Gender on Physician Attitudes Toward Advance Care Directives and Preferences for End-Of-Life Decision-Making." *Journal of the American Geriatrics Society* 47, no. 5 (May): 579–591. https://doi.org/10.1111/j.1532-5415.1999.tb02573.x.

Neiman, Susan. 2019. *Learning from the Germans: Race and the Memory of Evil.* New York: Farrar, Straus and Giroux.

Nelson, Daniel B., Michelle H. Moniz, and Matthew M. Davis. 2018. "Population-Level Factors Associated with Maternal Mortality in the United States, 1997–2012." *BMC Public Health* 18, no. 1 (August): 1007. https://doi.org/10.1186/s12889-018-5935-2.

NIH National Human Genome Research Institute. n.d. "Race." Accessed January 9, 2019, https://www.genome.gov/genetics-glossary/Race.

Obama, Michelle. 2018. *Becoming*. New York: Crown.

Olshansky, Jay S., Toni Antonucci, Lisa Berkman, et al. 2012. "Differences in Life Expectancy Due To Race And Educational Differences Are Widening, and Many May Not Catch Up." *Health Affairs* 31, no. 8 (August): 1803–1813. https://doi.org/10.1377/hlthaff.2011.0746.

Oregon Health Authority. 2018. "Oregon Death with Dignity Act 2017 Data Summary." February 2018. Accessed January 9, 2019. http://public.health.oregon.gov/ProviderPartnerResources/Evaluationresearch/deathwithdignityact/Pages/index.aspx.

Ortega, Maria. 2009. "Othering the Other: The Spectacle of Katrina for our Entertainment Pleasure." *Contemporary Aesthetics* no. 2 (July). https://contempaesthetics.org/newvolume/pages/article.php?articleID=531.

Payne, Keith. 2006. "Weapon Bias: Split-Second Decisions and Unintended Stereotyping." *Current Directions in Psychological Science*, 15, no. 6 (December): 287–291.

Proctor, Robert. 1988. *Racial Hygiene: Medicine under the Nazis*. Cambridge, MA: Harvard University Press.

Sanders, Justin, Maisha Robinson, Susan Block. 2016. "Factors Impacting Advance Care Planning among African Americans: Results of a Systematic Integrated Review." *Journal of Palliative Medicine* 19, no. 2 (February): 202–227.

Sharp, Shane. 2018. "Heaven, Hell, and Attitudes toward Physician-Assisted Suicide." *Journal of Health Psychology* (October): 1–12.

Smedley, Brian, Adrienne Stith, and Alan Nelson. 2003. *Unequal Treatment: Confronting Racial and Ethnic Disparities in Healthcare*. Washington DC: National Academies Press.

Spence, Lester. 2005. "A Perspective on Looters and Race." Interview by Ed Gordon, *NPR*. September 2, 2005. https://www-editor.npr.org/templates/story/story.php?storyId=4829538.

State Library of Oregon Digital Collections. n.d. "Eugenics in Oregon." Accessed July 8, 2019. https://digital.osl.state.or.us/islandora/object/osl%3Aeugenics?page=1&display=list.

Washington, Harriet. 2006. *Medical Apartheid*. New York: Anchor Books.

Washington State Department of Health. 2018. "Washington State Death with Dignity Act Report." March 2018. Accessed January 9, 2019. https://www.doh.wa.gov/Portals/1/Documents/Pubs/422-109-DeathWithDignityAct2017.pdf.

Chapter Eleven

Understanding the Role of Suffering in Legalized Physician-Assisted Dying

Robert A. Pearlman

Descriptions of suffering are ubiquitous. Newspapers report regions suffering from drought, societies suffering from the stress of war, and marine mammals suffering from forced captivity. Marketing advertisements often contribute to an indeterminate message about suffering, such as the late 1960s advertisement for medications to treat those suffering from the "heartbreak of psoriasis" (Stoughton 1974, 334).

Patient suffering is also an important theme in the practice of medicine—relief of suffering is one of several principal goals of medicine. As stated in a series of 1996 articles, "The Goals of Medicine," Callahan and colleagues discuss relief of pain and suffering caused by maladies (Allert et al. 1996, S9-S14). In the ensuing years, the discipline of palliative care has focused on improving patient quality of life through the prevention and relief of suffering (i.e., pain and other physical, psychosocial, and spiritual problems) (World Health Organization 2004).

In addition, patient suffering has become a major justification for health care providers' involvement in physician-assisted dying (PAD), which is also known as physician-assisted suicide in the United States and physician-assisted suicide and voluntary euthanasia in select European countries. The purpose of this chapter is to shed light on patient suffering and identify underlying challenges with using suffering as a justification for PAD. To do so, we will define subjective and objective suffering; review general limitations to these conceptualizations; examine the extensive use of patient suffering to justify PAD and specific challenges associated with the current use of patient suffering as justification for PAD; and show how these challenges undermine confidence in using patient reports of "suffering" as the sole justification for PAD.

CHARACTERIZING SUBJECTIVE
AND OBJECTIVE SUFFERING

Subjective Suffering. A well accepted theory of patient suffering comes from the work of Eric Cassell (2004, 29–61). According to Cassell, patient suffering is thoroughly personal, subjective, and meaningful. Suffering interferes with a person's agency and function, is associated with a negative affect or mood, and is a threat to or an injurious attack on a person's integrity that may involve physical, psychological, social, and existential elements. The personal nature of suffering explains why one individual may experience chronic pain of a certain intensity as an annoying symptom, while another suffers from the pain with preoccupying thoughts and fears as well as disruption to their interactions with friends and family.

Other similar conceptualizations of subjective suffering exist but are less well accepted. For example, one conceptualization anchors to "realized loss of the values that give a life integrity and make life meaningful and enjoyable, loss that is profound in the sense of being intensely felt and in the sense of being thoroughgoing" (Hoffmaster 2014, 37). Another characterization describes suffering as "a type of mental state or occurrence . . . consciously experienced, which is why it automatically lowers one's quality of life while it occurs" (DeGrazia 2014, 135).

A recent simplification of Cassel's model has been proposed (Tate and Pearlman 2019, 95–110). According to this framework, subjective patient suffering is a state in which a person experiences a loss of sense of self with an associated negative affect. This loss of sense of self may be the result of any one or combination of the following types of losses: relationship(s), role(s), and narrative. The loss of one or more relationships highlights that oftentimes another person, such as a parent or child, or intimate other, provides input and feedback that contributes to one's self-awareness (or sense of self). The relationship with one's community (social, cultural, or religious) can sometimes serve the same function. Similarly, a person's role or roles contribute to how they see themselves. Examples include, but are not limited to, being a parent, student, nurse, artist, or mechanic. Finally, most people have an idea of how they expect to live their lives in the future. For some, this may be living independently, retaining one's interests, living without financial concerns, living long enough to become grandparents, for example. The loss of this (usually comforting) narrative, this future sense of self, may lead to fear of one's future and cause subjective patient suffering. The negative affect associated with this type of suffering can range from a negative mood that colors all of one's perceptions, to a myriad of strong negative feelings, such as despair, alienation, emptiness, loneliness, fear, preoccupation about becoming/being a burden, and feeling tortured.

Objective Suffering. Whereas subjective suffering anchors to subjectively experienced loss, such as sense of self, objective suffering applies to those situations that undermine human flourishing and that others would report to cause suffering regardless of how the individual experiences it (van Hooft 1998, 125–131; Bozzaro and Schildmann 2018, 288–294). Thus, a strength of this conceptualization is that it can be applicable to situations in which persons do not perceive that they are suffering. For example, this formulation of suffering can apply to entire populations that live in poverty or without education, what some would refer to as social suffering. The notion of objective suffering can help identify situations that compromise human flourishing and motivate compassionate responses, such as food aid programs.

LIMITATIONS WITH SUBJECTIVE AND OBJECTIVE CONCEPTUALIZATIONS OF SUFFERING

Subjective Suffering. One major criticism of Cassell's theory of subjective patient suffering is that he describes suffering as having meaning. As a result, the theory does not address the suffering of many, such as those with severe dementia and very young children. Another objection to Cassell's theory is that clinicians find it challenging to incorporate it into their thinking, in part because many forms of suffering are not perceived by patients as threats or attacks. The theory also ignores objective suffering, or those situations that others would consider suffering regardless of how the patient experiences it. Thus, Cassell's theory addresses neither the suffering associated with children in abusive relationships that the children consider to be normal, nor comatose patients being kept alive through use of a mechanical ventilator and artificial hydration and nutrition.

Objective Suffering. When a group of individuals or a society has the ability to judge that others are suffering (even without their knowledge) or causing other members of society to suffer, this opens the gate to justify antisocial discrimination. For example, in their influential 1920 publication *Die Freigabe der Vernichtung lebensunwerten Lebens* (*Permitting the Destruction of Life Unworthy of Life*), German psychiatrist Alfred Hoche and jurist Karl Binding proposed criteria for euthanasia arguing that under certain conditions a life is not worthy to be lived. They invoked terms such as "useless eaters," and "empty human shells" in their discussion of the negative value of the disabled, their lack of contribution to the national community, and the expense of caring for such patients (Binding and Hoche 1920/1992, 231–265). German National Socialists, or Nazis, operationalized these values when they introduced the Law for the Prevention of Genetically Diseased Offspring, which permitted involuntary sterilization of persons suffering from illnesses, such as feeblemindedness, schizophrenia, manic depression, and insanity (Peter 1934, 187–191). Although this compulsory eugenic sterilization program caused many victims to experience a lifetime of emotional suffering, it was promoted to reduce "hereditary taint," an expression of social suffering (Joseph and Wetzel 2013, 1–30). Over time the regime extended this discriminatory, antisocial approach to eliminating "undesirables" from society through its involuntary euthanasia program, a program of mass killing designed to destroy the lives of people judged by Nazis to be unworthy of living.

Nazi propaganda emphasized the nation's health and the economic burden of diverting resources from healthy members of society—the good of the individual was relegated for the good of the larger whole (Gardella 1999, 132–135). The Nazi regime and its cultural propaganda, using terms such as "peoples' parasites" and "destroyers of culture," argued that the whole population suffered by spending money and resources for the support of socially inadequate people that perpetuated genetic deficiencies and threatened the quality of ensuing generations (Lifton 1986, 15–79; Proctor 1988, 95–117; Wunder 2015, 301–315). Nazi propaganda films also influenced cultural norms by powerfully portraying how inhumane and unnatural it was for society to keep those individuals with severe mental or hereditary illnesses alive to experience endless suffering (Schmidt 2002). Rather, it was better to relieve terrible individual suffering through a humane and gentle death.

THE ROLE OF PATIENT SUFFERING IN PHYSICIAN-ASSISTED DYING

In Oregon, Washington, Vermont, California, and Colorado, the statutes permitting one form of PAD, physician-assisted suicide, use suffering as a transitive verb; that is, to refer to a patient suffering from a terminal illness or suffering from a psychological or psychiatric disorder that causes impaired judgment (Oregon Health Authority 2017, 3.02–3.03; Washington State Department of Health 2018, 8; Steinbrook 2008, 2514; Vermont General Assembly 2014, 4; California Health and Safety Code 2015, 443.11; Colorado Statute 25–48, 2016). Similarly, in Hawaii House Bill 2739, if either the attending or the consulting physician refers a patient for counseling, the counselor must determine "that the patient is not suffering from a psychiatric or psychological disorder or depression causing impaired judgment" (2018).

Patients pursuing PAD in Oregon reported various aspects of suffering associated with terminal illness, including loss of independence and autonomy, loss of dignity, decreasing ability to engage in activities that make life enjoyable, readiness to die, and wanting to control the circumstances of death as reasons for their requests (Ganzini et al. 2000, 557–563; Hedberg and New 2017, 579–583). Similar concerns about loss of autonomy, loss of the ability to participate in activities that make life enjoyable, and loss of dignity were reported in Washington by more than 75 percent of patients participating in PAD (Loggers et al. 2013, 1417–1424; Washington State Department of Health 2018, 8).

It is important to recognize that patients' reasons for pursuing PAD could be influenced by their desire to "make their case" for PAD. However, interviews with patients pursuing PAD in Washington state *before* its legalization revealed that their reasons were similar to those of patients pursuing PAD *after* its legalization (Pearlman et al. 2005, 234–239).

In countries that permit PAD outside the United States, patient suffering assumes a more prominent role. For example, in Canada, having an illness, disease, or disability, or a state of decline that causes enduring physical or psychological suffering and is intolerable and cannot be relieved under conditions that the patient considers acceptable is a qualifying criterion for PAD (Bill C-14 Statutes of Canada 2016, 3).

PAD in the Netherlands, usually through voluntary active euthanasia (designated as euthanasia in the remainder of this chapter), is permitted when a patient is suffering unbearably and that the suffering is untreatable or "without prospect of improvement" (Regional Euthanasia Review Committees 2013). Thus, in the Netherlands the physician must be convinced that the patient's suffering is unbearable without prospect of improvement (Dees et al. 2012, 1–11). Suffering can be physical or psychological, and if psychological, it may be the result of a somatic or mental disorder. The basis for suffering being unbearable is:

> [the] patient's subjective evaluation given their prospects, their views on a good death, and considerations of the options that are available to them as alternatives. Unbearable can involve being unable to ensure living acceptably or continuing to live in unacceptable circumstances, as well as being unable to face the future. (Regional Euthanasia Review Committees 2013)

A qualitative study from the Netherlands (Dees et al. 2011, 727–734) suggests that multiple themes contribute to unbearable suffering including:

- medical—fatigue, pain
- psycho-emotional—loss of self, fear of future suffering
- socio-environmental—dependency, being a burden
- existential—pointlessness, loss of all that makes life worth living.

The Netherlands also has a protocol, the Groningen Protocol, that provides non-legal guidance for euthanasia of newborns with extremely poor quality of life due to severe handicaps or presumed unbearable suffering (Verhagen and Sauer 2005, 959–962; see chapter 5 in this book). A rationale for this ongoing PAD practice is that death is considered more humane than continued living. The projection of subjective suffering onto newborns is tantamount to a societally sanctioned (intersubjectively affirmed by physicians), objective measure of suffering, akin to the concept of "lives not worth living." Even though parental consent is required, consent by someone other than the patient may be just one step away from manipulation or coercion by social pressure. Although opposition to this protocol exists based on the historical precedent of Nazi euthanasia programs (Kodish 2008), the protocol continues to be used.

PAD practices in Belgium and Luxembourg also anchor to subjective patient suffering. In Belgium the criteria for obtaining PAD include suffering, defined as unbearable and untreatable somatic and psychological disorders that cannot be alleviated (constant) and results from a serious and incurable disease (The Belgian Act on Euthanasia of May 28, 2002, 182–188; Smets et al. 2010, 187–192). Reported suffering associated with cases of euthanasia in Belgium suggest that most patients experienced either "unbearable physical (96 percent) and/or psychological (68 percent) suffering." The nature of the former was reported to be pain, cachexia, gastrointestinal symptoms, dyspnea, etc. The latter included reports of loss of dignity and feelings of dependency (Smets et al. 2010, 187–192).

PAD in Luxembourg is offered only to those with terminal illness to "shorten the suffering and agony period" (Grand Duchy of Luxembourg 2009). In Luxembourg, the patient has to have an incurable condition with "constant, unbearable physical or mental pain" (Atwill 2008). Thus, in Canada and several countries in Europe, suffering plays a more prominent role in PAD decision-making than in the United States.

In summary, characterizations of patient suffering often seem to be either psychological responses to perceived losses, such as loss of dignity or being a burden, or as articulations of identifiable, functional losses, such as increasing dependency on others or inability to engage in meaningful activities. Of note, many of these issues identified as suffering characterize such a poor quality of life—circumstances sometimes referred to as "states worse than death"—that foregoing life-sustaining treatment is justified (Pearlman et al. 1993, 33–40). Furthermore, if suffering justifies not only foregoing life-sustaining treatment but also PAD, then what constitutes unbearable/ intolerable patient suffering that is not amenable to acceptable treatment is a critically important question.

CURRENT CHALLENGES WITH THE USE OF SUFFERING IN PHYSICIAN-ASSISTED DYING

Research has demonstrated that, according to patient interviews and physician reporting, patients' principal motivations for PAD include loss of autonomy and dignity, inability to enjoy one's life and activities, concerns about future circumstances, and physical and/or mental suffering (Pearlman et al. 2005, 235–239; Ganzini, Goy, and Dobscha 2009, 489–492; Emanuel et al. 2016, 79–97; Hedberg and New 2017, 579–583). To some degree, these particular patient responses may result from three limiting factors: the assumption by patients that these responses represent the best justifications to qualify for PAD, a limited number of check boxes describing patient motivations on forms reporting data about PAD, and a professional proclivity to focus on the causes of *dis-ease*. Because these motivations often represent sources of the patient's suffering experience, Spross has stated, "All providers must resist the temptation to reduce the human experience of suffering to the underlying sources of suffering" (Spross 1993, 71–79). In addition, as sources of suffering do not specify the patient's lived experience, professional assessments of whether the degree of suffering justifies PAD are susceptible to the projections and biases of the evaluators.

Much of the literature and our knowledge about patient suffering *excludes* learning about the highly personal experiences of suffering in the words of sufferers. For example, in one study investigators directly asked patients to talk about their suffering experience, but patients often did not have the words or language to easily describe their experiences (unpublished data, Back and Pearlman. 2000. Faculty Scholar Project on Death in America, "Patient Experiences with Life-Threatening Illness"). The paucity of descriptive language to communicate the patient's personal experience interferes with shared understanding and contributes to the indeterminate meaning of patient suffering in PAD. In addition, the absence of specific words that describe a patient's experience limits the ability of counseling to promote psychological flexibility and emotional regulation, and, thereby, potentially moderate the feelings of suffering being unbearable (Dewey 1894, 233, 245; Pine 1985, 139; Hayes et al. 2006, 1–30).

The relief of suffering is meant to promote holistic care and patient-centered well-being, yet the very nature of subjective suffering usually lacks an objective measure. Thus, the intrinsic quality of subjective patient suffering makes assessing therapeutic effectiveness difficult. This issue has direct implications for assessing the immutability criterion for PAD, as in the Netherlands.

Research describing why some providers have rejected patient requests for PAD offers insights into other challenges associated with the current role of patient suffering in PAD. According to one study in the Netherlands, some physicians rejected requests for PAD when patients claimed to be weary of living and not wanting to be a burden on their families. In addition, some physicians thought that there were more treatment options available, that the patients were depressed or had other psychiatric symptoms, or that the request was not well considered (Haverkate et al. 2000, 865–866). In another Dutch study, physicians rejected the status of unbearable suffering because of patient behavior thought to be incompatible with unbearable suffering. For example, the claim of unbearable suffering was rejected because a patient was still reading books or was able to ride a bicycle (Pasman 2009, 1235–1257). In a personal communication in April 2019 with a Canadian physician who participates in PAD, he reported that if a patient did not have a definitive timeline for dying from PAD, he denied the request, reasoning that if the suffering was unbearable, then a patient would have a definitive, short-term plan to address the unbearableness of the situation. These examples suggest that inter-provider variability in evaluating patients' claims of unbearable or intolerable suffering would inadvertently, but inevitably, lead to inequitable access to PAD. However, if providers shared similar views about what constitutes unbearable suffering without the prospect for improvement, they would be providing an intersubjective value judgment about the legitimacy of the patients' reporting of suffering. This intersubjectivity would provide a quasi-objective perspective that would somewhat validate or refute a patient's allegation. Thus, a patient's subjective suffering would be somewhat validated by an external perspective and no longer be purely subjective (see chapter 15 in this book).

CONCLUSION

This review of the role of suffering in legalized physician-assisted dying identifies that suffering is often indeterminate and subject to reporting requirements and interpretation. These attributes raise several implementation and policy concerns. First, widely variable interpretations and judgment about severity blur the legal boundary between bearable and unbearable suffering (Rietjens et al. 2009, 271–283). Second, the institutional process for obtaining and reporting PAD introduces reporting biases. Patients are essentially applying for PAD and will formulate their "best" case. Similarly, physicians may report only what makes sense to them and is justifiable to reporting boards/agencies. Finally, direct or indirect influence by others, including family, community, or society has the potential to unduly affect suffering and the pursuit of PAD.

In addition to general reporting concerns, the role of patient suffering as justification for PAD has significant intrinsic weaknesses. To review, when objective suffering is used, as in the Groningen Protocol, it relies on second-hand judgments of another's life. This either limits the analysis to observable characteristics, such as birth defects, cognitive disabilities, sensory deficits, and functional limitations, or involves value-laden projections about whether a life is not worth living. History attests to the potential abuses associated with this model.

Does subjective suffering do any better? As discussed earlier in this chapter, subjective suffering is often vague and poorly defined, can be applied to almost any condition, is not well understood, has unanswered questions about its mutability, and is not easily approached from a therapeutic perspective. In addition, when applied to PAD, subjective suffering may not be a pure reflection of an individual's values and autonomous preferences because it may be influenced by societal and family pressures and expectations. Consequently, at this time, "patient suffering" is too ambiguous to qualify as the sole basis for legislation supporting PAD. Before considering future physician-assisted dying legislation based exclusively on "patient suffering," more work is needed to refine our understanding of patient suffering, to reduce the possibilities of coercion, and to identify whether other options are available to relieve suffering without terminating life.

Acknowledgment: The author would like to thank Tyler Tate for both his generous and thoughtful feedback during the development of this manuscript and his lucid editorial suggestions.

Disclaimer: The opinions expressed in this article are the author's own and do not reflect the view of the Department of Veterans Affairs, the Veteran's Health Administration (VHA), the VHA National Center for Ethics in Health Care, or the United States government; nor those of the University of Washington.

BIBLIOGRAPHY

Allert, Gebhard, Bela Blasszauer, Kenneth Boyd, et al. 1996. "The Goals of Medicine: Specifying the Goals of Medicine." *Hastings Center Report* 26, no. 6 (Nov–Dec): S9–S14.

Atwill, Nicole. 2008. "Luxembourg: Right to Die with Dignity." *Global Legal Monitor*, March 2, 2008. http://www.loc.gov/law/foreign-news/article/luxembourg -right-to-die-with-dignity/.

Belgian Act on Euthanasia of May 28, 2002 (The). 2002. Translated by Dale Kidd. *Ethical Perspectives* 9, no. 2–3 (May): 182–188. https://alliance-primo.hosted.exli brisgroup.com/primo-explore/fulldisplay?docid=TN_medline15712447&context= PC&vid=UW&search_scope=all&tab=default_tab&lang=en_US.

Bill C-14 Statutes of Canada 2016 (chapter 3). Accessed December 3, 2019. https:// laws-lois.justice.gc.ca/PDF/2016_3.pdf.

Binding, Karl L., and Alfred E. Hoche. (1920) 1992. "Permitting the Destruction of Unworthy Life." Translated by Walter E. Wright. *Issues in Law and Medicine* 8, no. 2: 231–265.

Bozzaro, Claudia, and Jan Schildmann. 2018. "'Suffering' in Palliative Sedation: Conceptual Analysis and Implications for Decision Making in Clinical Practice." *Journal of Pain and Symptom Management* 56, no. 2 (August): 288–294.

California Health and Safety Code (Part 1.85), 2015. "End of Life Options Act." 443.11. Accessed December 3, 2019. https://leginfo.legislature.ca.gov/faces/codes_display Text.xhtml?lawCode=HSC&division=1.&title=&part=1.85.&chaper=&article=.

Cassell, Eric. 2004. *The Nature of Suffering and the Goals of Medicine*, 2nd ed. New York: Oxford University Press.

Colorado's End-of-Life Options Act (Statute 25–48). 2016. Accessed December 3, 2019. https://www.sos.state.co.us/pubs/elections/Initiatives/titleBoard/ filings/2015-2016/145Final.pdf.

Dees, Marianne, Myrra Vernooij-Dassen, Wim Dekkers, Kris Vissers, Chris van Weel. 2011. "Unbearable Suffering: A Qualitative Study on the Perspectives of Patients who Request Assistance in Dying." *Journal of Medical Ethics* 37, no. 12 (December): 727–734. https://doi.org/10.1136/jme.2011.045492.

Dees, Marianne, Myrra Vernooij-Dassen, Wim Dekkers, Glenn Elwyn, Kris Vissers, Chris van Weel. 2012. "Perspectives of Decision-Making in Requests for Euthanasia: A Qualitative Research Among Patients, Relatives and Treating Physicians in the Netherlands." *Palliative Medicine* 27, no. 1 (October): 1–11. https://doi .org/10.1177/0269216312463259.

DeGrazia, David. 2014. "What is Suffering and What Sorts of Beings Can Suffer." In *Suffering and Bioethics*, edited by Ronald M. Green and Nathan J. Palpant, 134–153. New York: Oxford University Press.

Dewey, John. 1894. *The Study of Ethics: A Syllabus*. Ann Arbor, MI: Inland Press.

Emanuel, Ezekiel J., Bregje D. Onwuteaka-Philipsen, John W. Urwin, and Joachim Cohen. 2016. "Attitudes and Practices of Euthanasia and Physician-Assisted Suicide in the United States, Canada, and Europe." *Journal of the American Medical Association* 316, no. 1 (July): 79–90. https://doi.org/10.1001/jama.2016.8499.

Ganzini, Linda, Heidi D. Nelson, Terri A. Schmidt, et al. 2000. "Physician Experiences with the Oregon Death with Dignity Act." *New England Journal of Medicine* 342, no. 8 (February): 557–563. https://doi.org/10.1056/NEJM200002243420806.

Ganzini, Linda, Elizabeth R. Goy, and Steven K. Dobscha. 2009. "Oregonians' Reasons for Requesting Physician Aid in Dying." *Archives of Internal Medicine* 169, no. 5 (March): 489–492. https://doi.org/10.1001/archinternmed2008.579.

Gardella, John E. 1999. "The Cost-Effectiveness of Killing: An Overview of Nazi 'Euthanasia.'" *Medical Sentinel* 4, no. 4 (July–August): 132–135.

Grand Duchy of Luxembourg. 2009. "Euthanasia and Palliative Care." Official Portal of the Grand Duchy of Luxembourg. Accessed December 3, 2019. http://www.luxembourg.public.lu/en/vivre/famille/fin-vie/euthanasie-soinspalliatifs/index.html.

Haverkate, Ilinka, Bregje D. Onwutgeaka-Philipsen, Agnes van der Heide, et al. 2000. "Refused and Granted Requests for Euthanasia and Assisted Suicide in the Netherlands." *British Medical Journal* 321(October): 865–866.

Hawaii House Bill 2739. 2018. Accessed December 3, 2019. https://health.hawaii.gov/opppd/files/2018/11/OCOC-Act2.pdf.

Hayes, Steven C., Jason B. Luoma, Frank W. Bond, Akihiko Masuda, and Jason Lillis. 2006. "Acceptance and Commitment Therapy: Model, Processes and Outcomes." *Psychology Faculty Publications.* 101: 1–30. https://scholarworks.gsu.edu/psych_facpub/101.

Hedberg, Katrina, and Craig New. 2017. "Oregon's Death with Dignity Act: 20 Years of Experience to Inform the Debate." *Annals of Internal Medicine* 167, no. 8 (October): 579–583. https://doi.org/10.7326/M17-2300.

Hoffmaster, Barry. 2014. "Understanding Suffering." In *Suffering and Bioethics*, edited by Ronald M. Green and Nathan J. Palpant, 31–53. New York: Oxford University Press.

Joseph, Jay, and Norbert A. Wetzel. 2013. "Ernst Rüdin: Hitler's Racial Hygiene Mastermind." *Journal of History of Biology* 46, no.1 (November): 1–30. https://doi.org/10.1007/s10739-012-9344-6.

Kodish, Eric. 2008. "Paediatric Ethics: A Repudiation of the Groningen Protocol." *Lancet* 371: 892–893.

Lifton, Robert J. 1986. *The Nazi Doctors: Medical Killing and the Psychology of Genocide*. New York: Basic Books.

Loggers, Elizabeth T., Helene Starks, Moreen Shannon-Dudley, Anthony L. Back, Frederick R. Appelbaum, and F. Marc Stewart. 2013. "Implementing a Death with Dignity Program at a Comprehensive Cancer Center." *New England Journal of Medicine* 368, no. 15 (April): 1417–1424. https://doi.org/10.1056/NEJMsa1213398.

Oregon Health Authority. 2017 Edition. *Oregon Revised Statute: Oregon's Death with Dignity Act* Section 3: 127.820§3.02 and §3.03. Accessed December 3, 2019. https://www.oregonlegislature.gov/bills_laws/ors/ors127.html.

Pasman, H. R. W., M. L. Rurup, D. L. Willems, and B. D. Onwutgeaka-Philipsen. 2009. "Concept of Unbearable Suffering in Context of Ungranted Requests for Euthanasia." *British Medical Journal* 339, no. 1349 (November 16): 1235–1237. https://doi.org/10.1136/bmj.b4362.

Pearlman, Robert A, Clarissa Hsu, Helene Starks, et al. 2005. "Motivations for Physician-Assisted Suicide: Patient and Family Voices." *Journal of General Internal Medicine* 20, no. 3 (March): 234–239. https://doi.org/10.1111/j.1525-1497.2005.40225.x.

Pearlman, Robert A., Kevin C. Cain, Donald L. Patrick, et al. 1993. "Insights into Treatment Preferences: States Worse Than Death." *Journal of Clinical Ethics* 4, no. 1 (February): 33–40.

Peter, W. W. 1934. "Germany's Sterilization Program." *American Journal of Public Health* 24, no. 3 (March): 187–191. https://doi.org/10.2105/AJPH.24.3.187.

Pine, Fred. 1985. *Development Theory and Clinical Process.* New Haven: Yale University Press.

Proctor, Robert N. 1988. *Racial Hygiene: Medicine Under the Nazis.* Cambridge, MA: Harvard University Press.

Regional Euthanasia Review Committees (Netherlands). 2013. "Annual Report 2013." Accessed December 3, 2019. https://www.euthanasiecommissie.nl/binaries/euthanasiecommissie/documenten/jaarverslagen/2013/nl-en-du-fr/nl-en-du-fr/jaarverslag-2013/annual-report-2013-tcm52-48.pdf.

Rietjens, Judith A. C., Paul J. van der Maas, Bregje D. Onwutgeaka-Philipsen, Johannes J. M. van Delden, and Agnes van der Heide. 2009. "Two Decades of Research on Euthanasia from the Netherlands: What Have We Learnt and What Questions Remain?" *Bioethical Inquiry* 6, no. 3 (September): 271–283.

Schmidt, Ulf. 2002. *Medical Films, Ethics and Euthanasia in Nazi Germany: The History of Medical Research and Teaching Films of the Reich Office for Educational Films/Reich Institute for Films in Science and Education, 1933–1945.* Husum, Germany: Matthiesen Verlag.

Smets, Tinne, Johan Bilsen, Joachim Cohen, Metta L. Rurup, and Luc Deliens. 2010. "Legal Euthanasia in Belgium. Characteristics of All Reported Euthanasia Cases." *Medical Care* 48, no. 2 (February): 187–192.

Spross, Judith A. 1993. "Pain, Suffering, and Spiritual Well-Being: Assessment and Interventions." *Quality of Life—A Nursing Challenge* 2, no. 3: 71–79.

Steinbrook, Robert. 2008. "Physician-Assisted Death—From Oregon to Washington State." *New England Journal of Medicine* 359, no. 24 (December): 2513–2514.

Stoughton, Richard B. "The Heartbreak of Psoriasis." *Journal of the American Medical Association* 229, no. 3 (July): 334. https://doi:10.1001/jama.1974.03230410058032.

Strang, Peter, Susan Strang, Ragnar Hultborn, and Staffan Arner. 2004. "Existential Pain—An Entity, a Provocation or a Challenge?" *Journal of Pain and Symptom Management* 27, no. 3 (March): 241–249. https://doi.org/10.1016/j:jpainsymman.2003.07.003.

Tate, Tyler, and Robert A. Pearlman. 2019. "What We Mean When We Talk about Suffering—And Why Eric Cassell Should Not Have the Last Word." *Perspectives in Biology and Medicine* 62, no. 1 (Winter): 95–110.

van Hooft, Stan. 1998. "Suffering and the Goals of Medicine." *Medicine, Health Care and Philosophy* 1 no. 2 (May): 125–131.

Verhagen, Eduard, and Pieter J. Sauer. 2005. "The Groningen Protocol—Euthanasia in Severely Ill Newborns." *New England Journal of Medicine* 352, no. 10 (March): 959–962.

Vermont General Assembly. 2014. *Chapter 113. Patient Choice at the End of Life*: 4. Accessed December 3, 2019. https://legislature.vermont.gov/statutes/chapter/18/113.

Washington State Department of Health, Disease Control and Health Statistics Division. 2018. *Washington State 2017 Death with Dignity Act Report*: 8.

World Health Organization. 2004. "WHO Definition of Palliative Care." Accessed December 3, 2019. https://www.who.int/cancer/palliative/definition/en/.

Wunder, Michael. 2015. "Learning with History: Nazi Medical Crimes and Today's Debates on Euthanasia in Germany." In *Science, Scapegoats, Self-Reflection: The Shadow of Nazi Medical Crimes on Medicine and Bioethics*, edited by Roelcke Volker, Etienne Lepicard, and Sascha Topp, 301–312. Germany: V&R unipress.

Chapter Twelve

Physician Countertransference and Patient Requests for a Hastened Death

Diane E. Meier

In May 2018, I went to Germany with the Center for Medicine After the Holocaust, an international organization based in Houston that challenges "doctors, nurses, and bioscientists to personally confront the medical ethics of the Holocaust and to apply that knowledge to contemporary practice and research." This trip was designed to explore the modern implications of Nazi physicians' justifications for the belief that some lives are "unworthy of life" and thus eligible for "mercy killing," or "euthanasia." The social process of prioritizing the greater good over the rights of individuals was conceptualized and led by German physicians and led directly to the Final Solution.

I had been unaware of this history and found it deeply disturbing, especially in the context of legalization of physician aid in dying (PAD) in both Canada and the United States. The behavior of physicians during the Third Reich casts doubt on the trustworthiness and reliability of present-day physicians, especially their willingness and ability to prevent either involuntary aid in dying or ending the lives of ineligible patients based on the judgment by others that certain patients' lives are no longer worth living.

In this chapter, I will argue that legalizing PAD is unwise. Three considerations lead me to this conclusion: (1) The safeguards purported to prevent misuse are unrealistic and demonstrably ineffective; (2) physicians are poor gatekeepers—we are imperfect and vulnerable humans, subject to internal and external pressures and, based on both past and recent evidence, not able to protect the most vulnerable patients from decisions made by others about the worthiness of their lives; and (3) public policy must rely not only on majority opinion but also on assurances that patients, especially the most vulnerable, will be protected from harm.

SAFEGUARDS PURPORTED TO PREVENT MISUSE ARE
UNREALISTIC AND DEMONSTRABLY INEFFECTIVE

As of 2019, eight states and the District of Columbia have legalized PAD and 14 more are considering similar legislation (Compassion & Choices 2019). Most of the ballot measures or legislation frame PAD this way: (1) PAD is a rational alternative to unbearable physical suffering; (2) patients must make a clearly autonomous request; (3) a physician must carefully evaluate each patient for potentially remediable causes of suffering; and (4) each patient ultimately self-administers a lethal dose of medication prescribed by the physician. Arguments for legalization include beneficence, the obligation of physicians to do good for patients, and a patient's right to control his or her life and death. As Brittany Maynard, a young and articulate terminally ill woman who advocated for and chose PAD, was widely quoted:

> But even with palliative medication, I could develop potentially morphine-resistant pain and suffer personality changes and verbal, cognitive and motor loss of virtually any kind . . . I would not tell anyone else that he or she should choose death with dignity. My question is: Who has the right to tell me that I don't deserve this choice? That I deserve to suffer for weeks or months in tremendous amounts of physical and emotional pain? Why should anyone have the right to make that choice for me? (Maynard 2014, 3)

Based on data from Oregon, the first state to legalize PAD, proponents assert that legislation will prevent misuse if it includes the following safeguards:

- Physicians determine patient eligibility for PAD.
- There must be a determination that the patient is of "sound mind."
- The patient must have a terminal illness.
- The patient must repeat the request to die over the course of his or her illness.
- The patient must self-administer the lethal prescription drug.

I argue that proponents of these safeguards make incorrect assumptions about a physician's ability to prognosticate, to determine a patient's decisional capacity, and to identify and treat depression and other psychiatric illnesses.

Physician prognostic assessments are often wrong (White et al. 2016). In Canada, Belgium, and the Netherlands, a prognosis of less than six months is not required (Wales et al. 2018; Ontario Ministry of Health n.d.; Buiting et al. 2009; Dierickx et al. 2016). The key variable is the patient's and physician's assessment of irremediable suffering, implying that elimination of suffering is a valid expectation and societal goal, and that suffering per se is sufficient justification for PAD, which would increase eligibility for multitudes. For example, in 2019, Oregon's legislature considered changing the definition of a terminal disease to include "a degenerative disease that will, at some point in the future, be the cause of the patient's death" (Oregon Legislative Assembly 2019).

The ability to determine a patient's decisional capacity requires training that many, if not most, physicians have never had. It also requires sufficient physician time to assess a patient's ability to communicate with others, and to listen, hear, and assess the patient's understanding of their medical circumstances, treatment options, fears, and rationales for considering PAD—no physician has sufficient time. The physician must also be aware that what sounds like a rational patient decision is often a cover for depression, hopelessness, rage, and fear (Quill 1993; Quill, Lee, and Nunn 2000), and must be both willing to invest the time and skilled in talking with patients about these complex issues. Shortcuts are inevitable given that most physicians lack the necessary training and time. For example, the Northern Territory in Australia committed to substantial, expensive regulatory protections for patients with mental health issues, including mandatory psychiatric evaluations. The psychiatrists recognized their inability to serve as gatekeepers (Kissane, Street, and Nitschke 1998), and the law was ultimately reversed (Fleming 2000).

Depression and other mood disorders have a higher prevalence among patients with serious and chronic medical illness compared to the general population (Kok and Reynolds 2017; Djernes 2006; Katon 2011). Physicians miss the diagnosis of depression in the majority of patients, and many are unaware that depression is a treatable and remediable disorder (Kok and Reynolds 2017). Even when depression is identified, doctors may wrongly assume that it is normal to be depressed or that they themselves would be depressed when faced with a serious progressive illness. Depressed or hopeless patients are much more likely to think about and request PAD (Hicks 2006).

Despite the regulatory requirement that doctors refer patients for psychiatric consultation if they suspect depression, such referral rarely takes place, either because the depression is unrecognized, referral is a hassle, the patient may be angry about the referral, the doctor feels a hastened death is appropriate given the circumstances, or other unknown reasons (Ganzini, Goy, and Dobscha 2008; Ganzini et al. 1993; Ganzini, Silveira, and Johnston 2002). Even in the instances where psychiatric evaluation occurs and establishes that the patient is not eligible for PAD, the hastened death sometimes still takes place. For example, in Oregon, at least one patient who was denied PAD because of dementia was able to "doctor shop" until they found an agreeable physician (Osler 1999). Furthermore, in Holland and Belgium, where patients with psychological suffering are eligible for both PAD and euthanasia, the evaluation and hastened death may be carried out by the patient's own psychiatrist (Naudts et al. 2006; Miller and Kim 2017; Thienpont et al. 2015).

Early proponents of PAD often painted an unrealistic or idealized portrait of the procedure:

> We are told to presume that decisions to commit assisted suicide would take place in the bosoms of loving families, that suicide would be facilitated by family doctors who have known the patient for decades and are intimately familiar with their values, and that assisted suicide would only be used as a last resort engaged in with great reluctance when nothing else could be done to alleviate intolerable pain. (Center for Bioethics and Culture Network 2006)

Perhaps because the initial eligibility criteria for PAD were unrealistic, there is evidence of what ethicists call eligibility creep; others might call it a slippery slope. As physician experience with PAD increases and more doctors become accustomed to helping people die, eligibility restrictions expand or are eliminated altogether, thereby affording a broader group of sufferers the same privilege.

Canada's parliament did not require the presence of a terminal illness for eligibility in its Medical Assistance in Dying law, and is considering extending this right to "mature minors," the mentally ill, and the cognitively impaired (Coletta 2018). In Holland, physician's growing willingness to help non-terminal patients die, including patients with dementia or mental illness and children, and documentation of euthanasia without consent suggest the real possibility of a slippery slope for PAD (Wunder 2014). In 2016, 141 euthanasia deaths were reported among people with mental illness or dementia (Doernberg, Peteet, and Kim 2016; Kim, De Vries, and Peteet 2016), leading one of its strongest initial proponents, a psychiatrist, to say, ". . . it really went off the tracks when the review committee concealed that incapacitated people were surreptitiously killed. I don't see how we can get the genie back in the bottle. It would already mean a lot if we'd acknowledge he's out" (Chabot 2017). These data indicate that regulatory safeguards are ineffective at protecting patients and society from misapplication of PAD to ineligible patients.

Existential distress about real or anticipated losses is universal, and it is not an adequate basis for expecting physicians to help to end a life. Fixing all suffering is not given to us. "Almost all lethal diseases will reduce life's pleasures and an individual's autonomy. Physicians cannot and should not be expected to use physician aid in dying to relieve that existential burden" (Dugdale and Callahan 2017).

WHY DOCTORS?

One possible reason for placing legal responsibility for eligibility decisions on doctors is that physician involvement lessens the stigma of suicide and legitimizes it as an acceptable medical decision. Another is that physicians can write prescriptions for lethal drugs that may seem to be a gentle, less terrifying method of hastening death. While legislators assume that physicians can safely assess and support suicidal patients, the evidence suggests that physicians are not objective, impartial, or uniformly skilled in communication and in identifying and treating depression and other sources of suffering (Miller and Kim 2017; Hicks 2006; Stevens 2006); nor do they uniformly provide the intensive and time-consuming attention that is required to care for patients in despair. Faith in physicians as wise and safe gatekeepers for socially sanctioned medical hastening of death is almost touchingly naïve, given the evidence to the contrary. If it is assumed that physicians represent the safe therapeutic frame (or holding space) for intense emotion, what does it mean if physicians, the safe frame, agree that the patient is better off dead? Wishful thinking? As surmised by Madelyn Hicks (Hicks 2006), perhaps ". . . society wishes doctors to be omnipotent and beneficent, providing reassurance, sanctioning its choices, and absolving it of responsibility for life and death decisions."

WHY NOT DOCTORS?

While all policies enabling PAD include criteria for patient eligibility and require physicians to serve as the decision-makers, none establish training or threshold competency criteria for the physicians charged with ensuring the safety and appropriateness of the decision. Here are two reasons to worry about this.

Family Coercion

Legislators legislate as if each and every patient requesting PAD acts with pure autonomy and self-determination. However, as a social animal embedded in and influenced by our family and society, no person's behavior is purely autonomous, and publications suggest that family and social coercion are real (Emanuel 1999), and physicians are not well trained to deal with these issues when patients request PAD. Physicians describe feeling intimidated and coerced ("I learned very quickly that the patient's agenda was to get the medication: When I try to talk them out of it, or to really assess their motivations, then they perceived me as obstructionist and became quite resentful . . .") (Stevens 2006, 196). Other physicians felt they had to accede to the request for PAD out of fear of disappointing the family ("If I backed out, they'd feel about me the way they had about their previous doctor, that I had strung them along, and in a way, insulted them")

(Stevens 2006, 194). Vulnerable patients, aware of the multidimensional burdens that their needs are imposing on their families, and their physicians, describe family coercion as a difficult-to-resist force (Stevens 2006; Hicks 2006). In these circumstances, access to a legal option that avoids prolonged and expensive end-of-life care may have undeniable appeal to the patient's family, but not necessarily to the patient.

I have personally witnessed family pressure on several occasions in New York where PAD is illegal. In one instance the wife of a patient with recurrent glioblastoma asked to discuss his care options. Because of his immobility, I visited them at home and discovered that the actual purpose of the request was for me to hasten his death. As I explored the patient's request and fears, he looked at his wife and did not answer; his wife did. I explained that palliative care could relieve many of the patient's symptoms and provide support for both the patient and his family for the rest of his life. The patient asked questions about home care options and the process of dying, and he seemed reassured by my answers. His wife, however, appeared irritated, saying, "We know all about hospice and we are not interested." When I asked to speak with him alone, she thanked me for coming and escorted me to the door. Had PAD been legal in NY at the time, I have no doubt that she would have found a willing prescriber to hasten her husband's death, even though he had months or years to live. When family members are stressed and burdened by their role, or when the illness is bankrupting the family, the patient gets the message.

Countertransference

Countertransference is defined as feelings arising in the physician occasioned by the care of the patient. These feelings may be conscious—"this patient reminds me of my daughter"—but are often unconscious—"this patient reminds me of my angry judgmental father; get me out of here." Because non-psychiatrist physicians are not usually aware of the normalcy and universality of countertransference, and because they are not trained to use it as a therapeutic tool, they ordinarily do not monitor the impact of their own feelings on the patient's thinking—"when I walk into this room, I feel angry and tense. I bet that's how the patient and his family are feeling,"—which may cause harm to the patient such as abandonment—"I just want to get out of this room as soon as I can." When these inevitable, natural, and appropriate feelings are heightened by the charged and pressured nature of a request for PAD, or by a patient's or a family member's angry insistence on the right to die with the physician's help, then physicians may have difficulty withstanding these pressures (Kelly, Varghese, and Pelusi 2003). Their understandable feelings of rage, irritation, and imposition are professionally unacceptable (Miles 1995), hence suppressed, and may lead them to withdraw, disengage, and/or abandon via acquiescence.

The countertransference feelings evoked in a physician by a request for PAD are likely to be powerful: anxiety in the face of the inevitability of death, disease, and decline; inadequacy for not being able to save or fix the patient; and hatred of the patient who won't try antidepressants or analgesics, who is not responding to treatment, and/or who demands too much time and attention. These unconscious feelings can influence a physician's decision to prescribe lethal medications without any awareness that the decision is driven by considerations other than the best interest of the patient.

The physician's own subjective evaluation of a patient's quality of life as unbearable—"I would want to die if I were facing this disease"—further underscores the risks of countertransference. The patient is now more vulnerable because he or she is subject to the physician's personal and unconscious fears about illness, disability, and death. Pseudoempathy, a physician's unconscious over-identification with the patient, may lead to affirmation of the patient's request because the doctor thinks the illness would be a fate worse than death for him or her. Such a patient may not hear the physician's assent to the prescription as expressive of the *physician's* own feelings of despair, fear, and failure. Rather, the patient may take the physician's assent as agreement with the patient's assessment that his or her life is not worth living and that he or she would be better off dead (Farber and Farber 2016).

The facility with which Nazi doctors and scientists accepted the eugenic notion that some lives are worthier than others and the rationality of eliminating the infirm or ill to achieve a healthier society should give us pause about empowering physicians as decision-makers. "The distinction between 'worthy to live' and 'unworthy to live' is inherent in the . . . medical thinking oriented only toward healing rather than alleviation and palliation. . . . The medical attitude to heal at any price is obviously close to the attitude to exterminate in cases of failure or incurability" (Wunder 2014, 304).

Physicians' unconscious fears of patient rage and of being pressured to fix the patient's despair is identified in the psychiatric literature as a common concomitant of psychiatric care for suicidal patients (Hendin et al. 2004). The patient's rage and anger toward the psychiatrist is hard to bear and evokes the clinician's own unconscious rage and shame about being overwhelmed by the patient's excessive and unmeetable demands. There is also shame at failing to restore the patient's will to live. Attempts to set limits on overwhelming patient demands may feel punitive or dangerous, especially if the patient is terminally ill, leaving clinicians feeling as if they must either abandon the patient or accede to extraordinary demands, up to and including helping the patient to die (Kelly and Varghese 2016). Contrary to the reality and universality of such physician countertransference, regulatory guidelines for PAD assume, based on no data, that physicians can objectively determine patient eligibility uninfluenced by their own unconscious feelings.

Professional attributes of doctors also heighten the power of countertransference and increase the likelihood that they may act unconsciously in response to their own needs, rather than to those of the patient. As professionals, we doctors have an unusually high and often rigid need for control, feel responsible even for things outside our immediate control, and have high levels of self-criticism, guilt, and perfectionism, all of which are threatened in the confrontation with a seriously ill patient facing death, the ultimate medical failure.

Physicians, by definition, are driven by a desire to help, to cure, to fix their patients. Some have argued that an unusually high fear of death and need to control it underlies career motivation for many physicians and leads to avoidance of dying patients, discomfort talking with these patients, and an inability to hear and allay patients' fears and worries (Corn 2013). As a profession, doctors seek control over the disease, and they may not tolerate the inevitable uncertainty, lack of control, and suffering associated with a serious illness (Kelly, Varghese, and Pelusi 2003; Kelly and Varghese 2016; Meier, Back, and Morrison 2001).

Legalization of PAD without acknowledging physician's limited ability to recognize, understand, and properly utilize countertransference for the patient's benefit carries risk:

> The failure of the clinician to be alert to psychiatric comorbidity such as depression, the inclination to minimize the psychosocial needs of the patient, or the failure to carefully assess such needs, may represent countertransference enactment of [physician] feelings such as hopelessness and nihilism about the terminally ill patient. . . . As Muskin [1998] has stated, the failure to explore the meaning and the basis of the patient's request for hastened death is the real violation of the rights of a dying patient. (Kelly, Varghese, and Pelusi 2003, 372)

The phrase "Don't just stand there—do something!" is commonly quoted in hospitals, alluding to doctors' need to act, even when the action is intentionally ending the patient's life. A better response is aggressive palliative care, being present, listening, and not abandoning the patient through this critical stage of life. Acting affirmatively, by helping the patient to die, restores the illusion of control for both, and the patient's death resolves the anxiety and distress that both had been feeling.

THE REQUEST TO DIE

The meaning of the request has a differential diagnosis: Quill et al. have argued that the etiology of most patients' requests to die is something treatable or remediable (Quill, Coombs Lee, and Nunn 2000; Quill, Cassel, and Meier 1992). Etiologies include fear of what is to come, poorly managed pain or other physical symptoms, unrecognized and/or untreated depression or other psychiatric illnesses, financial anxieties, anger (about the diagnosis, at God, at the doctors, at family members) and guilt (for failing treatment, letting down their doctor, or past behaviors). Patients harbor common and, sadly, realistic fears near the end of their lives, such as being a burden, dying alone, pain, indignity, distress, and abandonment by either their family or doctors—"Will you still be my doctor now that I have failed your treatments?" Exploring the differential diagnosis of a request for a hastened death requires training, supervision, wisdom, and the scarcest resource of all, time to explore the request.

The types of questions to ask and issues to raise when a patient requests PAD include:

- Why now?
- What has changed?
- Tell me about your fears about the future.
- Tell me about what has made your life worth living.
- What are you most proud of?
- What are you most worried about?
- Tell me about your family.
- What are your key relationships and their status?
- What gives you meaning and purpose?

Renee Katz writes: "Desire to die statements should trigger thoughtful, unhurried conversations with our patients and families in which we seek to understand the request without embedding it with our interpretations, assumptions, or projections" (Katz and Johnson 2016). Anyone who has been in a doctor's waiting or exam room recently will realize the impossibility of this idealized response—very few physicians have the training and the time. Basing a law on the assumption that an optimal or even adequate evaluation will reliably and routinely occur is fantasy.

What should happen when patients request help to die? When patients request help to die, their physicians should encourage discussion of patients' fears that life in the future will be unbearable. Chochinov has shown that terminally ill patients' desire to die can diminish, perhaps because of treatment of depression, resilience in adjusting to a new normal over time, or the reality not being as bad as the fantasy (Chochinov et al. 1995).

As with any suicidal patient, dying patients requesting PAD are sharing their fears or beliefs that their lives no longer have value and meaning for them or for others. Those people closest to dying patients may be overwhelmed by caregiving responsibilities and, consciously or unconsciously, give the impression that the patient's life is not worth living. Families may attempt to coerce patients and/or their doctors to hasten death to relieve their burdens. Physicians, on the other hand, are professionally obligated to advocate for sustaining a dying patient's life and for palliative care, regardless of the patient's or the family's opposition. In one description (Hamilton et al. 1998), a man with advanced chronic obstructive pulmonary disease asked his physician, "Can't you do something to just bring it to an end ? . . . Just put me out of my misery. It would save everyone a lot of trouble." The doctor replied, "Even though you feel like a burden, I can't do that." The patient asks, "Why not? You'd do it for your dog." The doctor answers "Because you aren't a dog. You're my patient and I'm your doctor, and I'm trying to help you. And I'll keep trying to help you as long as I have to." The patient took the doctor's hand in both of his and said, "Thank god, I thought everyone had given up on me." Confirming this case study, Barnard wrote, "The sting of illness and death is the specter of broken relationships and the loss of the world. Over and against this threat stand the efforts of caregivers and companions to embrace the sufferer and continuously reaffirm his or her capacity for relationship" (Barnard 1995).

THE ROLE OF PUBLIC POLICY

Legalizing PAD assumes that all licensed physicians are equally capable of responding appropriately, carefully, and patiently to patient requests. This assumption would be funny if it were not so absurd and frightening. A public policy, by definition, has to protect the public from harm but, in regard to PAD, such protection cannot be ensured by safeguards. In my view, the majority of physicians in practice have neither the training, the time, nor even the interest to help their distressed patients find reasons to live. Furthermore, society does not seem interested in paying for palliative care training and resources to support dying patients. Legalization also assumes that physicians are neutral about PAD and have no conscious or unconscious motivations to believe that not only the patient, but they themselves, would be better off if they hastened the patient's death. It is challenging and emotionally exhausting to accompany patients through a difficult illness (Katz and Johnson

2016). When dying patients ask or insist, when overwhelmed and burdened families pressure, when the law permits, when colleagues participate, and when the daily efforts to resist are exhausting, doctors might rationally conclude that writing a lethal prescription is the easiest and cheapest thing to do.

Our society, especially its patients and clinicians, needs to acknowledge the limits of human control over death. In the hospital where I trained, the obstetrics unit had a sign over the door that said, "No baby before its time." Perhaps we need similar signs that say, "No death before its time." Some things are not given to us: "Even in palliative care, not every health problem can be solved" (Müller-Busch 2018).

In closing, I will relate the story of Dr. Stu Farber, my former palliative medicine colleague, who died of leukemia in 2015. Bizarrely, his wife received the same diagnosis some months after he did. They both used the time before his death to reflect on and write about what they learned as patients (Farber and Farber 2016). First, living with a fatal illness taught them that "uncertainty is a given and control is an illusion." Second, they saw clearly how deeply invested their doctors were in that illusion of control, "Yet every clinician Annalu and I have interacted with is more afraid of death than we are; they focus on solving the problems of our illness with little awareness of how we want to live our lives. It is a paradox. The clinician is focusing on treating the illness that threatens life but the life of the person who is ill is invisible." Third, even when he expresses his grief and sadness to them:

> I have been amazed at the distance my providers keep from my grief, and when it is touched, how quickly they are bound to "fixing" it. Most of my clinicians are so busy protecting themselves that "being with me" is not possible. . . . As I sit with my medical caregivers, I see fear of failure at the center of their consciousness, with death being the ultimate defeat. (Farber 2015)

Stu published these reflections as a legacy to us, his colleagues. Perhaps he had the right prescription when there is no fix: a meaningful and committed human connection instead of a prescription for 2 grams of Seconal.

BIBLIOGRAPHY

Barnard, David. 1995. "The Promise of Intimacy and the Fear of Our Own Undoing." *Journal of Palliative Care* 11, no. 4 (December): 22–26.

Buiting, Hilde, Johannes van Delden, Bregje Onwuteaka-Philipsen, et al. 2009. "Reporting of Euthanasia and Phsycian Assisted Suicide in the Netherlands: Descriptive Study." *BMC Medical Ethics* 10, no. 18 (October): 18. doi:10.1186/1472 -6939-10-18.

Center for Bioethics and Culture Network. 2006. "The Dysfunctional Context in Which Assisted Suicide Would Be Practiced." October 15, 2006. http://www.cbc-network.org/2006/10/the-dysfunctional-context-in-which-assisted-suicide-would-be-practiced/.

Chabot, Boudewijn. 2017. "Worrisome Culture Shift in the Context of Self-Selected Death." NRC Handelsbad, June 16, 2017. Translated by Trudo Lemmens. https://trudolemmens.wordpress.com/2017/06/19/the-euthanasia-genie-is-out-of-the-bottle-by-boudewijn-chabot-translation/.

Chochinov, Harvey M., Keith G. Wilson, M. Enns, et al. 1995. "Desire for Death in the Terminally Ill." *American Journal of Psychiatry* 152, no. 8 (August): 1185–91.

Coletta, Amanda. 2018. "'The Right Time to Die': Canada's Law Allowing Physician-Assisted Suicide Faces Criticism over Restrictions." *Washington Post*. November 15, 2018. https://www.washingtonpost.com/world/2018/11/15/right-time-die-canadas-law-allowing-physician-assisted-suicide-faces-criticism-over-restrictions/?noredirect=on&utm_term=.0688b9f777de.

Compassion & Choices. 2019. "In Your State." Compassion & Choices website. Accessed November 22, 2019. https://compassionandchoices.org/in-your-state.

Corn, Benjamin. 2013. "Are Physicians More Afraid of Death Than the General Population?" KevinMD.com. (blog), April 1, 2013. https://www.kevinmd.com/blog/2013/04/physicians-afraid-death-general-population.html.

Dierickx, Sigrid, Luc Deliens, Joachim Cohen, and Kenneth Chambaere. 2016. "Euthanasia in Belgium: Trends in Reported Cases between 2003 and 2013." *Canadian Medicine Association Journal* 188, no. 16 (September): E407-E414. doi: https://doi.org/10.1503.cmaj.160202.

Djernes, Jens K. 2006. "Prevalence and Predictors of Depression in Populations of Elderly: A Review." *Acta Psychiatrica Scandinavica* 113, no. 5 (May): 372–87.

Doernberg, Samuel N., John Peteet, and Scott Y. H. Kim. 2016. "Capacity Evaluations of Psychiatric Patients Requesting Assisted Death in the Netherlands." *Psychosomatics* 57, no. 6 (June): 556–65.

Dugdale, Lydia, and Daniel Callahan. 2017. "Assisted Death and the Public Good." *Southern Medical Journal* 110, no. 9 (September): 559–61. doi: 10.14423/SMJ.000000000000690.

Emanuel, Ezekiel J. 1999. "What Is the Great Benefit of Legalizing Euthanasia or Physician-Assisted Suicide?" *Ethics* 109, no. 3 (April): 629–642. Accessed November 23, 2019. http://kcsschmidt.com/BME2016/Emanuel-whatisbenefit.pdf.

Farber, Annalu, and Stu Farber. 2016. "The Respectful Death Model." In *When Professionals Weep: Emotional and Countertransference Responses in Pallative and End-of-Life Care*, edited by Renee S. Katz and Therese A. Johnson, 177–187. New York: Routledge.

Farber, Stu. 2015. "Living Every Minute." *Journal of Pain and Symptom Management* 49, no. 4 (April): 796–800.

Fleming, John. 2000. "Death, Dying, and Euthanasia: Australia versus the Northern Territory." *Issues in Law & Medicine* 15, no. 3 (Spring): 291–305. Accessed November 23, 2019. https://www.ncbi.nlm.nih.gov/pubmed/10758701.

Ganzini, Linda, Elizabeth R. Goy, and Steven Dobscha. 2008. "Prevalence of Depression and Anxiety in Patients Requesting Physicians' Aid in Dying: Cross Sectional Survey." *British Medical Journal* 337, no. 7676 (February): a1682. DOI: 10.1136/bmj.a1682.

Ganzini, Linda, M. A. Lee, R. T. Heintz, and Joseph Bloom. 1993. "Depression, Suicide, and the Right to Refuse Life-Sustaining Treatment." *Journal of Clinical Ethics* 4 (Winter): 337–40.

Ganzini, Linda, Maria J. Silveira, and Wendy S. Johnston. 2002. "Predictors and Correlates of Interest in Assisted Suicide in the Final Month of Life Among ALS Patients in Oregon and Washington." *Journal of Pain and Symptom Management* 24, no. 3 (September): 312–17. https;//doi.org/10.1016/S0885-3924(02)00496-7.

Hamilton, N. Gregory, Pamela J. Edwards, James K. Boehnlein, and Catherine A. Hamilton. 1998. "The Doctor-Patient Relationship and Assisted Suicide: A Contribution from Dynamic Psychiatry." *American Journal of Forensic Psychiatry* 19, no. 2: 59–75.

Hendin, Herbert, Ann Pollinger Haas, John T. Maltsberger, Katalin Szanto, and Heather Rabinowicz. 2004. "Factors Contributing to Therapists' Distress after the Suicide of a Patient." *American Journal of Psychiatry* 161, no. 8 (August): 1442–46.

Hicks, Madelyn. 2006. "Physician-Assisted Suicide: A Review of the Literature Concerning Practical and Clinical Implications for UK Doctors." *BMC Family Practice* 7, no. 7 (June): 39.

Katon, Wayne J. 2011. "Epidemiology and Treatment of Depression in Patients with Chronic Medical Illness." *Dialogues in Clinical Neuroscience* 13, no. 1 (Mar.): 7–23.

Katz, Renee S., and Therese A. Johnson. 2016. "The Desire to Die: Voices from the Trenches." In *When Professionals Weep: Emotional and Countertransference Responses in Pallative and End-of-Life Care*, edited by Renee S. Katz and Therese A. Johnson, 153–60. New York: Routledge.

Kelly, Brian, and Francis T. N. Varghese. 2016. "The Seduction of Autonomy: Countertransference and Assisted Suicide." In *When Professionals Weep: Emotional and Countertransference Responses in Pallative and End-of-Life Care*, edited by Renee S. Katz and Therese A. Johnson, 137–51. NY: Routledge.

Kelly, Brian, Francis T. N. Varghese, and Dan Pelusi. 2003. "Countertransference and Ethics: A Perspective on Clinical Dilemmas in End-of-Life Decisions." *Palliative and Supportive Care* 1, no. 4 (January): 367–75.

Kim, Scott Y. H., Raymond G. De Vries, and John R. Peteet. 2016. "Euthanasia and Assisted Suicide of Patients with Psychiatric Disorders in the Netherlands 2011–2014." *JAMA Psychiatry* 73, no. 4 (April): 362–68. doi:10.1001/jamapsychiatry.2015.2887.

Kissane, David W., Annette Street, and Philip Nitschke. 1998. "Seven Deaths in Darwin: Case Studies Under the Rights of the Terminally Ill Act, Northern Territory, Australia." *Lancet* 352, no. 9134 (October): 1097–1102.

Kok, Rob M., and Charles F. Reynolds III. 2017. "Management of Depression in Older Adults: A Review." *Journal of the American Medical Association* 317, no. 20 (May): 2114–22. doi:10.1001/jama.2017.5706.

Maynard, Brittany. 2014. "My Right to Death with Dignity at 29." Posted November 2, 2014. http://scholar.google.com/scholar_url?url=http://fd.valenciacollege.edu/file/jcarpen1/Partner_Argument_Article2.docx&hl=en&sa=X&scisig=AAGBfm1XBuEbC_hkLkcfIG7nIMrYGxKLXg&nossl=1&oi=scholarr.

Meier, Diane E., Anthony L. Back, and R. Sean Morrison. 2001. "The Inner Life of Physicians and Care of the Seriously Ill." *Journal of the American Medical Association* 286, no. 23 (December): 3007–14. doi:10.1001/jama.286.23.3007.

Miles, Steven H. 1995. "Physician-Assisted Suicide and the Profession's Gyrocompass." *Hastings Center Report* 25, no. 3 (May–June): 17–19.

Miller, David G., and Scott Y. H. Kim. 2017. "Euthanasia and Physician-Assisted Suicide Not Meeting Due Care Criteria in the Netherlands: A Qualitative Review of Review Committee Judgements." *BMJ Open* 7, no. 10 (October): e017628. doi: 10.1136/bmjopen-2017-017628.

Müller-Busch, H. Christof. 2018. Lecture series at Center for Medicine after the Holocaust Berlin Seminar, May 18, 2018.

Muskin, Philip R. 1998. "The Request to Die: Role for a Psychodynamic Perspective on Physician-Assisted Suicide." *Journal of the American Medical Association* 279, no. 4 (January): 323–28.

Naudts, Kris, Caroline Ducatelle, Jozsef Kovacs, Kristin Laurens, Frederique van den Eynde, and Cornelis van Heeringen. 2006. "Euthanasia: The Role of the Psychiatrist." *British Journal of Psychiatry* 188 (May): 405–9.

Ontario Ministry of Health. n.d. "Medical Assistance in Dying." Accessed December 3, 2019. http://health.gov.on.ca/en/pro/programs/maid/#eligibility.

Oregon Legislative Assembly (80th). 2019. House Bill 2903. Accessed November 23, 2019. https://olis.leg.state.or.us/liz/2019R1/Downloads/MeasureDocument/HB2903/Introduced.

Osler, Kathryn Scott. (1999) 2015. "Physician-Assisted Suicide: A Family Struggles with the Question of Whether Mom Is Capable of Choosing to Die." *Oregonian*, originally published October 17, 1999; posted on Oregonian/Oregon Live, February 4, 2015. https://www.oregonlive.com/health/2015/02/physician-assisted_suicide_a_f.html.

Quill, Timothy E. 1993. "Doctor, I Want to Die. Will You Help Me? [see comments]." *Journal of the American Medical Association* 270, no. 7 (August): 870–73.

Quill, Timothy E., Christine K. Cassel, and Diane E. Meier. 1992. "Care of the Hopelessly Ill—Proposed Clinical Criteria for Physician-Assisted Suicide." *New England Journal of Medicine* 327, no. 19 (November): 1380–84.

Quill, Timothy E., Barbara Coombs Lee, and Sally Nunn. 2000. "Palliative Treatments of Last Resort: Choosing the Least Harmful Alternative." *Annals Internal Medicine* 132, no. 6 (March): 488–93.

Quill, Timothy E., Barbara C. Lee, and Sally Nunn. 2000. "Palliative Treatment of Last Resort and Assisted Suicide [Letter]." *Annals of Internal Medicine* 133, no.7 (October): 563.

Stevens, Kenneth R. Jr. 2006. "Emotional and Psychological Effects of Physician-Assisted Suicide and Euthanasia on Participating Physicians." *Issues in Law & Medicine* 21, no. 3 (Spring): 187–200.

Thienpont, Lieve, Monica Verhofstadt, Tony Van Loon, et al. 2015. "Euthanasia Requests, Procedures and Outcomes for 100 Belgian Patients Suffering from Psychiatric Disorders: A Retrospective, Descriptive Study." *BMJ Open* 5, no. 7 (June): e007454. doi: 10.1136/bmjopen-2014-007454.

Wales, Joshua, Sarina R. Isenberg, Pete Wegier, et al. 2018. "Providing Medical Assistance in Dying within a Home Palliative Care Program in Toronto, Canada: An Observational Study of the First Year of Experience." *Journal of Palliative Medicine* 21, no. 11 (November): 1573–79.

White, Nicola, Fiona Reid, Adam Harris, Priscilla Harris, and Patrick Stone. 2016. "A Systematic Review of Predictions of Survival in Palliative Care: How Accurate Are Clinicians and Who Are the Experts?" PLOS ONE 11, no. 8 (August 25): e0161407. https://doi.org/10.1371/journal.pone.0161407.

Wunder, Michael. 2014. "Learning with History: Nazi Medical Crimes and Today's Debates on Euthanasia in Germany." In *Silence, Scapegoats, and Self-Reflection: The Shadow of Nazi Medical Crimes on Medicine and Bioethics*, edited by Volker Roelcke, Sascha Topp, and Etienne Lepicard, 301–312. Göttingen, Germany: V & R unipress.

Chapter Thirteen

The Value of Life vs. the Principle of Autonomy

Avraham Steinberg

PERSONAL BACKGROUND

While I did not participate in the experience in Germany in 2018 as did many of the authors in this book, my background amply equips me to address the topic of physician-assisted suicide (PAS) and euthanasia after the Holocaust.

I was born in a Displaced Persons Camp in Germany, post–World War II, to parents who were Holocaust survivors. I am a descendant of a large Orthodox Jewish-Polish family. For generations, many of my ancestors served as rabbis in various towns in Poland and Ukraine.

My personal training is a combination of Jewish studies, primarily Jewish medical ethics, and secular studies—I am a rabbi, a practicing pediatric neurologist, and an ethicist with a primary interest in medical ethics. This scholarly background enables me to offer a perspective that carefully weighs both traditional and modern medical ethics. I teach and lecture on medical ethics, publish articles and books on modern medical ethics, such as the *Encyclopedia of Jewish Medical Ethics*, and have participated actively in the development of Israeli legislation regarding several medical ethics issues— for example, The Patient's Bill of Rights, The Dying Patient Act, and The Brain Death Act.

Given this background, I would like to begin this chapter by strongly rejecting the somewhat arrogant statements regarding traditional ethics that sometimes are made by secular medical ethicists, such as:

Although major writings in ancient, medieval, and modern health care contain a rich storehouse of reflection on the relationship between the professional and the

patient, these writings are inadequate for contemporary biomedical ethics. . . .
(Beauchamp and Childress 2001, 1)

With all due respect, philosophical ideas and ideologies come and go,
and a handful of current, talented philosophers should not take the liberty to
reject as "inadequate" the major writings of traditional and faith-based ethics
in ancient, medieval, and modern health care. These were formulated by not
less competent and talented individuals and cultural groups over many generations. It is highly reasonable to assume that the current trends in medical
ethics will be challenged and changed in the future. Philosophical ideas that
cannot be proven or disproven scientifically can and should be presented, argued, and justified, but they cannot be regarded as the only and absolute truth.

I strive to shed critical light on contemporary issues in medical ethics by
presenting both sides of arguments and suggesting a balanced approach that
draws upon all available sources, ancient and modern. It is in this spirit that I
examine the current ethical approaches to PAS and euthanasia.

DEFINITION

Physician-assisted suicide and euthanasia are euphemistic expressions for
acts of direct, deliberate, and intentional killing of disabled people, performed
by health care providers, justified by a perceived higher moral/social call than
the value of life.

I am opposed to any form of killing, including autonomously requested
"mercy" killing. My disapproval of end-of-life PAS and euthanasia is based
on religious and moral considerations both of the inherent immorality of these
acts and of their consequences. In the remainder of this essay, I will present
the arguments that support this conclusion.

HISTORICAL BACKGROUND

The debate about whether physicians should participate in euthanizing a dying patient dates back to antiquity. Hippocrates (c. 460–c. 370 BCE) in the
famous Oath stated, "I will not prescribe a deadly drug to please someone,
nor give advice that may cause his death" (Edelstein 1943).

In the early twentieth century, a euthanasia movement existed in the
United States, both for the relief of suffering by dying patients and for the
sake of eugenics. The moral justification of killing mentally and genetically
disabled people was to secure a healthier American society (Emanuel 1994).
Similarly, in the mid-twentieth century, the Nazis established euthanasia

programs to cleanse the German society of people with neuropsychiatric illnesses, sociopaths, homosexuals, and other "undesirables." Ideologically, eugenics and genocide all played a role in the Nazi euthanasia programs. Subsequently, it led to the atrocities of annihilating groups of people such as Jews and Gypsies, who were also deemed "undesirable." The origins of the Nazi euthanasia program, like those of the American euthanasia movement, predated the Third Reich and were intertwined with the history of eugenics and Social Darwinism and with efforts to discredit traditional morality and ethics ("Euthanasia Program," *Holocaust Encyclopedia*).

In a way, one can correlate these movements with capital punishment whereby society, through state legislation, kills certain criminals. The moral justification for capital punishment is that society punishes and protects itself from certain awful crimes—social needs take precedence over the value of life. One could even have a similar view of the killing of those labeled as heretics for not accepting certain religious beliefs, as Christians did in the Middle Ages during the Crusades and the Inquisition, and as ISIS, the Taliban, and other Islamic fundamentalists do today.

Currently, several Western countries and some ethicists and philosophers advocate, promote, and legislate PAS and/or euthanasia for terminally ill patients. The moral justification for these movements is the assumption that autonomy, freedom of choice, self-determination, and prevention of suffering override the value of life.

A COMPARISON OF CURRENT AND PAST PHYSICIAN-ASSISTED SUICIDE AND EUTHANASIA MOVEMENTS

The similarities between past and the current PAS and euthanasia movements are that: (1) The value of life is directly, deliberately, and intentionally overridden by other principles presumed to be of higher moral value, either personally or socially; and (2) PAS and euthanasia are applied to disabled people, whether physically, mentally, or socially.

There are, however, significant distinctions between early to mid-twentieth century euthanasia movements in the United States and the Third Reich, and the current end-of-life PAS and euthanasia movements. The first programs—whether only proposed, as in the United States, or implemented as in Nazi Germany—killed disabled people against their wishes, or at least without their consent. The current end-of-life PAS and euthanasia movements are generally and officially performed voluntarily with the explicit and autonomous request of the person. In addition, the ideological purpose of the first programs was the good of society, whereas the current end-of-life PAS and euthanasia movements are for the good of the individual person as he or she perceives it.

THE MORAL DEBATE CONCERNING
CURRENT PAS AND EUTHANASIA MOVEMENTS

The questions are: Are the above-mentioned distinctions morally sufficient and justifiable? And, unrelated to these historically, morally unacceptable, and unjustifiable actions, are contemporary end-of-life PAS and euthanasia inherently and practically morally justifiable?

There are two main moral justifications offered in favor of the current PAS and euthanasia programs for dying patients: (1) autonomy, the idea that respect for others demands the fulfillment of their competent wishes and respect for their freedom of choice and self-determination; and (2) beneficence, acting for patients' good as they perceive it and as they define their own quality of life and dignity (De Haan 2002).

There are, however, several reasons to reject these justifications. *Respect for autonomy is and ought to be restricted by several situations and considerations, including societal norms.* It is universally acceptable that the principle of autonomy is not an absolute and infinite one. It is certainly acceptable that an autonomous wish that harms others cannot be fulfilled. Similarly, the autonomous wish must be expressed by a fully competent person. There are additional limitations to autonomy (Steinberg 1993). One of the restrictions when fulfilling an autonomous wish is accepted social norms, which even current proponents of PAS and euthanasia acknowledge inasmuch as these procedures are restricted to dying and suffering patients. Proponents reject autonomous requests for PAS or euthanasia expressed by fully competent, non-dying persons. From a purely autonomous perspective, such limitation is senseless: If autonomy, self-determination, and respect for freedom of choice are morally binding, why accept an autonomous wish to perform euthanasia for a dying and suffering patient and not accept such an autonomous wish for a healthy person who lost his wife and children? Or who lost all his money? Or even without any explicit reason? A fully competent person who expresses a complete and competent autonomous wish to be killed just because he is sick and tired of living—why do we reject it? The clear answer is that societal norms value life over autonomy.

The counterargument might be that it makes sense to accept an autonomous wish of a dying and suffering person to be killed, but it does not make sense to accept an identical autonomous wish of a person who is suffering but is not dying. This counterargument, in fact, turns autonomy into a relative concept. If it makes sense from a societal point of view to kill a dying patient because of suffering, it should perhaps make even more sense to kill a non-dying, chronically suffering patient. The chronically ill are doomed to suffer for a long rather than a short period of time. If it makes sense to kill a dying person because of a perceived undignified *short* life, it should perhaps make even more sense to end a non-dying, *chronically* undignified life. Moreover, those who advocate PAS but reject euthanasia—how do they justify it based on the respect for autonomous decisions? Also, if only PAS is permissible, it might create discrimination when certain terminally ill patients cannot commit suicide either due to physical or emotional disability.

The decision of dying patients to be killed is not always undertaken in a fully autonomous way. There are numerous situations in which seemingly autonomous requests for PAS or euthanasia are made by partially competent patients, or non-competent ones. For example:

1. Severely disabled people may express their wish to be killed because of a real or perceived burden they impose on others, or because of economic considerations. Feeling this way may turn a "right to die" into a "duty to die."
2. Patients suffering from depression and/or anxiety, conditions that result in impaired decision-making ability, may request PAS or euthanasia. These patients cannot be regarded as fully competent.
3. Patients may express a wish to immediately terminate life due to physical pain and suffering, and sometimes due to emotional and cognitive suffering. Because their suffering may be effectively treated, leading patients to withdraw their initial request to die, the initial request may not be truly autonomous.
4. The decision to kill dying patients might be based on previous autonomous statements but, in "real time," they are no longer autonomous. When the patients made their autonomous statements, they may have had a view of their future quality of life, a very subjective and relative term, that is no longer applicable. For example, they might have believed that they would suffer if they developed a persistent vegetative state or dementia, but do patients with dementia or in a persistent vegetative state suffer? By definition, patients with these diagnoses are unaware of their "poor" quality of life as experienced by onlooking, cognitively able people.
5. Legitimizing the killing of severely disabled dying people may encourage patients to request PAS or euthanasia.
6. Societies occasionally promote killing severely disabled dying patients because of resource scarcity or other social concerns that are afforded a higher priority. They argue that it makes more sense to preserve resources such as highly skilled staff, equipment, hospital beds, and medications for those who wish to live, rather than those who do not.

There are several additional reasons for rejecting PAS and euthanasia. First, effective palliative care nowadays can relieve the pain and suffering of many dying patients who wish to be killed or to commit suicide because of their pain and suffering. Therefore, in most cases, more extreme acts should no longer be considered necessary.

Second, once the strict taboo against killing others is removed, it becomes almost impossible to restrain similar actions in more lenient situations, a slippery slope consideration. PAS and euthanasia weaken society's respect for the sanctity of life, leading to nonvoluntary and involuntary euthanasia because the same reason that allows us to accept the autonomously expressed wish of a competent dying patient to be killed—pain and suffering—is applicable to a non-competent patient as well. And, indeed, this has happened in the Netherlands where euthanasia has been legalized under strict conditions, but statistics show that in many instances these conditions are not adhered to (ten Have and Welie 1996; Jochemsen 1999). Reports reveal nonvoluntary euthanasia of depressed, psychiatric, and demented patients. Publications also state that physicians practicing euthanasia do not always adhere to the legal requirement for psychological evaluations of patients, do not report cases of euthanasia to the authorities as required by law, and do not obey other procedural demands. In Belgium, where euthanasia was initially legalized under similar strict conditions, it has been legally expanded to include infants and minors (Cohen-Almagor 2009; Saad 2017; Raus 2016).

Finally, assigning physicians and other health care providers to act as the "executioners" for society is diametrically opposed to the ethos of the medical profession. The goal of this profession is to cure, to heal, to support, but not to kill. Even when the principal aims of the medical profession become impossible to achieve because of the medical situation, there is still another very important goal of the medical profession—alleviating pain and suffering with palliative measures. Especially in our day and age, when palliation is so advanced and effective, and when spirituality, compassion, empathy, and sympathy are readily accepted in the relationship between dying patients and caregivers, there is no reason for the medical profession to violate the value of life.

THE MORAL POSITION TOTALLY REJECTING PAS AND EUTHANASIA

In my opinion, there is never an ethical justification to take a patient's life or to aid a patient in committing suicide directly, actively, deliberately, and intentionally—whether for eugenic, social, or racial reasons, or to fulfill a patient's autonomous wish to do so. This position, based on the inherent immorality of the act, is independent and unrelated to the consequences of the act or to past or future concerns about the slippery slope. Euphemistic and linguistic exercises cannot morally legitimize and substantiate such acts, including terms such as *euthanasia, mercy killing, death with dignity, death by physician's prescription, medical assistance in dying* (MAID), *physician aid in dying* (PAD), and others.

End-of-life decision-making ought to be balanced between two substantial values that occasionally conflict with each other, life and autonomy. Indeed, there are philosophers and ethicists who argue for absolute and imperative categories where one must adhere to some important moral dictates without any compromise. These, however, are theoretical assumptions that can hardly ever be materialized in real-life situations. If all values would run in parallel lines, it would have been morally right to always abide by the agreed upon imperative categories. However, in many real-life situations, when important values cross each other and oppose each other, there must be an appropriate way to balance opposing values, such as life and autonomy, based upon their relative and relevant moral weight and importance. Both are of utmost importance, but both are not absolute values. When there is a clash between them, it ought to be resolved in a balanced way. The debatable questions are where to place the dividing yardstick between these two values and by whom is it decided.

On the one hand, in thinking about the real-life situations of dying patients, we ought to respect their autonomous wishes. If their expressed desires and instructions are not to prolong their lives, it is morally justified and acceptable to withhold life-sustaining treatments and let the patients die of their illnesses, thus respecting their autonomy. On the other hand, we ought to respect the value of life. Physicians must never commit a direct, deliberate, and intentional act of killing or aiding in suicide, which are inherently wrong moral actions. As noted above, legalization of PAS and euthanasia in the Netherlands led to acts that violated true autonomy and exceeded legislative restrictions, acts that even proponents of PAS and euthanasia consider morally wrong—the slippery slope. This distinction between withholding life-sustaining measures and active killing is a sound moral viewpoint, which appropriately balances the two utmost important values, has strong holds in traditional moral teaching and medical practice and ethos, and avoids undesirable and unjustifiable slippery-slope situations.

Killing dying patients is certainly not the invention of the twenty-first century. Despite being well known since time immemorial, most ethicists and legislators have prohibited these acts. The moral justification for this prohibition since antiquity remains valid and appropriate today as well.

A JEWISH APPROACH

According to Jewish teaching, killing dying patients is not only inherently immoral and consequentially wrong, but it is totally wrong from a religious perspective as well, which is true from the perspective of almost all religions. On October 28, 2019, a position paper was signed in the Vatican by the heads of the three monotheistic religions—Jewish, Christian, Muslim—that rejects PAS and euthanasia and promotes palliative care and withholding life-prolonging measures (Times of Israel 2019).

In Judaism, the value of life is sanctified and of utmost importance. The biblical commandment "Thou shall not kill" (Exodus 20:13) applies to dying patients as well, and, therefore, PAS and euthanasia are forbidden (Gesundheit et al. 2006). Nonetheless, according to Jewish principles, there is a clear and justifiable difference between omitting and committing actions. According to most rabbinic authorities, although an act that directly and intentionally causes or hastens death is always prohibited, there is no obligation to actively prolong the life of a suffering, dying patient. Therefore, it is permissible to withhold life-prolonging measures such as cardiopulmonary resuscitation (CPR), ventilation, chemotherapy, and their like.

However, according to most rabbinic authorities, it is prohibited to withdraw life-sustaining treatments if the act of withdrawal will lead to death. But this prohibition is qualified in two ways. First, according to Jewish law, there is a clear distinction between continuous life-sustaining measures such as a ventilator or a cardiac pacemaker, and a cyclic, periodic, intermittent life-sustaining measure such as dialysis, chemotherapy, pressors, and the like (Steinberg 2003). In the first group of treatments, there is no point in time where there can be a passive, omitting stage, and therefore, the active withdrawal leads directly and inevitably to the demise of the patient. On the other hand, in the second group of treatments, once one cycle is completed, there is a stage where one can passively withhold the next cycle, which is permissible as it would have been permissible not to have started the treatment to begin with (Steinberg and Sprung 2006; 2007). Second, many rabbinic authorities accept the conversion of a continuous type of treatment, such as a respirator, into a cyclic type by introducing a timer on respirators that is set beforehand to terminate the function of the respirator at a specific time, after which it is permissible to withhold the reattachment of the respirator to the patient (Ravitsky 2005; Ravitsky and Steinberg 2019). This is a modern solution derived from traditional Jewish medical ethical principles to a complex, contemporary therapeutic problem, which satisfies a patient's autonomous wishes. In this circumstance, it appears that major writings in at least one ancient "storehouse of reflection on the relationship between the professional and the patient" is adequate for contemporary biomedical ethics (Beauchamp and Childress 1994).

A very important Jewish position is the requirement to alleviate pain and suffering, especially in the dying patient, even if it may hasten death, provided it is not done intentionally or unavoidably. The reason for this approach is the assumption that pain and suffering in a terminal condition becomes the "disease" that ought to be treated in the best professional manner. Any significant treatment of a serious disease has side effects, including mortality. This is the nature of medicine, and it should not be different concerning pain and suffering of a dying patient.

CONCLUSION

Some Western countries and ethicists are currently promoting a legal and ethical approach to the dying patient that permits physician-assisted suicide and euthanasia. In my view, this approach is wrong both from inherent moral and religious points of view as well as from practical and consequential points of view. The occasional conflict between the value and sanctity of life and the principle of autonomy ought to be resolved in a balanced way without resorting to the extreme total negation of the value of life.

BIBLIOGRAPHY

Beauchamp, Tom L., and James F. Childress. 2001. *Principles of Biomedical Ethics*, 5th ed. New York: Oxford University Press.

Cohen-Almagor, Raphael. 2009. "Belgian Euthanasia Law: A Critical Analysis." *Journal of Medical Ethics* 35, no. 7 (August): 436–39.

De Haan, Jurriaan. 2002. "The Ethics of Euthanasia: Advocates' Perspectives." *Bioethics* 16, no. 2 (April): 154–72.

Edelstein, Ludwig. 1943. *The Hippocratic Oath: Text, Translation and Interpretation*. Baltimore: Johns Hopkins University Press.

Emanuel, Ezekiel. 1994. "The History of Euthanasia Debates in the United States and Britain." *Annals of Internal Medicine* 121, no. 10 (November): 793–802.

"Euthanasia Program." n.d. *Holocaust Encyclopedia*. United States Holocaust Memorial Museum. Accessed October 28, 2019. https://encyclopedia.ushmm.org/content/en/article/euthanasia-program.

Gesundheit, Benjamin, Avraham Steinberg, Shimon Glick, Reuven Or, and Allan Jotkovitz. 2006. "Euthanasia: An Overview and the Jewish Perspective." *Cancer Investigation* 24, no. 6 (October): 621–29.

Jochemsen, Henk, and John Keown. 1999. "Voluntary Euthanasia under Control? Further Empirical Evidence from The Netherlands." *Journal of Medical Ethics* 25, no. 1 (February): 16–21.

Raus, Kasper. 2016. "The Extension of Belgium's Euthanasia Law to Include Competent Minors." *Journal of Bioethical Inquiry* 13, no. 2 (February): 305–15.

Ravitsky, Vardit. 2005. "Timers on Respirators." *British Medical Journal* 330 (February): 415–17.

Ravitsky, Vardit, and Avraham Steinberg. 2019. "Withholding and Withdrawing: A Religious–Cultural Path Toward a Practical Resolution." *American Journal of Bioethics* 19, no. 3 (March): 49–50.

Saad, Toni. 2017. "Euthanasia in Belgium: Legal, Historical and Political Review." *Issues in Law and Medicine* 32, no. 2 (Fall): 183–204.

Steinberg, Avraham. 1993. "A Jewish Perspective on the Four Principles." In *Principles of Health Care Ethics*, edited by Raanan Gillon, 65–73. Chicester: John Wiley & Sons.

Steinberg, Avraham. 2003. *Encyclopedia of Jewish Medical Ethics*, vol. 3. Jerusalem and New York: Feldheim Publishers.

Steinberg, Avraham, and Charles Sprung. 2006. "The Dying Patient: New Israeli Legislation." *Intensive Care Medicine* 32, no. 8 (August): 1234–37.

Steinberg, Avraham, and Charles Sprung. 2007. "The Dying Patient Act, 2005: Israeli Innovative Legislation." *Israel Medical Association Journal* 9, no. 7 (August): 550–52.

ten Have, Henk, and Joseph Welie. 1996. "Euthanasia in the Netherlands." *Critical Care Clinics* 12, no. 1 (January): 97–108.

Times of Israel (The). 2019. "Rabbis Join 'Historic' Interfaith Call at Vatican against Assisted Suicide." Accessed December 8, 2019. https://www.timesofisrael.com/chief-rabbis-join-interfaith-call-at-vatican-against-mercy-killings/.

Chapter Fourteen

The Distinction Between Voluntary and Involuntary Euthanasia and the Critical Role of Eugenics

James Downar

The fundamental problem with a discussion about physician-assisted suicide and euthanasia after the Holocaust (PASEATH), and even the terminology itself, is that it conflates concepts that are fundamentally different. There are clear differences between voluntary physician-assisted suicide and euthanasia (PASE) as it is currently practiced where it is legal and the eugenic genocide that marked the Holocaust. These differences relate mostly, but not entirely, to the identity of the person requesting PASE, the rationale underlying the request, the nature of the person's suffering, and the concept of the value of life. There are also important differences in the historical and philosophical circumstances under which voluntary PASE has been legalized and the circumstances under which the Holocaust occurred.

Please note that the purpose of this chapter is not to proselytize or to promote the practice of PASE. We can recognize the distinction between voluntary PASE and the Holocaust without concluding that PASE is morally acceptable. Rather, this chapter will address arguments that draw parallels between voluntary PASE and some of the antecedents and practice of involuntary euthanasia during the Third Reich including, for example, a slippery slope argument about the inevitability of state-driven eugenic programs and mass involuntary euthanasia of the vulnerable. At their core, these arguments overlook fundamental underpinnings of voluntary PASE, and they focus on superficial similarities or spurious claims that cannot be supported by data or experience.

No doubt, some will interpret this chapter as a justification for the legalization of PASE, which it is not. Rather it is an appeal to colleagues to consider a new approach to how they argue against the legalization of PASE. In the past two decades, more than a dozen jurisdictions have legalized voluntary PASE, sometimes by court decisions but typically with overwhelming public support (Ipsos 2014; Hanrahan 2019; ACT New Zealand 2019). It may be tempting to argue that these were naïve and short-sighted decisions made by a public and a judiciary that were functionally ignorant of the circumstances leading up to the Holocaust. A more likely explanation is that they saw vital distinctions between voluntary PASE and the Holocaust. As more jurisdictions contemplate laws permitting PASE, opponents of legalization may wish to better understand why so many members of the public and the judiciary reject analogies between voluntary PASE and the Holocaust.

EUGENICS AND THE ROOTS OF NONVOLUNTARY AND INVOLUNTARY EUTHANASIA IN NAZI GERMANY

The eugenic movement began long before the Third Reich. Eugenicists believe that individuals have an objective value, and that the quality of a population can be improved or diminished based on the objective value of the individuals within. As detailed in chapter 2 in this book, eugenicists attempted to improve the genetic makeup of a population either by "positive" acts such as encouraging childbearing by more desirable individuals, or by "negative" acts such as sterilization, abortion, or ending lives. As a rule, the eugenic argument was primarily an economic one—that individuals with a negative value would tend to proliferate faster than those with a positive value, placing an unsustainable economic burden on society. The argument of compassion—based on the presumption that individuals of negative value were experiencing suffering—was a secondary rationale which, like the economic argument, did not derive from the person in question.

The eugenic movement had many adherents in the medical community, including Nobel laureates (see chapter 2 in this book). Francis Galton first coined the term in the 1880s, and eugenic organizations, laws, and even scientific journals proliferated rapidly throughout Europe and North America. For example, involuntary sterilization was legal in at least a dozen countries before the Nazis came to power (Proctor 1988, 96–97).

The move to adopt euthanasia as a eugenic act in Germany gained momentum in 1920, when Karl Binding and Alfred Hoche proposed "beneficent euthanasia" in three scenarios:

- "those who, due to illness or after being severely wounded, are terminal cases, who fully understand their situation and urgently wish to be delivered from their agony and are able to somehow express this wish"

- "those who had been mentally healthy, but somehow lost consciousness and waking up, would suffer a nameless misery"
- the "incurable idiots who are the terrible image of real people and cause horror in each person who faces them." (Binding and Hoche quoted in Wunder 2014, 302)

The authors argued that in these scenarios these patients lost the "right to legal protection" due to their negative value to the community—a clear-cut eugenic argument. But it is clear that such logic only applies to the second and third scenarios, where the patients are incapable of advocating for themselves and require legal protection to prevent someone from ending their life for the supposed benefit of society. In the first scenario, the patients are terminally ill, suffering, and requesting euthanasia for their own self-perceived benefit. They can advocate for themselves; they do not want legal protection for their lives; and their requests are unrelated to any perception of their value to the community—they want to end their agony. It would not be a eugenic act.

In 1939, Hitler issued this decree regarding euthanasia:

Reichsleiter [Philipp] Bouhler and Dr. med. [Karl] Brandt are charged with responsibility to broaden the authority of certain doctors to the extent that [persons] suffering from illnesses judged to be incurable may, after a humane, most careful assessment of their condition, be granted a mercy death. (Hitler 1939)

The *Aktion* T4 program of large-scale involuntary and nonvoluntary euthanasia of patients in chronic care facilities (see chapter 3 in this book) began shortly after Hitler's decree and was well underway in 1940. Many were given overdoses of sedatives without their knowledge, while others were transported against their will to one of six euthanasia facilities equipped with gas chambers and crematoria. It is doubtful whether any of the victims had either "a humane, most careful assessment of their condition" or any idea of what was happening to them until it was too late. Therefore, *Aktion* T4 was not based on compassion or mercy, but on eugenics.

Because they had long embraced eugenic principles and flocked to join the Nazi party, many in Germany's medical community eagerly participated in *Aktion* T4. But they concealed their eugenic motivations and acts by producing false death certificates and misleading letters of condolence (Lifton 1986, 70, 75), indicating implicit acknowledgment that their actions were illegal. And as soon as the reality of *Aktion* T4 was revealed to the German public in a sermon by Bishop Clemens von Galen, the Nazi authorities effectively canceled the mass murder by gassing, but the decentralized, involuntary euthanasia using poisons, exposure, starvation, and neglect continued for the next four years, as described in chapter 3 in this book.

Notably, while eugenic principles were embraced by many nations, the practice of eugenic euthanasia was limited to Nazi Germany. In 1949, Leo Alexander described its development as follows:

> The beginnings at first were merely a subtle *shift in emphasis in the basic attitude of the physicians*. It started with the acceptance of the attitude, basic in the euthanasia movement, that there is *such a thing as life not worthy to be lived*. This attitude in its early stages concerned itself merely with the severely and chronically sick. Gradually the sphere of those to be included in this category was enlarged to encompass the socially unproductive, the ideologically unwanted, the racially unwanted and finally all non-Germans. But it is important to realize that the infinitely small wedged-in lever from which this entire trend of mind received its impetus was the attitude *toward* the nonrehabilitative sick. (Alexander 1949; italics mine)

In other words, a key development in Nazi Germany was the shift from accepting the idea of eugenics, to accepting the implementation of eugenic acts such as sterilization to prevent lives that would be considered "unworthy," to the ending of lives that were perceived as "unworthy," and the subsequent expansion of criteria for defining "unworthy." But the critical logic throughout this continuum is the longstanding attitude of physicians and society toward the incurably ill or disabled, rather than the view of the incurably ill of their own suffering. It was this attitude that led to enthusiastic participation and leadership by many in the medical community in *Aktion* T4 and the Holocaust; they not only carried out the acts themselves, but went to great lengths to conceal their acts. As Jan Menges explained in *"Euthanasie" in het Derde Rijk* (1972):

> *The interests of the patient did not count but only that of the state*. There was no thought of openness: fictitious organizations, the use of false names, the writing of repugnantly hypocritical letters of condolence and even misinforming from the supervising doctors put from the outset of the actions a veil of deception over the affair. Through all of these facts the "euthanasia" of the Nazis has condemned itself and proved that *one may speak more of murder than of a "saving act."* (Menges quoted in Kennedy 2014, 226; italics mine)

Menges highlights key behaviors seen in *Aktion* T4. Physicians and other authorities sought to obscure their acts, spread misinformation, and deceive the public. This is not the behavior of compassionate physicians who were respecting patient wishes. They clearly understood the distinction between what they were doing and what was acceptable and unacceptable to the public. They were motivated by a eugenic sense of duty to the state and acted outside the law to achieve their ends.

MODERN VOLUNTARY PHYSICIAN-ASSISTED SUICIDE AND EUTHANASIA FROM THE PERSPECTIVE OF A PATIENT, PROVIDER, AND SYSTEM

Several jurisdictions in North America, Western Europe, and Australia have now legalized physician-assisted suicide or euthanasia by legislative or judicial means, with very strong public support for their legalization. Although the rationale for legalization may have varied among the legislators, judges, and voters, it is logical to assume that all of them were aware of the Holocaust to some degree. Given the fact that every one of these countries fought against the Nazis during World War II, progressively repealed their eugenic laws, and signed international conventions prohibiting eugenic practices in the decades that followed (United Nations Treaty Series 1948; European Parliament 2012), it is difficult to maintain that the modern legalization of PASE is a manifestation of eugenics.

In Canada, where PASE was legalized by the Supreme Court in the *Carter* decision using the term *medical assistance in dying* (MAID), the rationale for legalization was provided in great detail. From an ethical perspective, the court felt that:

> while there is no clear societal consensus on physician-assisted dying, there is a strong consensus that it would only be ethical with respect to voluntary adults who are competent, informed, grievously and irremediably ill, and where the assistance is "clearly consistent with the patient's wishes and best interests, and [provided] in order to relieve suffering." (Carter v. Canada 2015)

The court also expressed concern that vulnerable persons might be "induced to commit suicide at a time of weakness." But the trial judge felt that: "After reviewing the evidence ... a permissive regime [that legalized voluntary MAID] with properly designed and administered safeguards was capable of protecting vulnerable people from abuse and error. While there are risks, to be sure, a carefully designed and managed system is capable of adequately addressing them." In other words, the court was aware of the potential for people to be killed for eugenic or other reasons, but this could be distinguished from voluntary MAID performed to relieve patient suffering based on the experience from other jurisdictions.

The first safeguard is that the request must come from a competent patient and must be contemporary and persistent. Secondly, the requesting individual must have severe suffering, or have an advanced and incurable illness, or both. Third, the person needs to be assessed by more than one clinician to ensure that they meet criteria, and cases must be reported to an oversight body for review.

For those who have never participated in an eligibility assessment, there are videos available on the internet that may help to give an image of what a typical assessment might look like (YouTube 2016). These videos also help convey the patients' rationales for their MAID request in their own words. Patients differ in their health status, the nature of their suffering, and their rationales for proceeding with MAID rather than continuing with palliative care and awaiting a natural death. The videos demonstrate that these patients are not acting out of impulse or desperation, that their decisions are clearly their own, and that there are no obvious reasons to suspect they are being pressured into requesting MAID.

Physicians generally spend a substantial amount of time assessing the patient for capacity and eligibility and consulting other specialists as needed. A substantial proportion of requests are not granted either because of ineligibility or because the patient becomes unconscious or dies a natural death before they can receive MAID. Data from Belgium show that in 2013, 23 percent of MAID requests were not granted (Chambaere et al. 2015). Data from the Netherlands show that more than half of MAID requests in 2010 were not granted (Onwuteaka-Philipsen et al. 2012). In Canada, 20 percent of patients who are found eligible for MAID die naturally before the MAID procedure takes place (Government of Canada 2019). Data from Oregon show that many who are found eligible ultimately are reassured by simply having the option of PAS available and do not go through with the actual procedure before they die of their underlying condition (Oregon Health Authority 2018).

A key feature of voluntary MAID is its transparency. In my experience, family members are aware of almost every MAID death well in advance, and are present when it takes place, even when they do not support the patient's decision to pursue MAID. The 2016 legislation authorized the federal Minister of Health to collect data on both requests for, and the provision of MAID (Government of Canada 2019). In my opinion, reporting rates in Canada are likely to be at or near 100 percent, simply because of the multiple checks and individuals involved in prescribing and dispensing the medication.

Of course, even if all cases of voluntary MAID are reported, it is possible that nonvoluntary euthanasia is practiced and unreported. Indeed, some have expressed a concern that legalizing voluntary MAID creates a permissive atmosphere where nonvoluntary euthanasia becomes more common (Peireira 2011). But this has been studied (to the degree that it is possible to study an illegal practice), and the data suggest that the opposite is true. The incidence of nonvoluntary euthanasia actually falls in jurisdictions that legalize voluntary PASE (Chambaere et al. 2015; Onwuteaka-Philipsen et al. 2012), and it is certainly no higher than it is in jurisdictions where voluntary PASE is illegal (van der Heide et al. 2003). Personally, I have never performed or witnessed nonvoluntary euthanasia, and I have only heard of anecdotes from family members who claimed that a physician performed euthanasia for an unconscious, terminally ill patient at the request of the family member. All of these anecdotes predated the legalization of voluntary MAID in Canada.

"UNWORTHY OF LIFE" VS "IT'S NOT WORTH IT FOR ME TO CONTINUE TO SUFFER"

The core justification of eugenic euthanasia is the notion that some people are unworthy of life, and so a central question for the study of PASEATH is whether the same justification is being used (or may be used) in voluntary PASE. Some suggest that a patient's decision to request PASE implies something about their worth or value, but, in my experience, this language appears totally alien to the patient requesting PASE. In a minority of cases in Oregon and Washington State, patients cite a fear of being a burden on family, friends, and relatives (Oregon Health Authority 2018; Loggers et al. 2013). I interpret this fear as a desire by patients to avoid others taking care of them, rather than a perception that incurable patients who require continuing and/or palliative care are unworthy of life.

Patients often make end-of-life decisions, including PASE and withholding or withdrawing life-sustaining therapies, with the logic that it is "not worth it to continue" because of the suffering involved. But there is an important difference between a eugenicist saying that lives are of no value or negative value—unworthy of living—and patients saying that the burden of their suffering *exceeds* the value of their remaining life—"it's not worth it for me to continue to suffer." When someone says that "it's not worth it," I interpret that to mean that the value of the joy they could derive from continuing to live is not sufficiently high to justify their degree of suffering. In that sense, patients' lives retain the same value they always had. Vitalists may argue that because the value of each life is infinite, no amount of suffering could justify PASE. There is a clear difference, however, between a nonvitalist position that all lives have a very high but finite value and a eugenic position that some lives have a negative value. Furthermore, because the nonvitalist position has been used for generations in Western society to justify withholding and withdrawing life-sustaining measures, it is not a novel concept when applied to PASE. In that sense, voluntary PASE is no more of a gateway to eugenic euthanasia than any of the more widely accepted end-of-life decisions that are made in jurisdictions where PASE is illegal. This is not to say that there is no difference between voluntary PASE and withholding or withdrawing life-sustaining measures, but merely to point out that if we are concerned about patients requesting PASE because they consider the value of their remaining life insufficient to justify the burden of their suffering, then we would need to be equally concerned about any other end-of-life decision that is justified on the same basis.

Some might point to the practice of MAID by advance directive for an incapable patient as an example of a eugenic practice, or at least something that resembles *Aktion* T4. But this modern practice cannot be easily compared with the eugenic, nonvoluntary euthanasia of *Aktion* T4 because the justification used in each case is different. For decades, some decisions to withhold or withdraw life-sustaining measures have been nonvoluntary in the sense that they are made by surrogates acting on behalf of patients at a time when they are no longer competent to make medical decisions (Silveira, Kim, and Langa 2010). We justify these decisions on the basis of respect for autonomy and try to re-create the decisions that patients would make if they were capable. In that sense, while we may not support the idea of MAID (or even withdrawal of life support) by surrogate decision-making, it is difficult to argue that these are eugenic practices. Of course, there is the possibility of forged advance directives; patients may not have been capable of understanding their options when preparing the advance directives; patients cannot predict the extent of their suffering in a hypothetical future state; and patients may change their minds but forget to update their advance directives. Indeed, any one of these concerns could justify prohibiting the practice of nonvoluntary PASE by advance directive, but jurisdictions that have chosen to legalize it are not acting out of a eugenic motive or a judgment that a person's life is of no value. Rather, they are simply applying the existing decision-making framework to another nonvoluntary end-of-life decision. I am not advocating for or defending the practice of nonvoluntary PASE. Rather, I argue that nonvoluntary PASE, when guided by a clear advance directive, says no more about the worth of a human life than nonvoluntary withholding or withdrawal of life support, which are routine practices throughout the Western world.

Members of the disability community are particularly concerned about attempts to assign value or worth to human life, given that they were the principal targets of eugenic programs in the past. But those who support legalization of PASE actually turn the question of value on its head. For example, the late physicist Stephen Hawking, a famous member of the disability community, said that "To keep someone alive against their wishes is the ultimate indignity" (Elgot 2015). Canadian politician Steven Fletcher, another prominent member of the disability community, put it this way:

> Some argue that doctor-assisted dying devalues the lives of those with disabilities; I argue the opposite. [Legalization of voluntary PASE] will allow people who are physically unable to end their lives on their own terms to decide how

they wish to die—just as any able-bodied Canadian can. A competent adult Canadian who is disabled should have all the tools available to any Canadian to live well or to die well. Allowing other people to suffer hopelessly in no way increases the value of my life as a disabled person. (Fletcher 2015)

SUMMARY

As outlined above, the conflation of voluntary and nonvoluntary euthanasia is not a recent phenomenon. It was clearly evident in Binding and Hoche's essay published almost a century ago and continued throughout the *Aktion* T4 program. But beyond the most superficial similarities between voluntary and involuntary/nonvoluntary euthanasia (namely, the ending of a person's life by a clinician), numerous differences are apparent.

Aktion T4 and the Holocaust were the products of a eugenic philosophy that had been prevalent, particularly in the medical community, for generations. The belief that some lives were not worthy of living (or, indeed, a threat to society) led to a series of programs in many countries aimed at preventing those lives from being lived. In Germany, the rise of the Nazis led to extreme efforts to end lives. While Binding and Hoche argued for legalization of both voluntary and nonvoluntary euthanasia on the basis of either eugenics or compassion, *Aktion* T4 and the Holocaust involved almost exclusively involuntary and nonvoluntary euthanasia. From a eugenic perspective, the programs were effective largely because they found strong support among the medical community, even if the physicians appeared to understand that what they were doing was illegal and unacceptable to many. They went to great lengths to obscure their acts, spread misinformation, and deceive the public.

Euthanasia programs during the Third Reich stand in sharp contrast to contemporary, voluntary PASE. Eugenic philosophies are not prevalent and, indeed, not tolerated in polite company throughout most of the world. There has been great progress worldwide toward ending forced sterilizations and abortions and providing support for the physically and mentally disabled, the primary targets of *Aktion* T4. Modern PASE begins with the patient's capable request and includes transparency and, in my view, thorough and reliable documentation as required by law in most jurisdictions. A substantial proportion of those who request PASE are refused by physicians (Chambaere et al. 2015; Onwuteaka-Philipsen et al. 2012), and even among those who are approved, a large minority never complete the procedure before dying of natural causes (Government of Canada 2019). While some individual physicians are willing participants, many are not, and groups of physicians in Canada have taken legal action to avoid referring eligible patients to providers for PASE (*Christian Medical and Dental Society of*

Canada v. College of Physicians and Surgeons of Ontario 2018). Physician organizations have typically opposed the legalization of PASE (De Lima et al. 2017), and some continue to oppose the practice of PASE even when it becomes legal in their jurisdiction (AMA Victoria n.d.). Although support for the legalization of voluntary PAS appears to have grown within the Oregon medical community (Ganzini et al. 2001), it remains far below that of the general public in all countries studied by Emanuel et al. (2016). Nobody could argue that, as a group, physicians have been leaders and eager participants in the practice anywhere in the world.

Hence, there is a fundamental problem with conflating the practice or the justification of voluntary PASE with that of eugenic, state-sponsored, involuntary euthanasia. Aside from the involvement of a clinician in the death of a patient, the two practices share almost nothing in common. Voluntary PASE is no more eugenic in nature than any other end-of-life decision made today by incurably ill patients, such as the withdrawal of life-sustaining measures or stopping dialysis. The concept that a person is not "worthy of life," which is so central to eugenic acts, is absent from patients' decisions in PASE. Indeed, for physicians and patients involved in the practice of PASE, the discussion of "worth" seems contrived, an attempt by opponents of PASE to discredit the practice by co-opting the language of eugenics.

SO WHY SHOULD ANYONE STUDY PASEATH?

Clearly, we have a lot to learn from the Holocaust. But we do not honor the memory of the millions of people who were murdered by drawing spurious analogies or superficial comparisons to modern events. The Holocaust was not an accidental by-product of well-intentioned but naïve physicians who put too much faith in safeguards. The Holocaust was a deliberate attempt at genocide and mass murder by a eugenic society, decreeing, or ignoring laws as needed to further their political goals. There have been many other examples of genocide throughout history, right up to the present day, and none of them involved PASE. Believing that the legalization of voluntary PASE would lead to genocide is as naïve as believing that the criminalization of PASE would prevent genocide. To be clear, we are likely to see more genocides but, based on data and experience, they will not be the result of legalizing voluntary PASE.

So perhaps the lesson is not to focus our energy on drawing analogies that cannot be sustained, but rather to understand and appreciate how National Socialist euthanasia and contemporary legal PASE are different, so that we can recognize signs that indicate an impending shift toward eugenic euthanasia or outright genocide. When discussing current PASE, we need to be alert to arguments that shift the focus from the self-perceived interests of the person to the perceived benefits of the community. We need to be alert to eugenic ideologies.

BIBLIOGRAPHY

ACT New Zealand. 2019. "New Poll: Euthanasia Support Overwhelmingly Strong." *Scoop Independent News*, May 9, 2019. https://www.scoop.co.nz/stories/PA1905/ S00088/new-poll-euthanasia-support-overwhelmingly-strong.htm.

Alexander, Leo. 1949. "Medical Science under Dictatorship." *New England Journal of Medicine* 241 (July 14): 39–47.

AMA (Australian Medical Association) Victoria. n.d. "AMA Victoria statement on the Voluntary Assisted Dying Bill." Accessed December 5, 2019. https://amavic .com.au/media/Archived-Media-Releases/2017-media-releases/ama-victoria-state ment-on-the-voluntary-assisted-dying-bill.

Binding, Karl, and Alfred Hoche. 1920. *Die Freigabe der Vernichtung lebensunwerten Lebens: Ihr Mass und ihre Form.* Leipzig: Felix Meiner.

Carter v. Canada (Attorney General). 2015. 2015 SCC 5 (Supreme Court of Canada). Case no. 35591.

Chambaere, Kenneth, Robert Vander Stichele, Freddy Mortier, and Joachim Cohen. 2015. "Recent Trends in Euthanasia and Other End-of-Life Practices in Belgium." *New England Journal of Medicine* 372, no. 12 (March 19): 1179–1181.

Christian Medical and Dental Society of Canada v. College of Physicians and Surgeons of Ontario. 2018 ONSC 579. Ontario Superior Court of Justice Divisional Court. Court File No. 499/16/500/16.

De Lima, Liliana, Roger Woodruff, Katherine Pettus, et al. 2017. "International Association for Hospice and Palliative Care Position Statement: Euthanasia and Physician-Assisted Suicide." *Journal of Palliative Medicine* 20, no. 1 (January): 8–14.

Elgot, Jessica. 2015. "Stephen Hawking: 'I would consider assisted suicide.'" *Guardian*. June 3, 2015.

Emanuel, Ezekiel, Bregje Onwuteaka-Philipsen, John Urwin, and Joachim Cohen. 2016. "Attitudes and Practices of Euthanasia and Physician-Assisted Suicide in the United States, Canada, and Europe." *Journal of the American Medical Association* 316, no. 1 (July): 79–90.

European Parliament, Council of the European Union. 2012. *Official Journal of the European Union.* C 326, Volume 55, October 26, 2012. Charter of Fundamental Rights. https://eur-lex.europa.eu/legal-content/EN/TXT/?uri=OJ:C:2012:326:TOC.

Fletcher, Steven. 2015. "Doctor-Assisted Dying: Personal View—Steven Fletcher." *Economist.* June 24, 2015. https://www.economist.com/international/2015/06/24/ personal-view-steven-fletcher.

Ganzini Linda, Heidi D. Nelson, Melinda A. Lee, et al. 2001. "Oregon Physicians' Attitudes about and Experiences with End-of-Life Care since Passage of the Oregon

Death with Dignity Act." *Journal of the American Medical Association* 285, no. 18 (May): 2363–2369.

Government of Canada. 2019. *Fourth Interim Report on Medical Assistance in Dying in Canada.* Accessed July 20, 2019. https://www.canada.ca/en/health-canada/services/publications/health-system-services/medical-assistance-dying-interim -report-april-2019.html.

Hanrahan, Catherine. 2019. "Euthanasia Support Strengthens to Nearly 90pc, Vote Compass Data Shows." ABC News (Australia), May 8, 2019. https://www.abc.net .au/news/2019-05-08/vote-compass-social-issues-euthanasia-transgender-republic -drugs/11087008.

Hitler, Adolf. 1939. Decree cited in "Euthanasia Program." United States Holocaust Memorial Museum website. Accessed November 18, 2019. https://collections .ushmm.org/search/catalog/pa15074.

Ipsos. 2014. "Most (84%) Canadians Believe a Doctor Should Be Able to Assist Someone Who Is Terminally Ill and Suffering Unbearably to End Their Life," October 8, 2014. https://www.ipsos.com/en-ca/most-84-canadians-believe-doctor -should-be-able-assist-someone-who-terminally-ill-and-suffering.

Kennedy, James. 2014. "The Legacy of National Socialism for the Dutch Debate." In *Silence, Scapegoats and Self-Reflection: The Shadow of Nazi Medical Crimes on Medicine and Bioethics,* edited by Volker Roelcke, Etienne Lepicard, and Sascha Topp, 213–229. Gottingen: V and R unipress.

Lifton, Robert. 1986. *The Nazi Doctors: Medical Killing and the Psychology of Genocide.* New York: Basic Books.

Loggers, Elizabeth, Helene Starks, Moreen Shannon-Dudley, Anthony Back, Frederick Appelbaum, and Marc Stewart. 2013. "Implementing a Death with Dignity Program at a Comprehensive Cancer Center." *New England Journal of Medicine* 368, no. 15 (April): 1417–1424.

Menges, Jan. 1972. *'Euthanasie' in het Derde Rijk.* Haarlem: De Erven Bohn.

Onwuteaka-Philipsen Bregje, Arianne Brinkman-Stoppelenburg, Corine Penning, Gwen de Jong-Krul, Johannes van Delden, and Agnes van der Heide. 2012. "Trends in End-of-Life Practices before and after the Enactment of the Euthanasia Law in the Netherlands from 1990 to 2010: A Repeated Cross-Sectional Survey." *Lancet* 380, no. 9845 (September): 908–915.

Oregon Health Authority. 2018. *Oregon Death with Dignity Act Annual Reports.* cited in Death with Dignity website. Accessed November 20, 2019. https://www .deathwithdignity.org/oregon-death-with-dignity-act-annual-reports/.

Pereira, J. 2011. "Legalizing Euthanasia or Assisted Suicide: The Illusion of Safeguards and Controls." *Current Oncology* 18, no. 2 (April): e38–45.

Proctor, Robert N. 1988. *Racial Hygiene: Medicine Under the Nazis.* Cambridge, MA: Harvard University Press.

Silveira, Maria J., Scott Y. H. Kim, and Kenneth M. Langa. 2010. "Advance Directives and Outcomes of Surrogate Decision Making before Death." *New England Journal of Medicine* 362, no. 13 (April): 1211–1218.

United Nations: Treaty Series. 1948. "No. 1021 Convention on the Prevention and Punishment of the Crime of Genocide." Adopted by the General Assembly of the

United Nations on 9 December 1948. Accessed December 5, 2019. https://treaties
.un.org/doc/publication/unts/volume%2078/volume-78-i-1021-english.pdf.

van der Heide, Agnes, Luc Deliens, Karin Faisst, et al. 2003. "End-of-Life Decision-
Making in Six European Countries: Descriptive Study." *Lancet* 362, no. 9381
(August 2): 345–350.

Wunder, Michael. 2014. "Learning with History: Nazi Medical Crimes and Today's
Debates on Euthanasia in Germany." In *Silence, Scapegoats, Self-Reflection: The
Shadow of Nazi Medical Crimes on Medicine and Bioethics*, edited by Volker Ro-
elcke, Etienne Lepicard, and Sascha Topp, 301–312. Gottingen: V & R unipress.

YouTube. 2016. "Full Interview: A Patient Discusses Her Decision to Seek Medical
Assistance in Dying." Video. October 30, 2016. Accessed July 20, 2019. https://
youtu.be/Mg-EHDvZ8Z4.

Chapter Fifteen

Euthanasia Old and New

Lives Not Worth Living and Unequal Respect for Autonomy

Scott Y. H. Kim

Comparing the Nazi era euthanasia regime with the modern practice of "physician-assisted death" or "medical assistance in dying," as it is called in Canada, can have adverse consequences. On June 6, 2014, Harvey Schipper, a distinguished Canadian oncologist, wrote an opinion piece against the legalization of euthanasia and assisted suicide (EAS) in *The Globe and Mail*. "I am an oncologist, and I am Jewish," he wrote, enumerating ethical, clinical, and policy reasons. He made one reference to the Nazi era:

> Similar arguments about relieving suffering were used by the Nazis to justify first exterminating the weakened and disabled, then the mentally ill, and then non-Aryans on the regime's hell-bent descent into depravity. In order to execute the policy, a cohort of licensed killers was created. This, in a society once considered the world's most sophisticated and cultured.

That there was no public outcry at the time is not surprising; after all, there was nothing novel about citing the Nazi experience as a cautionary note in debates about EAS. However, in May of 2017, about a year after the enactment of the Canadian "Medical Assistance in Dying" (MAID) law, Schipper was forced to step down from chairing one of three working groups of a government-sponsored expert panel examining the potential expansion of EAS in Canada for those with mental disorders, by advance request, and for mature minors (Council of Canadian Academies 2018). The expert panel was convened to fulfill a requirement of the Canadian law.

Schipper's resignation followed a public campaign labeling him as a "strident" and "vocal" opponent of assisted dying—the centerpiece of the attack being his reference to the Nazi era several years earlier (Bryden 2017a;

Bryden 2017b). The media faithfully featured EAS advocates who questioned the impartiality of the panel and called for a new chair "who has at least been publicly neutral on the issue of assisted dying" (Bryden 2017b). So it came to pass that in the name of impartiality, Schipper was replaced by a philosopher named Jennifer Gibson who was known to be openly critical—not, it must be said, "publicly neutral"—of the three restrictions in the MAID law, the very topics of the panel's work (Gibson 2016).

What the above episode shows is that EAS is a highly controversial, sensitive, and divisive topic. But that hardly seems a justification for avoiding a legitimate topic of inquiry. Of course, there are obvious and deep differences between the old and new regimes of EAS. But our tendency to think that there are no morally relevant similarities at all between the two regimes is, I think, mistaken. Indeed, I will argue that the old involuntary EAS regime motivated by eugenics and the new voluntary EAS regime motivated by "relief" of suffering share two morally relevant features.

First, both regimes imply that some lives are not worth living. It is a noticeable feature of the EAS debates that an individual can, without causing offense, say things like "my life is not worth living." It seems, however, to cause offense when someone says of another person or persons—or of a class of persons—that "their life is not a life worth living." No doubt a part of that reaction is due to the historical residue attached to phrases such as "life unworthy of life" (Proctor 1988). The old eugenics-based EAS regime was explicit about its view that some lives were not worth living, and it might be assumed that modern regimes do not imply such views. I argue that the old and new regimes both imply that, from a societal, intersubjective point of view, some lives are not worth living. Both regimes create a class of persons whose lives are deemed by society as not worth living.

Second, the old and new EAS regimes share another feature in that both regimes have difficulty with equal respect for autonomy. This is, of course, not surprising regarding the old regime. But I will argue that a voluntary, autonomy-based modern EAS regime incurs, by the legalization of EAS, a societal obligation that is unlikely to be met, and this failure results in discriminatory treatment of some people.

Some caveats are in order at the outset. First, in arguing for these two claims, I will focus mostly on EAS for non-dying persons, such as persons with disabilities and psychiatric illnesses, where EAS means termination of a life of a person who would have gone on living. Such a practice has been permitted in Belgium and the Netherlands for years (Kim, De Vries, and Peteet 2016). It is being debated in Canada following a court decision (*Truchon c. Attorney General of Canada* 2019), and advocates in the US are arguing to expand the practice of "physician aid-in-dying" to include non-dying patients (Nicolini, Gastmans, and Kim 2019). How my arguments apply to EAS for the end-of-life situation will require a separate discussion. Second, I do not here provide *arguments* to show that regarding others' lives as not worth living is morally wrong or problematic. I tend to think it is problematic, but I do not argue for it here. Third, my argument is not a psychological claim about how people in a society with legal EAS will feel or will be made to feel about the worth of their lives. It is an argument about what moral judgments are implied from various perspectives when EAS for the non-terminally ill is made legal.

DETERMINATION OF LIVES NOT WORTH LIVING

The modern practice of EAS supports individual choice (not state coercion) to relieve suffering (not to improve the gene pool). Since these two differences are the core differences between the modern and old regimes and, therefore, the only possible reasons why a modern regime might not imply that some lives are not worth living, my argument will proceed by examining each of these two differences.

Suffering-Based Euthanasia and Lives Not Worth Living

The "old" eugenics-based EAS regime was inherently discriminatory. Its central thesis was that some human lives are worth more than others, measured by the yardstick of eugenic potential. It might be thought that when we move from a eugenic justification to a suffering-based justification for EAS, the issue of judging the "worth of human lives" no longer comes into play. The language of suffering seems different; indeed, the motivation to relieve suffering hardly seems discriminatory and, in fact, it is intended to evoke what is noble in us. But the appeal to relief of suffering in EAS regimes rests on an equivocation.

EAS does not strictly speaking provide relief of suffering in the ordinary sense where non-suffering replaces suffering in the continuing life of the person, like quenching a thirst. Rather, EAS removes the ground of suffering. To say that this amounts to true relief of suffering is akin to claiming that one can quench a person's thirst by ending that person's life. EAS does not relieve someone's suffering but eliminates the possibility of it. Because of the way in which suffering is erased, rather than relieved, by terminating the life of the person, EAS inevitably raises the question of the worth of that person's life in the following way: if we justify ending the life (that would otherwise go on) of a person with a disability state (D) because death is better than a life with D, then that is a judgment that a life with D is not worth living.

One might object that this does not show that the modern practice of EAS for persons with D implies a judgment about the lives of *all* persons with D as not worth living. The modern autonomy-based regimes of EAS might not imply judgments of worth of human lives beyond each individual with D who receives EAS: a person with D who voluntarily seeks EAS is saying *his* life is not worth living, as a purely private matter that engages no one else's values except his own.

Are Individuals' Judgments of Their Lives as Not Worth Living Entirely a Private Judgment?

An individual might argue, "I'm not saying that living with D makes every life with D not worth living. I'm only saying that life with D is not worth it *for me*. It is my choice and no one else has a right to interfere with my choice." Autonomy is thus proposed as a shield against interpersonal judgments that some other lives are not worth living.

But is the claim that one's life is not worth living purely private in this sense? Consider the following passage written by a man with Parkinson's disease as he observes a fellow patient with more advanced disease:

> Crouched like a frightened bird, he ate his sauerkraut mash while keeping his mouth close to the plate and drooling. From time to time some of the food fell back from his fork or from his raw, red swollen lower lip. When his plate was half empty, a nurse mercifully fed him a few more bites. His chin sagged on to the plate, his gray beard dipping in the cold sauerkraut mash.

He then goes on, "My God [. . .] I thought, this is what lies ahead of me. And it won't even kill me" (Blanken 2018).

This writer describes an actual patient who has the same disorder as his, and he does so skillfully, clearly evoking an evaluative perspective in the reader: "Crouched," "frightened," "drooling," "raw, red swollen lip," "mercifully," "sagged," "cold." To be clear, I am not debating whether these descriptors are in some sense accurate. There is no doubt that the patient being portrayed is in a difficult state. Although the writer may have intended to illustrate why he himself does not want to live like the man portrayed, that illustration works by way of evoking in us a reaction about the life of the man portrayed as a standard.

Our first thought in reading the above is not: "Oh, you are talking only about your own subjective valuation of your own state of disability—you are saying, for you only and for no one else, not even for the man you portray, you wished the disorder would kill you instead of leaving you in such a state." The writer is judging the life before him as not worth living and *that* is why he does not want that life. Judgments about whether a certain *kind* of life is worth living is logically prior to, and serves as the purported justification for, even one's own judgments about whether one's life is worth living. What this author shows the reader is his belief that a life like the one he so skillfully portrays is not worth living. The author's language is evocative, an attempt to persuade. Both the effort to justify and the need to persuade imply that the author's judgment is universal for all rational persons considering a life under such circumstances rather than an idiosyncratic judgment of a single individual.

Of course, having such a view need not commit the writer to anything like endorsing state-sponsored involuntary euthanasia of such persons or even an attitude that the person being described should choose to die voluntarily. And it need not imply a disrespectful attitude toward that person. Indeed, in a liberal society, we respect people's choice not to request EAS even when others consider their lives not worth living. But permitting EAS does imply that we share the view that a person's life is not worth living.

Some readers will continue to resist this conclusion. They may want to insist that their valuations of their lives as not worth living are indeed private. Perhaps what they mean when they say they have a right to end their lives is simply: Do not *interfere* with my life, my choice, and my values; how I see the worth of my life is my business, not yours.

Is Euthanasia Only a Matter of Not Interfering with Someone's Freedom?

It is somewhat surprising that some philosophers continue to portray EAS as based on a right to noninterference (Cholbi 2013). If it were truly a right to noninterference, the controversy over physicians' conscience right not to participate in EAS would have no meaning. A person's EAS request is a claim on at least one other human being. Indeed, when the EAS request comes from someone who is not dying, then usually the claim involves (for example, in the Netherlands or in Belgium) at least two or three trained experts: the doctor who manages the evaluation and performs the EAS, and one or two other medically trained consultants (The Belgian Act 2002; Regionale Toetsingscommissies Euthanasie [RTE] 2018). The requestor is asking these others to affirm the requestor's judgment that his or her life is not worth living and asking at least one of them to *act* on that *shared* judgment. Whether one performs voluntary or nonvoluntary euthanasia, the judgment expressed by the performer of EAS is the same: in both, the person who provides the EAS expresses a value judgment about the person's life as not worth living.

Of course, people who provide euthanasia might reply, "I'm not making a judgment about the worth of this person's life with D; I am only doing what he wants—it is up to him to decide that his life is not worth living." This indeed is the sort of thing that people might say. Let's see if such a response is an option for the person who performs euthanasia.

First, it is worth noting that in the case of nonvoluntary EAS, because the person receiving EAS is not requesting it, the person performing EAS cannot offer the response that one is "only doing what he wants." What about in the case of voluntary euthanasia? I do not think the response is available in that context either. By itself, an informed request is insufficient to establish eligibility for EAS in any jurisdiction. If a jurisdiction did accept an informed request as the sole criterion for eligibility for EAS, then at least legally, the provider of EAS could possibly offer the response that one is "only doing what [the recipient of EAS] wants." Such a jurisdiction would in fact be promoting a purely voluntarist basis for determining that some lives are not worth living. Some may point to Switzerland here, but the actual norms of practice and other supporting legal considerations make it clear that assisted suicide purely on demand is not endorsed there (Black, 2012).

Consider the Netherlands, one of the most liberal regimes of EAS in the world, where the doctor and the patient *together* must determine that "there is no reasonable alternative" to the EAS (Regionale Toetsingscommissies Euthanasie 2018). If death by EAS is the only reasonable alternative left for the person, then death is also the best option; any alternative (that is, continuing to live) is worth less than death. This rationale is built into the Dutch law on euthanasia.

The Dutch law also requires that the person is "suffering unbearably." The Dutch Regional Euthanasia Review Committees (Regionale Toetsingscommissies Euthanasie, or RTE) say that such suffering, of course, must be seen as a subjective phenomenon in light of an individual's history, personality, etc. (RTE 2018). However, the RTE is quite clear that a patient merely believing and asserting that he is suffering unbearably is not sufficient. One can mistakenly believe one has hopeless and unbearable suffering; in that case, the doctor may find that the person is not suffering unbearably nor in a state where EAS is the only alternative.

The objective—that is, societally sanctioned, interpersonal—perspective of the judgement of whether a person's life is worth living is clearly demonstrated by the requirement that the patient be unbearably suffering even if he lacks the capacity to evaluate and judge the quality of his or her life. As one report regarding a patient noted, "The geriatric specialist and the entire treatment team unanimously agreed that the patient's suffering was objectively unbearable" (RTE, Case 2016-18). It is clear from the Dutch practice that even if a person had written an advance directive saying that he desired EAS if he were admitted to the nursing home, an admission to a nursing home would not by itself be enough to judge that he was suffering unbearably. The patient's suffering at the time of EAS must be objectively verified by experts (RTE 2018, Cases 2016-62 and 2017-103).

Thus, whether a patient's life is worth living is not a wholly private assessment. By law, the doctor who provides EAS as well as the patient making the request must *both* be convinced of it. In turn, the committee who monitors and reviews the doctor must ascertain that the doctor is convinced and, in fact, has a sufficient basis for that conviction. The Dutch system is quite clear that what makes a life not worth living—from a societal, intersubjective point of view, not merely a private judgment regarding the worth of one's own life—is a determination that must be made by a medical doctor. It requires an expert. It is intended to be, in that sense, an objective judgment.

The Function of Autonomy in Euthanasia Regimes: Informed Consent

Legalizing EAS brings into existence a practice of classifying persons as having lives that are not worth living. In the Netherlands (and in other jurisdictions with similar laws), the law also designates the doctor as the only expert who can, together with the patient, determine whether a person's life is worth living.

What is the role of autonomy then? It is precisely the difference between the modern and old regimes of EAS. Unlike the historical National Socialist EAS regime that is based on eugenics, the modern regime of EAS is liberal: *It respects even those persons who choose against their own best interests.* Thus, even persons whose lives are objectively, that is, socially and interpersonally, deemed not worth living are given the respect and the protection of informed consent as a requirement for EAS, at least in theory. (See second part of this chapter.)

Consider how a liberal society handles the tension between the promotion of socially valuable health research with the autonomy of research participants. There are many more eligible persons for clinical research than there are people who volunteer. But in a liberal state, even crucially important clinical research cannot justify coercing people into it. Likewise, from a societal perspective, there are many more people who are, in a modern euthanasia regime, living lives not worth living than who actually voluntarily opt for EAS—yet, they are protected from being coerced into it by the requirement of informed consent.

Informed consent does not make a research protocol ethical, nor does it change the social value of the science performed. It only makes permissible the involvement of the particular individuals. It serves to protect the autonomy of an individual; his or her choice matters. Likewise, informed consent for EAS does not change the assessment of the value of the person's life from a societal perspective. Legally, informed consent makes an otherwise eligible person's EAS permissible. It shows respect for the person's autonomy. But whether or not a person provides informed consent for EAS does not change the fact that, from a societal perspective, that person's life is deemed a life not worth living.

UNEQUAL RESPECT FOR AUTONOMY IN EUTHANASIA REGIMES

In the old eugenic EAS regimes, the state did not respect the autonomy of those coerced into EAS. Since only some people—eugenically inferior people—were coerced into euthanasia, it meant that only some people's autonomy was seen as not worth respecting. Thus, it would seem that in a modern regime in which only voluntary EAS with informed consent is allowed, there is no question of unequal treatment of people's autonomy.

But respecting someone's autonomy is not only a matter of not coercing the person, of leaving that person alone. The exercise of our capacity to make choices, build relationships, and engage in activities—the exercise of our autonomy—requires more. Among other things, there is an expectation that the state will play *some* active role in ensuring resources necessary for its citizens to live as autonomous persons. Of course, the level of such resources that are deemed necessary for the state to provide its citizens varies between societies and is the subject of perennial debate. But for a liberal democratic state, it would be fair to assume that on matters of life or death, the state bears a significant responsibility of treating its citizens equally.

Euthanasia Is Not a Demand for Noninterference (Again): Negative and Positive Autonomy

Because EAS involves making available a service, an expertise-based service, along with mobilizing the necessary resource to oversee its practice, it is not only a matter of not interfering with someone's choice. Thus, when someone says that EAS should be legal "because the government has no business interfering with my freedom," they are in fact asking the government to not simply leave them alone but to provide them with sufficient resources to exercise their positive autonomy. It is an acknowledgment that we are all connected, and we need each other, and that, in order for us to exercise our individual freedoms, we need others' help. It is, in fact, a demand for respect for *positive* autonomy, not merely respect for their right to be left alone (Beaudry 2018).

The fact that EAS is a significant demand for resources should not surprise any advocate of EAS since the very point of EAS is that being left alone to commit suicide is not what they want. What they want—demand—is help. What they are demanding are sufficient resources to broaden their options and they are claiming that it is the obligation of society and the state to provide them.

Unequal Respect for Autonomy?

Imagine two women, Ana and Rose, with severe, recurrent depression. Both are in their late forties. They have suffered from depression on and off for nearly 15 years. Their current episodes of depression have lasted several long, difficult years. Both have attempted suicides in the past. They have both tried many medications; both have received electroconvulsive therapy in the past.

There are two features about these cases of which the reader should be aware. First, there likely are physicians in the Netherlands or Belgium who could be convinced—and could convince the review committees that they have sufficient basis for being convinced—that both Ana and Rose, if they requested it, would be eligible for EAS for depression. Second, there is also evidence that with proper treatment, both patients have at least a 60 to 70 percent chance of remission from their current episode of depression (Fekadu et al. 2012; Rush et al. 2006). Furthermore, although there are characteristics that correlate with outcomes, they are not robust enough for individual clinicians to make reliable predictions about individual patients. Indeed, even if someone goes through a treatment program and initially does not respond, no one really knows what the chances of response would be if another attempt is made with therapeutic adjustments based on the failed course of treatment. How the above two facts are compatible in a regime that requires that EAS be the last resort ("no reasonable alternative") is a complex discussion, but suffice it to say, doctors are allowed considerable clinical discretion in these regimes (Kim, De Vries, and Peteet 2016).

Now suppose that there is a specialty program in a nearby clinic. It would begin with an inpatient admission followed by outpatient care. Ana has private means and excellent insurance that will cover the costs of this program but after hearing about and researching the details of the program, she declines. She is fed up with her situation. She is despondent but is deemed competent to make her own medical decisions, including the decision to seek EAS. When asked why, she says, "My life is not worth living. I don't want to fight anymore. I'm ready for euthanasia."

Rose is different. She does not want to die and, at first, is not interested in EAS. Prior to her current depressive episode, she worked as an architect but now has no job and no private insurance. She resorts to the state-sponsored insurance pool that is unwilling to pay for the specialty program. However, they will pay for her EAS should she choose it. Rose would much prefer to try the specialty clinic; she is not ready to give up. But when she is denied access to the specialty clinic, she begins to wonder if it is better to die than to go on living. With the specialty program closed to her, she feels she has *no other option* but to choose EAS.

At least in theory, Ana is free and autonomous to choose EAS; Rose is not. Does the state bear some responsibility for correcting this inequitable state of affairs? People's views will vary, just as people vary in their politics. But it may be useful to recall that the *Carter* decision in Canada contains the following reasoning to justify its decision to make EAS available as an option: the prohibition on physician-assisted dying "ha[s] the effect of *forcing* some individuals to take their own lives prematurely, for fear that they would be incapable of doing so when they reached the point where suffering was intolerable" (Carter v. Canada 2015; italics mine). Although the court sees this reasoning as engaging the right to life, it is obvious that such reasoning enhances the positive autonomy of Ana but, unless equal opportunities are provided, not for Rose.

What this example points out is the extraordinary degree of responsibility that a modern regime of EAS takes on when it legalizes EAS. Those who advocate for EAS often criticize their opponents as "paternalistic," and invoke a negative freedom argument. However, when people invoke the right to be left alone as they go off the grid, the state need not do anything further to respect their right to do so. On the other hand, when EAS is legalized, the state must create systems of control and access; professional societies must create guidelines and training programs; hospitals must procure medications and develop standard operating procedures; and review systems must be set up and administered. If a state takes on the responsibility of providing EAS as a means of promoting and respecting autonomy, it should be ready to meet the demands of equality of respect that such a policy requires (Beaudry 2018).

Conclusion: Positive Autonomy and Lives Not Worth Living

If we use the language developed in the first part of this chapter to describe Ana and Rose, we can see from the state's perspective that neither Ana's nor Rose's life is a life worth living. Their lives meet the objective, social criteria for what makes a life not worth living in an EAS regime: Physicians becoming convinced, within the bounds of discretionary judgment accorded them, that they can endorse the patients' views of their lives as not worth living. The difference between the old and the new EAS regimes is in the yardstick used to judge a life not worth living—eugenic potential versus quality of life. But they both make judgments of the worth of a life.

Of course, in the National Socialist regime, if a life was not worth living, there was no commitment to liberal ideals of freedom and autonomy—it was a regime in which the needs of the collective took precedence over the individual. There was no such thing as informed consent as a prerequisite for EAS. But in a modern, liberal regime where individual freedom and autonomy are highly valued, even persons who choose to live lives that are not worth living are not to be coerced or unduly influenced. Informed consent is seen as inviolable and necessary so that people are permitted to continue living even against their best interests.

The story of Ana and Rose points out that the commitment to liberal ideals cannot stop at mere non-coercion. In an EAS regime that is truly liberal, there must be support for the equal positive autonomy rights of those whose lives are deemed not worth living. Such a society therefore must be committed to mobilizing a large amount resources for the benefit of those who are seen by society as having lives not worth living and yet are choosing to live contrary to their own best interests. Is such an idealistic society realizable and sustainable?

One cannot help wonder whether such a utopian vision could well end up a dystopian reality.

This work was supported in part by the Intramural Research Program of the National Institutes of Health, Bethesda, Maryland. The ideas and opinions expressed are the author's own; they do not represent any position or policy of the National Institutes of Health, the Department of Health and Human Services, or the U.S. government.

Portions of this chapter on modern euthanasia regimes and lives not worth living have been adapted from: Kim, SYH. 2019. "Lives Not Worth Living in Modern Euthanasia Regimes," *Journal of Policy and Practice in Intellectual Disabilities* 16, no. 2 (June): 134–136.

BIBLIOGRAPHY

Beaudry, Jonas-Sébastien. 2018. "The Way Forward for Medical Aid in Dying: Protecting Deliberative Autonomy is Not Enough." *Supreme Court Law Review, Second Series, Vol. 85*. https://ssrn.com/abstract=3189417.

"The Belgian Act on Euthanasia of May, 28, 2002." 2002. Reprinted in *Ethical Perspectives* 9, no. 2–3 (June–September): 182–188.

Black, Isra. 2012. "Suicide Assistance For Mentally Disordered Individuals in Switzerland and the State's Positive Obligation To Facilitate Dignified Suicide: Haas c. Suisse, Cour européenne des droits de l'homme, 1re section (20 janvier 2011) (Unreported)." *Medical Law Review* 20, no. 1 (Winter): 157–166. doi:10.1093/medlaw/fwr033.

Blanken, Henk. 2018. "My Death Is Not My Own: The Limits of Legal Euthanasia." *Guardian.* August 10, 2018. Accessed September 20, 2018. https://www.theguardian.com/news/2018/aug/10/my-death-is-not-my-own-the-limits-of-legal-euthanasia.

Bryden, Joan. 2017a. "Strident Opponent of Assisted Dying to Chair Review of Advance Requests." *Globe and Mail.* April 28, 2017. Accessed May 11, 2018. https://www.the globe and mail.com/news/national/strident-opponent-of-assisted-dying-to-chair-review-of-advance-requests/article34852825/.

Bryden, Joan. 2017b. "Vocal Opponent of Assisted Dying No Longer Leading Advance Request Review. *Globe and Mail.* May 11, 2017. Accessed May 11, 2018. https://www.the globe and mail.com/news/national/vocal-opponent-of-assisted-dying-no-longer-leading-advance-request-review/article34953834/.

Carter v. Canada (Attorney General). 2015. Report 1 SCR 331, Case no. 35591. Accessed September 9, 2015. https://scc-csc.lexum.com/scc-csc/scc-csc/en/item/14637/index.do.

Cholbi, Michael. 2013. "The Terminal, the Futile, and the Psychiatrically Disordered." *International Journal of Law and Psychiatry*, 36, no. 5–6 (July): 498–505. doi:10.1016/j.ijlp.2013.06.011.

Council of Canadian Academies. 2018. The Expert Panel on Medical Assistance in Dying. Accessed November 8, 2019. https://www.scienceadvice.ca/reports/medical-assistance-in-dying/.

Fekadu, Abebaw, Lena Rane, Sarah Wooderson, Kalypso Markopoulou, Lucia Poon, and Anthony Cleare. 2012. "Prediction of Longer-Term Outcome of Treatment-Resistant Depression in Tertiary Care." *British Journal of Psychiatry*, 201, no. 5 (November): 369–375. doi:10.1192/bjp.bp.111.102665.

Gibson, Jennifer. 2016. Testimony before the Justice and Human Rights Committee on May 5, 2016. Accessed September 7, 2018. https://openparliament.ca/committees/justice/42-1/14/jennifer-gibson-1/.

Kim, Scott Y. H., Raymond De Vries, and John Peteet. 2016. "Euthanasia and Assisted Suicide of Patients with Psychiatric Disorders in the Netherlands 2011 to 2014." *Journal of American Medical Association Psychiatry* 73, no. 4 (April): 362–368. doi:10.1001/jamapsychiatry.2015.2887.

Nicolini, Marie E., Chris Gastmans, Scott Y. H. Kim. 2019. "Parity Arguments for 'Physician Aid-in-Dying' (PAD) for Psychiatric Disorders: Their Structure and Limits." *American Journal of Bioethics* 19, no. 10 (September): 3–7.

Proctor, Robert. 1988. *Racial Hygiene: Medicine Under the Nazis.* Cambridge, MA: Harvard University Press.

Regionale Toetsingscommissies Euthanasie (RTE) [Regional Euthanasia Review Committees]. 2018. "EuthanasieCode 2018." The Hague. Accessed November 8, 2019. https://www.euthanasiecommissie.nl.

Rush, A. John, Madhukar Trivedi, Stephen Wisniewski, et al. 2006. "Acute and Longer-Term Outcomes in Depressed Outpatients Requiring One or Several Treatment Steps: A STAR*D Report." *American Journal of Psychiatry* 163, no.11 (November): 1905–17. doi:10.1176/appi.ajp.163.11.1905.

Schipper, Harvey. 2014. "With Assisted Suicide, Context Is Everything." *Globe and Mail*. June 6, 2014. Accessed May 11, 2018. https://www.the globeand mail.com/opinion/with-assisted-suicide-context-is-everything/article19012073.

Truchon c. Attorney General of Canada, 2019 QCCS 3792 (CanLII).

Chapter Sixteen

Can a Person Ever Be "Not Useful"?

A Critical Analysis of the Anthropological Roots of Euthanasia under National Socialism and Today

Ashley K. Fernandes

Between 1933 and 1945, under National Socialism, one's right to life was justified in many circumstances by its "usefulness." Those considered "not of use" (*unbrauchbar*) for the state due to their racial, hereditary, or even "moral" makeup were targeted for death in the Third Reich's euthanasia programs. Today, this concept of *usefulness* bears critical philosophical examination, as justification for both physician-assisted suicide (PAS) and euthanasia is often made on this basis. The critical difference in contemporary medical ethics is that, under the banner of autonomy, patients may choose for *themselves* that they are useless. This choice is then thought to be unassailable, thereby dismissing comparisons of justifications for Nazi and contemporary euthanasia. But does the fact that one *chooses* to call oneself "not of use" simply make it so?

In this chapter, I argue that the dogmatic acceptance of autonomy is based on a flawed anthropology that is particularly harmful to the most vulnerable patients contemplating PAS or euthanasia. This flawed anthropology removes the possibility that people may be challenged in their assessment of others' value, and also, that patients themselves might be challenged in their assessment of their own value. I also argue against the unassailability of autonomy by showing how, both clinically and professionally, physicians are often obligated to correct and improve patient's perceptions of self and value. Finally, I offer an alternative concept of person—one based on the personalism of writers such as Jacques Maritain, Emmanuel Levinas, and Karol Wojtyla—that offers another way of conceptualizing personhood that better upholds the dignity of persons, rejects the concept of *usefulness* as a criterion for personhood, and grounds dignity in a relational community of persons.

On this basis, both the historic and contemporary designation of patients as *unbrauchbar* to justify PAS or euthanasia ought to be rejected.

NAZI EUTHANASIA AND THE LINK TO *UNBRAUCHBAR*

The role of physicians in planning and implementing medical abuses of patients during the Third Reich has been well documented—perhaps most notably by Robert J. Lifton (1986) and Robert N. Proctor (1988)—shattering the myth that physicians were coerced to utilize knowledge and skill against those considered unfit for existence. Central in all discussions has been the Nazi doctors' role in involuntary euthanasia. In October 1939, Adolf Hitler authorized euthanasia of the "incurably sick," which, in practice, meant patients he and physicians considered *unbrauchbar*. Patients' right to life now had to be justified to avoid being euthanized as a "life unworthy of life." That phrase, made infamous in 1920 by Alfred Hoche and Karl Binding in *Die Freigabe der Vernichtung lebensunwerten Lebens* (*The Authorization of the Destruction of Life Unworthy of Life*), demonstrates that euthanasia was a culmination of a cultural and moral shift set in motion before Hitler became chancellor in 1933. Because of these shifts, the physician leaders of the Nazi euthanasia programs were actively supported by nurses, midwives, research scientists, and administrative personnel, and benefited from the passive and active cooperation of the ordinary enculturated populace (Foth 2014).

The euthanasia program began secretly with disabled children. Between 1939 and 1945, physicians organized and implemented more than 30 euthanasia centers that killed at least 5,000 children. Between 150,000 and 200,000 adults were murdered in the adult euthanasia programs, the centrally coordinated *Aktion* T4 carried out in gas chambers until 1941 and the decentralized euthanasia "carried out through starvation, medication, and neglect" until 1945 (Foth 2014). Michael Burleigh's sobering volume, *Death and Deliverance* (1994), and chapters 1 and 3 by Gerrit Hohendorf in this book describe the origins and impact of the Nazi domestic euthanasia program on further developments of the Holocaust.

EUTHANASIA AND PHYSICIAN-ASSISTED SUICIDE: THE DIFFERENCE AUTONOMY MAKES

Hohendorf noted that beyond the obvious primacy of state and racial interests over individual interests, National Socialism justified euthanasia through "more subtle moral gateways." These included:

1. the demand for a "right to death" the *autonomous individual* is said to have, including the right to decide about one's own life and body,
2. the idea that in situations of incurable illness and unbearable suffering humans and in particular physicians should provoke death out of pity, and
3. the idea that the value of human life cannot only be defined subjectively by somebody being concerned him/herself but that it may also be defined from the outside, according to the degree of his/her *usefulness for society* and after having dropped out of societal relations. (Hohendorf 2014, 278; italics mine)

It should be noted that while the first and second justifications are often cited in contemporary bioethical and empirical literature as justificatory reasons for PAS and euthanasia (Blanke et al. 2017; Pearlman et al. 2005; Jansen-van der Weide, Onwuteaka-Philipsen, and van der Wal 2005) and have strong appeal both among academics and in Western culture, the third justification, usefulness for society, is scarcely found in the adult literature. Steven Pinker, however, has defended early infanticide on the basis of usefulness to the mother (1997). Alberto Giubilini and Francesca Minerva have argued that killing a newborn is justified on the same moral grounds as abortion and are explicit as to the reason why:

> To bring up such children might be an *unbearable burden on the family and on society as a whole, when the state economically provides for their care*. . . . In spite of the oxymoron in the expression, we propose to call this practice "after-birth abortion," rather than "infanticide," to emphasise that the moral status of the individual killed is comparable with that of a fetus. . . . Accordingly, a second terminological specification is that we call such a practice "after-birth abortion" rather than "euthanasia" *because the best interest of the one who dies is not necessarily the primary criterion for the choice*, contrary to what happens in the case of euthanasia. (Giubilini and Minerva 2013; italics mine)

Contemporary justifications for pediatric euthanasia seem to be a combination of (1), (2), and (3)—that is, the mother (or family) has an autonomous right to euthanize a child, often for compassion's sake, and that life's value may be judged by an external person or entity weighing the benefits and burdens of existence as a way of calculating another's usefulness.

In adults, however, autonomy is the principal ethical difference between euthanasia in the Nazi era and the current practice of PAS and euthanasia. Dan W. Brock outlined the centrality of autonomy in this way:

> two fundamental ethical values supporting the . . . permissibility of euthanasia . . . are individual self-determination or autonomy and individual well-being. By self-determination as it bears on euthanasia, I mean people's interest in

making important decisions about their lives for themselves according to their own values or conceptions of a good life, and in being left free to act on those decisions. . . . A central aspect of human dignity lies in people's capacity to direct their lives in this way. The value of exercising self-determination presupposes some minimum of decision-making capacities or competence, which thus limits the scope of euthanasia supported by self-determination. . . . (Brock 1992, 11)

More recently, Ronit D. Leichtentritt and his co-authors (1999) interviewed 15 Holocaust survivors and asked them what they perceived to be the differences between euthanasia then and now. Utilizing a qualitative phenomenological approach, the authors reported that participants identified only one similarity—the outcome of death—and several other dissimilarities, which they felt were crucial in demonstrating that euthanasia today is unlike that during the Nazi era. In a closer review of themes extracted from these perspectives, however, a common thread emerges—that of choice.

One survivor stated: "In one case, the physician's intentions are to kill, or to use one's body for some crazy experimental procedures, while the other, the intention is completely different, it is to help *you* die; You became the center of the process." Another said:

Give people the right to choose; That is what democracy is all about . . . I should have the final decision about my and my own body, my own life and death; In the concentration camps someone else was in charge of all these domains; In some cases, someone else was also in charge of other people's souls. . . . If a person chooses euthanasia as the way he wishes to die, why call it Nazi Germany? Why not call it democracy?

Still another elderly survivor summarized the difference this way:

Summarize my life in the camps, summarize the main idea of the Nazi torturing process: Take control away from people, "leave them in the dark" . . . I did not know if I am going to be dead or alive tomorrow morning, I did not know if I am going to be alive in the next seven minutes; This is exactly the opposite from mercy killing, where the person gains control over one of the processes in human life that tends to be the least in our control—that is exactly the opposite; Regardless of one's moral attitudes toward gaining control over death and dying, how can you say they are the same? (Leichtentritt, Rettig, and Miles 1999, quotes on 191–192)

These poignant and powerful testimonies should be taken to heart but still subject to critical analysis. In Nazi Germany, where euthanasia was involuntary, a person acting for the state interest would judge another person's usefulness. In my view, it would be a mistake to conclude that simply *choos-*

ing PAS and euthanasia negates all historical comparisons, warnings about parallels, or critiques of the practice. Yet, as James Kennedy has shown in his paper describing the impact of National Socialism on the twentieth century Dutch euthanasia debate:

> Dutch policy-makers and the Dutch public in the course of the 1970s and early 1980s decisively moved in a direction that, at least at the discursive level, eliminated the tension [between "greater human autonomy" and the desire to "release" all those suffering from a "meaningless" life] by insisting that "euthanasia" was—by definition—voluntary. (Kennedy 2014, 215)

Early proponents of PAS and euthanasia in the Netherlands understood the parallel between euthanasia under the Nazis and now and intentionally confronted it head on, separating the practices of the past from contemporary euthanasia by elevating the moral decisiveness of choice.

Can an autonomous person judge himself or herself to be *unbrauchbar*? That is, can a supporter of PAS and euthanasia legitimately say, "Only I can value myself—whether wrong or right—my judgment is my own, and that is enough"? Is such a judgment ethically acceptable simply because it comes from within the person? In my view, the answer is no.

In the remainder of this chapter, I will explain my answer by making the case that autonomous choices are tied to a criterion outside oneself and embrace a relational element. In clinical medicine, physicians know that patients and families often make mistakes about small things, as we all do. But it is a disastrous mistake to assign unassailability to the self-assessment of our own value, let alone that of others. The option that best safeguards the inherent dignity of the person requires a more inclusive philosophical anthropology, one which replaces unassailability of autonomy with the inviolability of person; only then will we avoid the devastating mistakes of the past.

HOW CAN PERSONS JUDGE THEMSELVES "NOT USEFUL"?

Elsewhere, I have described the importance of philosophical anthropology to questions in bioethics, and specifically to the question of PAS and euthanasia:

> unlike abortion or brain-death discussions, the euthanasia argument does not turn on "questions" of whether the human is a person. The patient who requests suicide is considered by all parties to be a rational agent with full moral standing in the community. But what does it *mean* to be a moral agent? Proponents of euthanasia frequently cite, for example, patient autonomy and compassion as justifications for their point of view, but without justifying a corresponding notion of the patient as *person*." (Fernandes 2001, 381)

The anthropological question is, thus, critical to any discussion of PAS and euthanasia. The late Dr. Edmund Pellegrino rightly noted that:

> We must know the nature of ourselves, others, and the world, otherwise there is no template against which to measure the moral status of our thought and action. The persistence of the anthropological question is a reminder of both our continuing puzzlement and our need to base our moral lives on some concept of the good for humans, that which advances our humanity. (2006, 250)

The near-absolutist framing of autonomy in contemporary Western bioethics infers a type of anthropology in which a rational person cannot (should not) be challenged about decisions made by him or her. Suffering at the end of life—its value and reason for being, for example, becomes subject to our autonomous choice. Stanley Hauerwas described how the nature of modern medicine has continued to reinforce this idea by disconnecting suffering from anything but the processes of the body:

> Medicine can be interpreted as the attempt to have us view our suffering as pointless, thus making it subject to therapeutic intervention. In other words, medicine tends to break the moral link between our suffering and our projects by suggesting that our suffering is pointless. Medicine thus schools us to think of our suffering in a mechanical model. (Hauerwas 1986, 33)

An autonomist anthropology also has implications for the question of dignity. As I have pointed out in a previous work (Fernandes 2010), both Ruth Macklin (2003) and Steven Pinker (2008) have criticized the concept of *human dignity* as "useless" or "stupid," respectively, since they argued that what actually provides dignity is autonomy. Macklin's ultimate conclusion was that dignity adds nothing to debates in bioethics that *cannot be found outside the principle of respect for autonomy*, and as such, ought to be eliminated as a factor altogether (2003). Later, she refined the argument, stating that dignity is not a "useless concept"—since everyone uses it in one way or another—but it is perhaps better characterized as "an infinitely elastic" concept, making it just as meaningless outside of its attachment to autonomy (Macklin 2004). For contemporary Western mainstream bioethics, the concept of autonomy and the concept of dignity are one and the same. Another person cannot restrict one's choices about oneself, since there are no objective criteria on which to justly restrict it. The only truly "bad" thing is to deny another's choice, which would be akin—if Macklin and Pinker are right—to harming the dignity of a person. Thus, when it comes to the choice for PAS or euthanasia, we may come back to Dan Brock's contention that "A central aspect of human dignity lies in people's capacity to direct their lives in this way" (1992, 11).

The autonomist anthropology also has profound implications for how members of society relate to one another. If my dignity and value are bound to the autonomous choices I make, then noninterference in the choices of another becomes an act of caring, a concept PAS supporter Timothy Quill, describes as *nonabandonment* (Quill and Cassel 1995). When the autonomist anthropology is embraced, it is, therefore, possible that physician noninterference when patients ultimately choose PAS or euthanasia leads patients to believe that they are "not of use" to others, and that no one else has standing to challenge this belief. Empirical evidence indicates that many patients at the end of life perceive themselves as burdens to others, which further reinforces a perception of worthlessness and hopelessness and a desire for suicide (Wilson, Curran, and McPherson 2005). Such "self-perceived burden" was a substantial problem for 19 to 65 percent of terminally ill patients in one study, and correlated with patients' perceptions of "loss of dignity, suffering, and a 'bad death.'" According to Alisa Carse, suffering shatters "the *myth* of the 'in-control agent,'" and Western philosophical thought has underplayed our natural vulnerability in favor of "self-sufficiency, independence, a capacity for deliberation and rational transcendence of emotion"—with drastic moral consequences (Carse 2006, 34–35). Therefore, it is not surprising that 48.9 percent of patients who committed suicide in 2016 under the Oregon Death With Dignity Act did so, in part, because they felt they were a burden; 65.4 percent felt a loss of dignity; and 89.5 percent cited a loss of autonomy as primary end-of-life concerns (Oregon Health Authority 2017). These reasons underscore that for some, value is tied to what they see themselves able to do or not do—a functional criterion—rather than whom they intrinsically are, a criterion of being. It is impossible to quantify how many patients would describe themselves as *unbrauchbar*, but the soft evidence in the empirical literature is abundant.

Harder evidence can be found in the slip from self-perception of uselessness to societal perception of the same. A recent review noted ominously, "The right to die is leading to a duty to die," (Sprung et al. 2018) and demonstrates a growing number of documented cases throughout the developed world in which involuntary and nonvoluntary euthanasia have occurred, despite guidelines and safeguards to prevent abuse. Sprung and colleagues also offered substantial evidence that vulnerable populations such as the elderly, women, the less educated, and those in nursing homes are at greater risk of being pressured to accede to PAS or euthanasia (2018). Another survey in the Netherlands showed that 550 patients were killed without express consent, and in the majority of these cases, pressure from relatives played a significant role (van der Heide 2007). These abuses are evidence that the value of life is now being defined, not by autonomous individuals, but "from the outside" as Hohendorf suggested was the case under National Socialism (Hohendorf 2014, 278). This is not merely a benign side effect of extant laws—for each loss of life without consent is an irrevocable, infinite loss of a person, a loss to a family, a loss to a community—and the undermining of the very concept of autonomy.

Worse still, there are now cases of euthanasia being granted or proposed for patients with severe dementia (Sheldon 2005), depression and schizophrenia (Kim, DeVries, and Peteet 2016), autism (Cheng 2018), addiction (Hall and Parker 2017), and even transgenderism (Heylens, Verschelden, and De Cuypere 2016). Cases in which mental illness plays a role are perhaps the most disturbing and lay bare the negative effects of the unassailability of autonomy. First, it is hard to imagine how these select cases promote dignity as autonomy. They would seem to undercut it, since ill or anxious patients are permitted to conclude themselves useless, without dignity and, therefore, unworthy of life. But, second, even if these were truly autonomous decisions (a big if)—should they be absolute? Because these are purely subjective decisions, we are not even permitted to dissuade patients from considering themselves not of use, and ultimately prohibit their action.

PERSONALISM: AN ALTERNATIVE ANTHROPOLOGY

In the middle of an otherwise blistering medical and empirical critique of the Netherlands' Groningen Protocol for euthanasia for pediatric patients, T. H. Rob de Jong quoted Emmanuel Levinas: "Ethos cannot be founded in scientific facts; it is founded in the human relationship itself. Mutual dependency, which is characteristic for 'human being,' makes us responsible just by itself and therefore defines 'the disposition of ethos' as a rational fact. This relationship always precedes facts themselves" (2008, 15). This startling summation of a personalist conclusion is where we can begin to see an alternative to the autonomist model. Levinas, known for his notion of "the face of the Other," stated that "Subjectivity is not for itself; it is, once again, initially for another" (1985, 96). Levinas believed that we have responsibilities to another person that cannot be separated from the nature of our own personhood.

Elsewhere I have defended the use of a personalistic anthropology in bioethics, based on the philosophical writings of Karol Wojtyla, who would later become St. Pope John Paul II, as an alternative to the autonomist view (Fernandes 2001). Wojtyla identified four specific characteristics that define what it means to be a person (Modras 1982).

First, *a person is one who thinks* (has a rational nature) and creates by "extracting truths from reality" (Modras 1982, 123). A person who considers himself or herself useless is not making a harmless mistake in judgment that cannot be challenged. Instead, since thinking involves abstraction from an objective reality, a person cannot only be wrong, but can be seriously wrong. And when the consequence of allowing a mistake about self-value is death, a "moral shrug" is simply unacceptable.

Second, *a person is a creature who acts in freedom*, but this is not merely a freedom to choose. Freedom is authentic only when one chooses what is objectively true. For this to happen, there must exist, outside subjectivity, a criterion of correctness that is discernible by both reason and experience.

Third, *a person is one who loves*. Loving oneself, loving another, and being loved are part and parcel of existence; it is self-giving through love—both as a terminally ill patient and a physician—that is the key to overcoming suffering, uselessness, and hopelessness at the end of life. In loving, we continue the path to perfect our being for which we were created.

Finally, and critical to our discussion, *a person is one who acts within a community* for the common good of other persons. The relational element of personhood can also be found in Wojtyla's influences such as Martin Buber (1986), Gabriel Marcel (1963), and, in particular, Jacques Maritain (1985). Maritain, writing in the immediate post–World War II era, acutely saw the consequences of any other good obscuring the good of the individual person. In National Socialism, Maritain saw the danger of having a concept of *person* that is not absolute. Nazi physicians had, in fact, a robust concept of *person* that required contributions to the German *Volksgemeinschaft* (people's community). The elimination of the *unbrauchbar* made perfect sense, for society was merely a collection of individuals who lived together out of convenience or self-interest. Then, as now, the consequences of a disordered philosophical anthropology necessarily have an impact on relationships to others and to society. Euthanasia today can threaten the trust and solidarity found in the physician-patient relationship (Kass 1989); some patients desiring PAS or euthanasia are motivated by a "loss of their sense of self" and feelings of being a burden to others (Pearlman et al. 2005).

Wojtyla claimed that solidarity is contained in the actions for the common good, which elevate both the person who acts and the object(s) of action (Wojtyla 1969). In support of Wojtyla's claim about solidarity, Alasdair MacIntyre called for a society that incorporates dependence into its social fabric (1999, 130). Thus, the sick person, while perhaps not even able to exercise thought, act in freedom, or perceive love, is still integrated fully into the human community and has objective value through the participation and love of the other.

For personalists, the *communio personarum* (communion of persons) arises out of human dignity itself, dignity contained within each person.

Therefore, the community functions both as the mechanism for discovering and the product of intrinsic human dignity. Wojtyla noted that "the matter of the dignity of the human person is always more of a call and a demand than an already accomplished fact, or rather it is a fact worked out by human beings, both in the collective and the individual sense" (Wojtyla 1969, 179).

The community is the vehicle by which we experience our own dignity and the dignity of others. On a deeper level, the connectedness of persons with dignity—and the value of each person discovered through their interdependence—is what makes a community possible and gives the community a dignity all its own. However, if the intersubjective experience of dignity is ignored, then the opposite occurs, and the person is at risk of isolation and alienation, and the community is shattered (Wojtyla 1969).

By contrast, a society that permits PAS or euthanasia distorts the notion of *community*. By permitting them, society sends several messages to the dependent and vulnerable patient: (1) the patient's experience is understood but alien; (2) perhaps there is empathy but not sympathy; (3) if the patient perceives his or her dependency or "un-usefulness" as an intolerable burden, then society will, too, simply because the patient says it is so. Instead, we ought to view vulnerability as an inseparable part of living in a communion with others—not a condition to fear or to escape from by permitting PAS or euthanasia. It is in the vulnerable patient that we realize our own vulnerabilities, and in doing so, learn something of the value of humanity.

IS AN AUTONOMOUS CHOICE ALWAYS UNASSAILABLE?

National Socialism posited that certain individuals were not of use and could, therefore, be eliminated. Gerrit Hohendorf has also argued that, both then and now, PAS and euthanasia require "a value judgment on certain states of life." The fact that such a judgment is required poses a danger "this judgment will be extended also on people who are no longer capable of an autonomous decision," and that such legal and medical practices may "make feel patients with severe disablement or in states of suffering urged to express such a desire [to die] because they do not want to be a burden for themselves, for others, or for society" (Hohendorf 2014, 301). I have averred that we should be profoundly troubled whether an external force, be it the state or a physician, decides that a patient is not of use. I would also assert that we should be equally troubled if the patient reaches the same conclusion. I would argue further that the bright red line between an external force and an individual making such a decision is often not so bright and that, as a result, so-called voluntary PAS and euthanasia has already begun a troubling slide that should not be tolerated.

A dogmatic acceptance of any patient's autonomous choice of PAS or euthanasia should be rejected on the philosophical grounds I have laid out above. Such a view risks exposing the patient to more harm and is at odds with the human experience of the moral life and community. Importantly, empirical evidence also suggests that many patients requesting PAS and euthanasia are ambivalent in their requests (Johansen et al. 2005)—all the more reason to question their decisions rather than accept them as unassailable. Isabelle Marcoux and colleagues found that Dutch patients who changed their minds after making an explicit request for PAS or euthanasia had poorer mental health status overall and were more likely to have anxiety or depression before the request (Marcoux et al. 2005).

Personalism values all individuals despite their vulnerability and seeks to heal through a community. The relational element of persons is key to their protection from harm—we need others to protect ourselves. We must be able to say that one can be wrong about one's self-assigned value and that the inherent dignity of that person requires protection.

As a doctor, I do not affirm my patients' wishes for suicide when they are clinically depressed, hate themselves, and/or see themselves as not of use. I try to persuade them of the opposite, judiciously using antidepressants to treat what I view as a pathology. Doctors should encourage patients with low self-esteem or self-worth to see their worth rather than affirm their self-perception of worthlessness.

Even at the end of life, clinicians have attempted to change their patient's minds about their self-perceived burden. Harvey Chochinov's ingenious study of "dignity therapy" is an example of such a successful innovation (Chochinov et al. 2005). Short-term psychotherapeutic interventions have been proposed and tried successfully in patients with cancer and amyotrophic lateral sclerosis (commonly referred to as ALS), two of the primary diagnoses leading to PAS in the United States (Oberstadt et al. 2018). In sum, patients can be incorrect about their assessment of their own and others' usefulness, and physicians are professionally obligated to affirm the dignity and worth of their patients, particularly in the face of serious or terminal illness.

FUTURE CHALLENGES

The autonomist view is deeply troubling in at least two senses. First, it takes a passive view of the truthfulness of patients' wishes and perceptions, an impractical and dangerous posture in clinical medicine that ultimately allows patients to wrongly devalue their own lives. Second, it allows patient autonomy to reflexively override crucial issues, such as the doctor-patient relationship, the conscience of the physician, the meaning of suffering, and the relational elements of personhood (solidarity). Are we, as a medical community and as a society, willing to accept the extreme autonomist view?

There will be great challenges if the crass form of utilitarianism that equates utility with social usefulness leads to legalization of PAS or euthanasia in more of the developed world. The conflict between population-based ethics and population-based care on the one hand, and medical ethics and patient-centered care on the other, will increase. Also, we risk exposing more people, especially those with mental illness, to increased rates of non-assisted suicide (in one study, by 6.3 percent) that follow legalization of PAS and euthanasia, the "social contagion" effect (Jones and Paton 2015).

However, the greatest challenge will be to an authentic, inclusive anthropology that retains our sense of community in the face of increasing individualism and isolation. We must remember what happened when National Socialist physicians were empowered to kill patients believed to be *unbrauchbar* by a state and a culture saturated with eugenics, and acknowledge that we are now doing the same when patients believe it about themselves. In this chapter, I have tried to show that we must consider alternatives to the presumed unassailability of individual autonomy, and that solidarity with another is our solution to preserving our grasp of human dignity. Medicine must recommit to healing by our presence as healers rather than killing by our capitulation to the dogma of choice.

BIBLIOGRAPHY

Blanke, Charles, Michael LeBlanc, Dawn Hershman, Lee Ellis, and Frank Meyskens. 2017. "Characterizing 18 Years of the Death with Dignity Act in Oregon." *Journal of the American Medical Association Oncology*, 3, no. 10 (October): 1403–1406.

Brock, Dan W. 1992. "Voluntary Active Euthanasia." *Hastings Center Report* 22, no. 2 (March–April): 10–22.

Buber, Martin. 1986. *I and Thou*, 2nd ed. Translated by Ronald Smith. New York: Scribners.

Burleigh, Michael. 1994. *Death and Deliverance: "Euthanasia" in Germany 1900–1945*. Cambridge: Cambridge University Press.

Carse, Alisa. 2006. "Vulnerability, Agency and Human Agency." In *Health and Human Flourishing: Religion, Medicine, and Moral Anthropology*, edited by Carol R. Taylor and Roberto Dell'Oro, 33–52. Washington, DC: Georgetown University Press.

Cheng, Maria. 2018. Associated Press News. "Belgium Investigates Doctors Who Euthanized Autistic Woman." November 27, 2018. Accessed July 8, 2019. https://www.apnews.com/249a8067af6740d2af22ed66fc9e1a90.

Chochinov, Harvey, Thomas Hack, Thomas Hassard, Linda J. Kristjanson, Susan McClement, and Mike Harlos. 2005. "Dignity Therapy: A Novel Psychotherapeutic Intervention for Patients Near the End of Life." *Journal of Clinical Oncology* 23, no. 24 (August 20): 5520–5525.

de Jong, T. H. Rob. 2008. "Deliberate Termination of Life of Newborns with Spina Bifida, a Critical Appraisal." *Child's Nervous System* 24, no. 1 (January): 13–28.

Fernandes, Ashley K. 2001. "Euthanasia, Assisted Suicide, and the Philosophical Anthropology of Karol Wojtyla." *Christian Bioethics* 7, no. 3 (December): 379–402.

Fernandes, Ashley K. 2010. "The Loss of Dignity at the End of Life: Incommunicability as a Call and a Demand." *National Catholic Bioethics Quarterly* 10, no. 3 (Autumn): 529–546.

Foth, Thomas. 2014. "Changing Perspectives: From 'Euthanasia Killings' to the 'Killings of Sick Persons.'" In *Nurses and Midwives in Nazi Germany: The "Euthanasia Programs,"* edited by Susan Benedict and Linda Shields, 218–242. New York: Routledge.

Giubilini, Alberto, and Francesca Minerva. 2013. "After Birth Abortion: Why Should the Baby Live?" *Journal of Medical Ethics* 39, no. 5 (May): 261–263.

Hall, Wayne, and Malcolm Parker. 2017. "The Need to Exercise Caution in Accepting Addiction as a Reason for Performing Euthanasia." *Addiction*, 113, no. 7 (October): 1178–1180.

Hauerwas, Stanley. 1986. *Suffering Presence: Theological Reflections on Medicine, the Mentally Handicapped, and the Church.* Notre Dame, IN: University of Notre Dame Press.

Heylens, Gunter, Els Elaut, Gerd Verschelden, and Griet De Cuypere. 2016. "Transgender Persons Applying for Euthanasia in Belgium: A Case Report and Implications for Assessment and Treatment." *Journal of Psychiatry* 19, no. 1 (January): 347.

Hoche, Alfred, and Karl Binding. 1920. *Allowing the Destruction of Life Unworthy of Life: Its Measure and Form.* Translated by Cristina Modak. 2012. Greenwood, WI: Suzeteo Enterprises.

Hohendorf, Gerrit. 2014. "The National Socialist Patient Murders Between Taboo and Argument: Nazi Euthanasia and the Current Debate on Mercy Killing." In *Nazi Ideology and Ethics*, edited by Wolfgang Bialas and Lothar Fritze, 276–306. Cambridge: Cambridge Scholars Publishing.

Jansen-van der Weide, Marijke, Bregje Onwuteaka-Philipsen, and Gerrit van der Wal. 2005. "Granted, Undecided, Withdrawn, and Refused Requests for Euthanasia and Physician-Assisted Suicide." *Archives of Internal Medicine* 165, no. 15 (August 8–22): 1698–1704.

Johansen, Sissel, Jacob Chr. Hølen, Stein Kaasa, Jon H. Loge, and Lars Johan Materstvedt. 2005. "Attitudes Toward, and Wishes for, Euthanasia in Advanced Cancer Patients at a Palliative Medicine Unit." *Palliative Medicine* 19, no. 6 (September): 454–460.

Jones, David Albert, and David Paton. 2015."How Does Legalization of Physician-Assisted Suicide Affect Rates of Suicide?" *Southern Medical Journal*, Volume 108, no. 10 (October): 599–604.

Kass, Leon. 1989. "Neither for Love nor Money: Why Doctors Must Not Kill." *Public Interest* 94, no. 94 (Winter): 24–46.

Kennedy, James. 2014. "The Legacy of National Socialism for the Dutch Euthanasia Debate." In *Silence, Scapegoats and Self-Reflection: The Shadow of Nazi Medical Crimes on Medicine and Bioethics*, edited by Volker Roelcke, Etienne Lepicard, and Sascha Topp, 213–229. Gottingen: V and R unipress.

Kim, Scott Y. H., Raymond De Vries, and John R. Peteet. 2016. "Euthanasia and Assisted Suicide of Patients with Psychiatric Disorders in the Netherlands 2011–2014." *Journal of the American Medical Association Psychiatry* 73, no. 4 (April): 362–368.

Leichtentritt, Ronit D., Kathryn D. Rettig, and Steven H. Miles. 1999. "Holocaust Survivors' Perspectives on the Euthanasia Debate." *Social Science & Medicine* 48, no. 2 (January): 185–196.

Levinas, Emmanuel. 1985. *The Ethics of Infinity*. Pittsburgh: Duquesne University Press.

Lifton, Robert J. 1986. *The Nazi Doctors: Medical Killing and the Psychology of Genocide*. New York: Basic Books.

MacIntyre, Alasdair. 1999. *Rational Dependent Animals: Why Human Beings Need the Virtues*. Chicago: Harcourt Press.

Macklin, Ruth. 2003. "Dignity is a Useless Concept." *British Medical Journal* 327, no. 7429 (December 20–27): 1419–1420.

Macklin, Ruth. 2004. "Reflections on the Human Dignity Symposium: Is Dignity a Useless Concept?" *Journal of Palliative Care* 20, no. 3 (Autumn): 212–216.

Marcel, Gabriel. 1963. *The Existential Background of Human Dignity*. Cambridge, MA: Harvard University Press.

Marcoux, Isabelle, Bregje Onwuteaka-Philipsen, Marijke Jansen-van der Weide, and Gerrit van der Wal. 2005. "Withdrawing an Explicit Request for Euthanasia or Physician-Assisted Suicide: A Retrospective Study on the Influence of Mental Health Status and Other Patient Characteristics." *Psychological Medicine* 35, no. 9 (September): 1265–1274.

Maritain, Jacques. 1946. *The Person and The Common Good*. Trans. John J. Fitzgerald. (reprint 1985) South Bend, IN: University of Notre Dame Press.

McPherson, Christine J., Keith G. Wilson, and Mary Ann Murray. 2007. "Feeling Like a Burden to Others: A Systematic Review Focusing on the End of Life." *Palliative Medicine* 21, no. 2 (March): 115–128.

Modras, Ronald. 1982. "The Thomistic Personalism of John Paul II." *Modern Schoolman* 59, no. 2 (January): 117–127.

Oberstadt, Moritz Caspar Franz, Peter Esser, Joseph Classen, and Anja Mehnert. 2018. "Alleviation of Psychological Distress and the Improvement of Quality of Life in Patients with Amyotrophic Lateral Sclerosis: Adaptation of a Short-Term Psychotherapeutic Intervention." *Frontiers in Neurology* 9, no. 231 (April): 1–6.

Oregon Health Authority, Public Health Division, Center for Health Statistics. 2017. *Oregon Death with Dignity Act, Data Summary 2016*. February 10, 2017. https://www.oregon.gov/oha/ph/ProviderPartnerResources/EvaluationResearch/DeathwithDignityAct/Documents/year19.pdf.

Pearlman, Robert A., Clarissa Hsu, Helene Starks, et al. 2005. "Motivations for Physician-Assisted Suicide: Patient and Family Voices." *Journal of General Internal Medicine* 20, no. 3 (March): 234–239.

Pellegrino, Edmund. 2006. "Toward a Richer Bioethics: A Conclusion." In *Health and Human Flourishing: Religion, Medicine, and Moral Anthropology*, edited by Carol R. Taylor and Roberto Dell'Oro, 247–269. Washington, DC: Georgetown University Press.

Pinker, Steven. 1997. "Why They Kill Their Newborns." *New York Times Magazine*, November 2, 1997. https://www.nytimes.com/1997/11/02/magazine/why-they-kill-their-newborns.html.

Pinker, Steven. 2008. "The Stupidity of Dignity," *New Republic Online*, May 28, 2008:1–6. http://www.tnr.com/story.html?id=d8731cf4-e87b-4d88-b7e7-f5059cd0bfbd.

Proctor, Robert N. 1988. *Racial Hygiene: Medicine under the Nazis*. Cambridge, MA: Harvard University Press.

Quill Timothy E., and Kristen C. Cassel. 1995. "Nonabandonment: A Central Obligation of Physicians." *Annals of Internal Medicine* 122 (April): 368–374.

Sheldon, Tony. 2005. "Dutch Approve Euthanasia for Patient with Alzheimer's Disease." *British Medical Journal* 330, no. 7499 (May): 1401.

Sprung, Charles L., Margaret A. Somerville, Lukas Radbruch, et. al. 2018. "Physician-Assisted Suicide and Euthanasia: Emerging Issues from a Global Perspective." *Journal of Palliative Care* 334, no. 4 (October): 197–203.

van der Heide, Agnes, Bregje Onwuteaka-Philipsen, Mette L. Rurup, et. al. 2007. "End-of-Life Practices in the Netherlands under the Euthanasia Act." *New England Journal of Medicine* 356, no. 19 (May): 1957–1965.

Wilson, Keith G., Dorothyann Curran, and Christine J. McPherson. 2005. "A Burden to Others: A Common Source of Distress Among the Terminally Ill." *Cognitive Behaviour Therapy* 34, no. 2: 115–123.

Wojtyla, Karol. 1969. *Osoba i Czyn* (The Acting Person). Edited by Anna-Teresa Tymieniecka, Translated by Andrzej Potocki. 1979. Dordrecht, Holland: D. Reidel Publishing.

Chapter Seventeen

The Best Physicians Are Destined for Hell

Kenneth Prager

In May 2018, I traveled with medical ethics colleagues from the United States and Canada to Germany to learn about the collaboration of German physicians with the Nazis between 1933 and 1945. This experience brought to mind the puzzling statement of Rabbi Yehuda almost two millennia ago: "The best physicians are destined for Hell" (Babylonian Talmud, Kiddushin 200 CE, 82: a).

This seemingly inexplicable statement took on new meaning after my trip. In this chapter, I will show how German physicians were, in fact, the best of their time, and how a combination of arrogance, historical circumstances, pseudo-scientific principles, anti-Semitism, and racism led them to betray the most basic principles of medical ethics, thereby deserving the torments of Hell.

THE STATEMENT

Approximately 1,800 years ago, Rabbi Yehuda, a Jewish scholar residing in Israel, made some cryptic generalizations about the characteristics of people in various occupations. His observations were recorded in the Babylonian Talmud, an enormous body of Jewish law and lore compiled over a 500-year period. He stated: "Most donkey drivers are evil; most camel drivers are righteous; most sailors are pious; the best physicians are destined for Hell . . ." (Babylonian Talmud, Kiddushin 200 CE, 82: a).

His statement was baffling not only for singling out physicians for damnation but for specifying "the best." After all, the medical profession was then, and has always been, considered by Jews to be among the noblest and most respected of all callings. Some of Judaism's greatest personalities, such as Maimonides, were physician-scholars.

Jewish commentators offered a variety of explanations for Rabbi Yehuda's puzzling and disconcerting statement. In the eleventh century, Rashi, the foremost Jewish commentator on the Torah and Talmud, wrote: "The best of doctors do not fear sickness; they do not act humbly before God; sometimes they kill; sometimes they refrain from healing a poor person because they won't be paid" (Rashi, Babylonian Talmud, Kiddushin 200 CE, 82: a). A thirteenth century Catalonian Talmud scholar, Menachem son of Solomon Meiri, stated: "Physicians often shed blood because they give up and do not attempt as they should in order to heal; or they sometimes do not understand the cause of the illness but act as if they are experts" (quoted in Brown 2016). A sixteenth century Jewish scholar in Prague, Judah ben Bezalel Leviah, explained: "A physician who is not influenced by God's Bible will view his subjects as nothing but material things; therefore he is destined for hell" (quoted in Brown 2016). A common thread running through these and other explanations is that it is precisely the *best* physicians who are most likely to be arrogant, incautious, and disrespectful of their patients, which could lead to immoral and harmful behavior deserving of Hell.

What are the characteristics of the medical profession that make a breach of trust so evil as to warrant eternal damnation? Physicians are entrusted by society to examine their patients, to operate on them, to subject them to painful and dangerous treatments, and to explore the most private facts of their lives. With these privileges comes the obligation to practice medicine skillfully, humbly, humanely and, most importantly, ethically. This trust, however, can be violated in many ways, intentionally and unintentionally, with disastrous consequences for the patient—a physician's errors of omission or commission can cause suffering, disability, or death.

WHAT ARE THE CHARACTERISTICS OF THE BEST PHYSICIANS?

Why might the best physicians be more likely to betray their calling and merit the severest of punishments? Broadly speaking, we attribute two skills to the best physicians. The most important is proficiency in diagnosing and treating a sick patient. The best diagnostician is the one to whom other doctors refer patients with difficult to diagnose illnesses, and the best surgeon is the one who can operate on the most challenging surgical patients. The second, critically important skill, often referred to as a doctor's bedside manner, includes empathy, understanding, insight, and the ability to communicate effectively with a patient. The doctors blessed with these skills are venerated by their patients, receive awards and gifts, and attract the rich and famous. And so, it is not surprising that some of them lose sight of their fallibility and, as Judah Loew ben Bezalel Leviah stated, treat their patients "as nothing but material beings" rather than human beings, which is precisely what characterized so many of the best physicians in the Nazi era.

German medicine in the late nineteenth and early twentieth centuries was, indeed, the best in the world. "Nazism took root in the world's most powerful scientific culture boasting half of the world's Nobel Prizes and a sizeable fraction of the world's patents. German science and medicine were the envy of the world" (Proctor 1999, 15). Michael Kater, author of the authoritative *Doctors Under Hitler*, noted that German medical school faculties were the most successful and revered of all university faculties before Hitler came to power, and their power increased under Hitler. From 1923 to 1932, almost 36 percent of all university rectors were physicians, and, during the Third Reich, the figure was 59 percent (Kater 1989, 111).

Many leading American physicians and educators went to Germany for training, including William Osler in the 1870s (National Library of Science NIH n.d.) and Michael DeBakey in the 1930s during the Third Reich (DeBakey 2008). The most impactful visitor was Abraham Flexner, a highly regarded American educator commissioned by the Carnegie Foundation to evaluate and modernize the sorry state of American medical education in the early twentieth century. His "Flexner Report," profoundly influenced by German scientific medicine, revolutionized medical education in the United States, and its impact continues to this day:

> The Flexner Report of 1910 transformed the nature and process of medical education in America . . . and established the biomedical model as the gold standard of medical training. This transformation . . . embraced scientific knowledge and its advancement as the defining ethos of a modern physician. Such an orientation had its origins in the enchantment with German medical education. (Duffy 2011, 269)

Duffy also analyzed the dangers of scientific medicine:

> The advancement of knowledge was to trump all other involvements in the academic physician's life. . . . Did the Flexner Report overlook the ethos of medicine in its blind passion for science and education? . . . The profession appears to be losing its soul at the same time its body is clothed in a luminous garment of scientific knowledge. . . . Patients were primarily viewed as serving the academic purposes of the professor . . . doctors had become neutered technicians with patients in the service of science rather than science in the service of patients. . . . The profession's infatuation with the hyper-rational world of German medicine created an excellence in science that was not balanced by a comparable excellence in clinical caring. (Duffy 2011, 269–276)

His analysis of the Flexner Report and scientific medicine opens a window on the unfeeling, hyperrational nature of German medicine at the turn of the twentieth century that contributed to the ultimate corruption of the profession several decades later. The physicians that wrote Nazi medical textbooks, conducted inhumane medical experiments, sterilized and euthanized hundreds of thousands of patients without their consent, and designed gas chambers that would ultimately kill 4,500,000 Jews were not ordinary physicians, physiologists, and anatomists—they were the best in their fields. Unconstrained by religious or Hippocratic scruples, they opportunistically advanced German medical science, their own academic careers, and Nazi health care policy.

PERVERSION OF GERMAN MEDICINE UNDER THE NAZIS

We may never have a complete answer to the question of how a substantial percentage of the world's best physicians chose to participate in, and frequently formulate, Nazi health care policies and practices. The perpetration of mass murder, torture, and heinous medical experiments on non-consenting human beings by cultured and educated products of Western society is, however, a scrupulously documented fact. Documented, yes; well-known, no.

Few physicians today, much less the lay public, are aware that thousands of German physicians participated in the medical horrors of this period. To the extent that people are aware of Nazi physicians, it is only Josef Mengele, MD, PhD, the notorious and diabolical "Angel of Death" of Auschwitz, who comes to mind. The many practicing physicians who referred patients for forced sterilization and euthanasia, and the academic physicians who devised Nazi health care policies (see chapter 3 in this book) and provided ethical justifications for them (see chapter 4 in this book), were often not prosecuted for their medical crimes and, therefore, remain unknown. Nearly 50 percent of physicians were members of the Nazi party by the end of World War II, and 7 percent were in the dreaded paramilitary *Schutzstaffel* (SS), or Protection Squad, the highest percentages of any profession (Proctor 1988, 66).

Hitler recognized the importance of physicians in the development and implementation of his political programs. While in prison for his failed Munich putsch, Hitler was given a copy of *Menschliche Erblichkeitslehre und Rassenhygiene* (*Human Heredity and Racial Hygiene*) authored by Erwin Baur, Eugen Fischer, and Fritz Lenz in 1921. Hitler must have appreciated the applicability of negative eugenics, which German (and many other) physicians had been advocating for decades, to his political philosophy. In a speech to the Nazi Physician League that was established four years before Hitler came to power, he flattered and recruited doctors to his cause, telling them that, if necessary, he could do without builders, engineers, and lawyers but that "you, you National Socialist doctors, I cannot do without you for a single day, not a single hour. If not for you, if you fail me, then all is lost. For what good are our struggles, if the health of our people is in danger?" (Proctor 1988, 64).

The Nazi government offered economic incentives, power, and prestige to encourage cooperation by a German medical profession already inclined toward the government's murderous health care policies. Nearly 1,000 physicians took a two-week course at the Leadership School of German Physicians at Alt-Rehse, the "character school of the German doctor" and a model for continuing medical education in the Nazi Weltanschauung (Kater 1989, 67). Eliminating Jewish practicing physicians, who comprised approximately 13 percent of all German physicians and 60 percent of Berlin's physicians in 1933, provided Aryan practicing physicians an opportunity to enlarge their practices at a time when there was an oversupply of physicians during a depression (Proctor 1988, 90, 147, 154). New employment opportunities were created for physicians, such as:

- surgeries to sterilize 400,000 German citizens between 1934 and 1944 (see chapter 3 in this book)
- 181 genetic health courts, each with two doctors (and a lawyer) were established in 1934 to settle disputes arising from the Sterilization Law (Proctor 1988, 102)
- "genetic doctors" decided who was a Jew according to the 1935 Nuremberg Laws (Proctor 1988, 102)
- physicians were required to examine people who wished to marry and issue a certificate affirming they were "fit to marry" (Proctor 1988, 139)
- a host of positions in the Nazi health care bureaucracy, SS, euthanasia programs, and concentration camps

These last two positions also included an unlimited supply of human subjects and cadavers for research, publications, and academic advancement. Finally, eliminating the substantial number of Jewish academic physicians from Germany's medical schools—138 at Berlin's famous Charité University Hospital, for example—provided opportunities for Aryan academic physicians to advance their careers (Proctor 1988, 92).

A ROSTER OF SOME OF THE "BEST" NAZI PHYSICIANS

In addition to Dr. Ernst Rüdin, who is described in detail by Roelcke in chapter 2 of this book, here are some other academic Nazi physicians who advocated for, sometimes participated in, and profited from the sterilization, torture, and murder of many innocents.

Eugen Fischer published an important field study in 1913, *Die Rohoboter Bastards und das Bastardierungsproblem beim Menschen* (The Rehoboth Bastards and the Problem of Miscegenation among Humans), which greatly influenced subsequent German legislation, particularly the 1935 Nuremberg Laws (Friedlander 1995, 11). He coauthored, with Baur and Lenz, the influential textbook on genetics and eugenics and, in 1927, became director of the newly founded research institute, the Kaiser Wilhelm Institute for Anthropology, Human Genetics, and Eugenics, where Josef Mengele studied and sent specimens from his experiments at Auschwitz on twins (Proctor 1988, 40). Fischer and scientists working under him at his institute adjudicated the 1933 Sterilization Law in Berlin's Appellate Genetic Health Courts (Proctor 1988, 41).

Fritz Lenz edited, from 1913 to 1933, *Archiv für Rassen- und Gesellschafts-biologue* (*Journal of Racial and Social Biology*) that was founded in 1904 by Ploetz, his mentor who was considered the "father" of German eugenics or racial hygiene. In 1923, Lenz was named Germany's first professor of racial hygiene at the University of Munich, and shortly thereafter, he published his influential textbook on eugenics and genetics with Eugen Fischer and Erwin Baur; Lenz took pride in the fact that Hitler quoted from it in his speeches (Weigmann 2001). Although Lenz did not join the Nazi party until 1937, he strongly advocated Nazi policies, stating in 1933, "It is the will of the Führer, that the demands of racial hygiene should be put into practice, without delay" (Proctor 1988, 46). Lenz also served on government bodies that drafted the Nazi sterilization and castration legislation (Proctor 1988).

Julius Hallervorden was head of the Neuropathology Department of the prestigious Kaiser Wilhelm Institute for Brain Research, co-discovered the eponymous Hallervorden-Spatz syndrome and did extensive research on the brains of executed prisoners (Shevell 1992, 2214). In addition, he was an active participant in the notorious "T4" program in which German citizens with physical or mental disabilities were involuntarily euthanized (Kondziella 2009, 59). Hallervorden told the following to Dr. Leo Alexander, a Jewish Austrian neurologist who advised the prosecution at the Nuremberg Medical Trial: "Look here now, boys. If you are going to kill all those people, at least take the brains out so that the material can be utilized. They asked me, 'How many can you examine?' And so I told them . . . the more the better." Indeed, he personally selected victims with interesting neurological problems for involuntary euthanasia and then removed their brains for examination (Kondziella 2009, 61). After World War II, he became president of the German Neuropathological Society and continued his research at the Max Planck Institutes, the new name given to the former Kaiser Wilhelm Institutes.

Incidentally, debates continue over the use of eponyms when the scientist involved was an unethical Nazi researcher like Hallervorden or Hans Reiter (Lu and Katz 2005). Some have suggested removing the name if the person was involved in medical crimes (Strous and Edelman 2007), while others recommend preserving the eponyms with an asterisk for a teachable moment (Keynan and Rimar 2008; Ackerman 2009; Siegel-Itzkovich 2014; Ben David, Solt, and Fox 2019).

Eduard Pernkopf was an Austrian physician and anatomist who joined the paramilitary *Sturmabteilung* (SA), or Storm Troopers, in 1934. When Germany invaded Austria in 1938, he became Dean of the Medical Faculty of the University of Vienna. One of his first acts as dean was to rid the University of Vienna faculty of all Jews. *Pernkopf's Topographische Anatomie des Menschen* (*Pernkopf's Topographical Atlas of Man*) is considered one of the greatest and most beautiful works of its kind. Research has shown that the atlas included paintings of bodies of prisoners executed by the Nazis, brain illustrations derived from children euthanized in a Vienna hospital, and illustrators' signatures with swastikas or the letters *SS*. These facts have raised ethical issues as to its use (Atlas 2001, 51–58).

CAN ANYTHING BE LEARNED FROM THIS HISTORY THAT IS RELEVANT TODAY?

The history of Nazi medicine makes plain that physicians are not immune to either being influenced by or generating ideologies that could pervert the practice of medicine. In a review of the *Deadly Medicine* exhibit about Nazi medicine at the United States Holocaust Memorial Museum, Dr. Sherwin Nuland quoted polymath physician Oliver Wendell Holmes Sr.:

> The truth is, that medicine . . . is as sensitive to outside influences, political religious, philosophical, imaginative, as is the barometer to the changes of atmospheric density. . . . The danger in this lies . . . in the inability of society and the community of scientists to recognize the pervading influence of such an unpalatable reality, which flies in the face of the claims that form the groundwork for our worship of the scientific enterprise. . . .(Nuland 2004, 37)

Nuland continued, "There is good reason for so many wags and wise men down the centuries to have repeatedly observed that the road to hell is paved with good intentions" (2004, 38). He added this honest but most disturbing observation: "To my startled dismay, I found myself understanding why so much of the German medical establishment acted as it did. I realized that, given the circumstances, I might have done the same" (2004, 32).

Haque et al. posed this question, "Why did so many German doctors join the Nazi Party early?" and answered that physicians' "professional vulner-abilities, motives and rationalizations," and traits such as "valuing conformity and obedience to authority, valuing the prevention of contamination . . . and a basic interest in biomedical knowledge and research" may have predisposed German physicians to follow the Nazi banner (Haque et al. 2012, 473–479).

Michael Grodin highlighted other aspects of medicine that make physi-cians particularly vulnerable to becoming perpetrators:

> The motivation for choosing a career as a physician is often a fantasy of power, either sadistic or voyeuristic, as medicine gives license to look, touch, and con-trol. Doctors medicalize and dehumanize their patients so that they can more easily process what they have to do and deal with the suffering to which they are daily exposed—using science to objectify their work, they heal by attacking and killing disease with surgery or therapy or whatever tools they have avail-able. (Grodin 2009, 58)

The fantasy of power and scientific objectification described by Grodin is reminiscent of explanations offered by the rabbis for why it is the best of doctors that are most vulnerable. Extremely fluent in scientific medicine, they may view their patients as nothing but material things and, fueled with fantasies of power, they may arrogantly act as experts even when their sci-entific knowledge fails them, rather than humbly admitting that they do not understand the cause of an illness.

Could German physicians, ideologically aligned with the Nazi health care policy, have resisted Nazi enticements and incentives? On the one hand, Leo Alexander cited the successful medical resistance in Holland in the early 1940s that led to incarceration of more than 100 physicians and some deaths: "It is obvious that if the medical profession of a small nation under the conqueror's heel could resist so effectively, the German medical profession could likewise have resisted . . ." (Alexander 1949, 45). On the other hand, Kater postulated that it is difficult to conclude:

> whether the fate of doctors and medicine under Hitler . . . has had a salutary effect on the practice of medicine in our modern world. The not altogether heartening answer could partially be the result of the immutability of human nature, but also because a study dealing with the gradual decline of a culturally developed nation's medicine has never been presented before and certainly not for universal dissemination. (Kater 1989, 6)

Because of its history of racism and slavery, malevolent treatment of Na-tive Americans, and robust but barely acknowledged embrace of eugenics, the United States, in general, and American medicine, in particular, have a heavy responsibility to study and learn from medicine during the Third Reich (Neiman 2019). American physicians, arguably the best in the world today, need to study and learn from the behavior of Nazi physicians, the best in the world in their time.

THE SLIPPERY SLOPE IN NAZI MEDICINE

Dr. Leo Alexander gave his view of how it all began with a:

> subtle shift in emphasis in the basic attitude of the physicians. It started with the attitude, basic in the euthanasia movement, that there is such a thing as life not worthy to be lived. This attitude in its early stages concerned itself merely with the severely and chronically sick. Gradually the sphere of those to be included in this category was enlarged to encompass the socially unproductive, the ideologically unwanted, the racially unwanted, and finally all non-Germans. (Alexander 1949, 44)

Wald et al. noted that most medical trainees do not have the knowledge or sophistication to recognize or appreciate the importance of the subtle early shift in the basic attitude of German physicians that ultimately led them down the slippery slope. Therefore, trainees typically dismiss the possibility of committing similarly egregious medical crimes themselves. Yet,

> If our trainees were to consider the Holocaust as "End Stage Disease," the horrific culmination of incremental injustices, they might be able to better grasp how such events could occur and engage in preventive strategies to maintain medical professionalism and avoid transgressions that marked Nazi medicine. (Wald, Rubenfeld, and Fins 2016)

With the important caveat that there is a fundamental ethical difference between the euthanasia policies of the Third Reich and those in some European countries today, as discussed in other chapters in this book, there is a slippery slope in both instances. In the Netherlands and Belgium, voluntary adult euthanasia led to nonvoluntary (a patient lacking capacity and not objecting) euthanasia, and then to a reported case of involuntary (patient objecting) euthanasia (Crouch 2017). Voluntary child euthanasia evolved into nonvoluntary child euthanasia (Verhagen and Sauer 2005). While only patients with physical suffering were initially euthanized, patients with untreatable mental suffering are now being euthanized (Klugman 2016). Once physicians are empowered to kill, even for the best of reasons, the slide toward ever-wider applications of physician-assisted suicide and euthanasia may be inevitable, as suggested by the following two examples from North America.

In 2019, Oregon passed legislation allowing its citizens to bypass its previously legislated 15-day waiting period (*Oregonian* 2019). Its 2019 legislative assembly also considered House Bill 2903 that would expand the definition of terminal disease to include individuals who have "a degenerative disease that will, at some point in the future, be the cause of the patient's death," thereby eliminating the current requirement of a prognosis of less than six months to live (Oregon Legislative Assembly 2019, Section 1. ORS 127.800).

Also in 2019, a Superior Court judge in Canada—where euthanasia is legal—invalidated previous restrictions on medical assistance in dying that required a natural death be "reasonably foreseeable" and that eligible persons must "be at the end of life." The case was brought by two people with debilitating chronic illnesses with prognoses of living at least two or three additional years, but they claimed that suffering, not imminent death, was the original law's most important consideration (Marin 2019). If this decision stands, then many more people will be eligible for physician-assisted suicide and euthanasia in Canada.

ARE THE BEST PHYSICIANS TRULY DESTINED FOR HELL?

So, is Rabbi Yehuda's assertion about the best physicians relevant today? I suspect the rabbi's pithy statement about the destiny of the best physicians was meant to shock and, thereby, deliver a cautionary warning to those who appeared to hold a unique power of life and death by virtue of their technical skills alone.

By the *best*, he could not have meant empathetic and humane physicians with technical skills and excellent judgment—these physicians would clearly merit the highest eternal rewards. He was clearly referring to those *best* physicians that view their patients as sick organs rather than as suffering human beings, a view that is encouraged by modern technology, increasing specialization, and a growing distance between doctor and patient. These physicians are highly skilled technicians rather than healers of body and soul. If they are not imbued with a belief in the sanctity of each human life, no matter how compromised physically or mentally, and with a humble recognition that "For of the Most High cometh healing" (Ecclesiasticus 38:2, KJV), these *best* physicians may be most subject to arrogance, cruelty, and the lure of societal ideologies that are divorced from the foundational ethics of the medical profession.

The extreme representatives of this paradigm were those Nazi physicians who were the best in their fields: bright, academically recognized, original thinkers unconstrained by millennia of medical ethics, who sought to purify the German *volk* (people) and cleanse the world of human pathogens guided by the new pseudoscience of eugenics and a pervasive racist and anti-Semitic ideology. They sought to expand the horizons of medical knowledge with research that treated humans as inanimate objects.

The lesson for physicians today is that the Oath of Hippocrates and millennia of normative medical ethics do not immunize them against well-intentioned but wicked ideologies. And given their unique power over the life and death of trusting patients, when these physicians accept societal norms that promote evil, the best of them can perpetrate the worst violations of human rights. Surely these are the physicians referred to by Rabbi Yehuda.

BIBLIOGRAPHY

Ackerman, A. Bernard. 2009: "Reiter Syndrome and Hans Reiter: Neither Legitimate." *Journal of the American Academy of Dermatology* 60, no. 3 (March): 517–518. doi:https://doi.org/10.1016/j.jaad.2008.09.062.

Alexander, Leo. 1949. "Medical Science Under Dictatorship." *New England Journal of Medicine* 241, no. 2 (July): 39–47.

Atlas, Michel. 2001. "Ethics and Access to Teaching Materials in the Medical Library: The Case of the Pernkopf Atlas." *Bulletin of the Medical Library Association* 89, no.1 (January): 51–58.

Babylonian Talmud, Art Scroll Edition. 200 CE. Kiddushin 82: a.

Baur, Erwin, Fritz Lenz, and Eugene Fischer. 1921. *Menschliche Erblichkeitslehre und Rassenhygiene (Human Heredity and Racial Hygiene)*. Munich: J. F. Lehmann.

Ben David, C. Ido Solt, and Mathew Fox. 2019. "Is It Appropriate to Change the Names of Surgical Procedures and Examinations in the Field of Obstetrics and Gynecology which Give Eponyms Distinction to Nazi Doctors?" *Harefuah* 158, no. 8 (August 2019): 511–14. https://www.ncbi.nlm.nih.gov/pubmed/31407539.

Brown, Jeremy. 2016. "The Best Doctors go to Hell." Accessed October 15, 2019. http://www.talmudology.com/jeremybrownmdgmailcom/2016/5/22/kiddushin-82a-the-best-doctors-go-to-hell?rq=best%20doctors%20go%20to%20hell.

Crouch, Giulia. 2017. "Female Dutch doctor drugged a patient's coffee then asked her family to hold her down as she fought not to be killed–but did not break the country's euthanasia laws." *Daily Mail*, January 27, 2017. https://www.dailymail .co.uk/news/article-4166098/Female-Dutch-doctor-drugged-patient-s-coffee.html ?offset=0&max=100&jumpTo=comment-175426032#comment-175426032.

DeBakey, Michael. 2008. Interview of Michael DeBakey, by Sheldon Rubenfeld, May 16, 2008. Distinguished Speaker Videos. http://www.medicineaftertheholo caust.org/interview-of-dr-michael-e-debakey-may-16-2008/.

Duffy, Thomas. 2011. "The Flexner Report—100 Years Later." *Yale Journal of Biology and Medicine* 84, no. 3 (September): 269–76.

Flexner, Abraham. 1910. "Medical Education in the United States and Canada: A Report to the Carnegie Foundation for the Advancement of Teaching." Bulletin Number Four. New York: Carnegie Foundation.

Friedlander, Henry. 1995. *The Origins of Nazi Genocide: From Euthanasia to the Final Solution.* Chapel Hill: University of North Carolina Press.

Grodin, Michael. 2009. "Mad, Bad, or Evil: How Physician Healers Turn to Torture and Murder." In *Medicine After the Holocaust: From the Master Race to the Human Genome and Beyond*, edited by Sheldon Rubenfeld, 49–67. New York: Palgrave Macmillan.

Haque, Omar Sultan, Julian De Freitas, Ivana Viani, Bradley Niederschulte, and Harold Bursztajn. 2012. "Why Did So Many German Doctors Join the Nazi Party Early?" *International Journal of Law and Psychiatry* 35, no. 5–6 (September–December): 473–79.

Kater, Michael H. 1989. *Doctors Under Hitler.* Chapel Hill: University of North Carolina Press.

Keynan, Yoav, and Doron Rimar. 2008. "Reactive Arthritis—The Appropriate Name." *Israel Medical Association Journal* 10, no. 4 (April): 256–58.

Klugman, Craig. 2016. "Euthanasia for Reasons of Mental Health." Bioethics.net. Posted May 12, 2016. Accessed November 8, 2019. http://www.bioethics.net/2016/05/euthanasia-for-reasons-of-mental-health/.

Kondziella, Daniel. 2009. "Thirty Neurological Eponyms Associated with the Nazi Era." *European Neurology* 62, no. 1 (May): 56–64.

Lu, Dave, and Ken Katz. 2005. "Declining Use of the Eponym 'Reiter's Syndrome' in the Medical Literature, 1998–2003." *Journal of the American Academy of Dermatology* 53, no. 4 (October): 720–23. doi:10.1016/j.jaad.2005.06.048.

Marin, Stephanie. 2019. "Quebec Court Invalidates Parts of Medical Aid in Dying." *Montreal Gazette*, September 11, 2019. https://montreal.ctvnews.ca/a-quebec-court-has-invalidated-parts-of-the-medical-aid-in-dying-laws-1.4588622.

National Library of Science. National Institutes of Health. n.d. William Osler Profile. Accessed November 8, 2019. https://profiles.nlm.nih.gov/spotlight/gf/feature/biographical.

Neiman, Susan. 2019. *Learning from the Germans: Race and the Memory of Evil.* New York: Farrar, Straus and Giroux.

Nuland, Sherwin. 2004. "The Death of Hippocrates." *New Republic*, September 12, 2004.

Oregon Legislative Assembly. 2019. House Bill 2903. Section 1. ORS 127.800. Section 1. https://olis.leg.state.or.us/liz/2019R1/Downloads/MeasureDocument/HB2903/Introduced.

Oregonian. 2019. "New Law Shortens 'Death with Dignity' Waiting Period for Some Patients." Posted July 24, 2019. https://www.oregonlive.com/politics/2019/07/new-law-shortens-death-with-dignity-waiting-period-for-some-patients.html.

Proctor, Robert. 1988. *Racial Hygiene: Medicine Under the Nazis.* Cambridge: Harvard University Press.

Proctor, Robert. 1999. *The Nazi War on Cancer.* Princeton: Princeton University Press.

Shevell, Michael. 1992. "Racial Hygiene, Active Euthanasia, and Julius Hallervorden." *Neurology* 42, no. 11 (November): 2214–19.

Siegel-Itzkovich, Judy. 2014. "Israeli Researcher: Nazi Doctors Should Be Remembered Alongside Diseases Named for Them." *Jerusalem Post.* Israel News,

July 14, 2014. https://www.jpost.com/Health-and-Science/Israeli-researcher-Nazi
-doctors-should-be-remembered-alongside-diseases-named-for-them-362669.

Strous, Rael, and Morris Edelman. 2007. "Eponyms and the Nazi Era: Time to Remember and Time for Change." *Israel Medical Association Journal* 9, no. 3 (March): 207–14.

Verhagen, Eduard, and Pieter Sauer. 2005. "The Groningen Protocol—Euthanasia in Severely Ill Newborns." *New England Journal of Medicine* 352, no.10 (March): 959–62.

Wald, Hedy, Sheldon Rubenfeld, and Joseph Fins. 2016. "The Holocaust as End Stage Disease: Medical Education as a Moral Imperative." Hektoen International (Spring). https://hekint.org/2017/01/29/the-holocaust-as-end-stage-disease-medi cal-education-as-a-moral-imperative/.

Weigmann, Katrin. 2001. "In the Name of Science." *EMBO Reports* 21, no. 10: 871–75.

Chapter Eighteen

Pediatric Euthanasia

A Call for Civil Disobedience

Eric Kodish

It is time to speak out. In 2008, I published a short article in the *Lancet* entitled: "Pediatric ethics: A repudiation of the Groningen protocol." In the decade since then, my own thinking has evolved and my opposition to pediatric euthanasia has become more resolute. My experience in Germany and Houston as part of the Physician-Assisted Suicide and Euthanasia after the Holocaust program (PASEATH) sponsored by the Center for Medicine after the Holocaust (CMATH) provided new intellectual and emotional insights, which reinforced my view that pediatricians should exercise civil disobedience and resist the prospect of euthanizing infants and/or children. Involvement in such activity is antithetical to pediatric ethics, and failure to protest implies complicity. In this chapter, I will build on the arguments set forth in the 2008 paper and incorporate observations and lessons from PASEATH.

In Germany, we studied eugenics, sterilization, euthanasia, and genocide in addition to visiting relevant historical sites. While sterilization and eugenics are commonly analyzed in the domain of reproductive ethics, they are also relevant to pediatric ethics. Pediatricians commonly care for impaired children with congenital anomalies, most of whom would have been murdered by Nazi physicians.

This chapter is personal, combining a detached philosophical analysis with a sense of urgency created by greater acceptability of infant and child euthanasia in Europe, by euthanasia in Canada, by physician-assisted suicide (PAS) in the United States, and by a sense of vulnerability as a Jew in the twenty-first century, all of which culminated in a primal need to call out a warning: pediatricians must not kill.

We landed in Berlin on May 13, 2018, and my time in Germany, my conversations with fellow scholars, my readings, and my writing this chapter have changed and galvanized me. While walking in Berlin, I witnessed a neo-Nazi march that evoked a déjà vu moment. Although I was born 15 years after the end of the Holocaust, years of reading about it had created a false memory of personally experiencing its horrors, which was reactivated by the neo-Nazi march. Of all the planned tours, lectures, and discussions in Germany, this real-time event provoked the loudest and clearest alarm for me. The murder of 11 elderly Jews at prayer in Pittsburgh later in 2018 only reinforced my fear (Robertson, Mele, and Tavernis 2018).

Could it happen again? In the first decades of the twentieth century, German and American medicine proposed eugenic theories that were considered scientifically advanced at the time (Proctor 1988, 46–63). When Hitler became chancellor, he empowered physicians to implement policies they had advocated for decades, policies aligned with his worldview. Might twenty-first century doctors become complicit in well-intentioned PAS and euthanasia programs that could, someday, be used for evil purposes by a resurgent nationalistic European, Canadian, American, or other government? Where this all ends is not clear, but rather than living in fear of another Holocaust aided and abetted by the medical profession, I prefer optimism coupled with action to prevent further spread of PAS and euthanasia.

FROM REPUDIATION TO RESISTANCE

Our focus in Germany was on the history of medicine during the Third Reich and the impact of current European trends in end-of-life treatment on the increasing acceptability and legalization of PAS and euthanasia in North America. One reason for their increased acceptability is the evolution of the terminology for ending lives with medical assistance. Ten years ago, the phrase commonly used to describe the procedure legislated by Oregon's 1997 Death with Dignity Act was *physician-assisted suicide*, whose strength is the precision with which it places *agency*. Because actions and agency matter in ethical analysis, the question of who is administering the lethal drug is morally relevant (Brudney and Lantos 2011). There is no doubt that the patient is committing suicide when we call the practice physician-assisted suicide. Physician aid in dying (PAD), by contrast, introduces a morally problematic ambiguity by conflating patient-administered and doctor-administered death. Whether this is the strategic intention of those who advocate for this position or simply an innocent and improved characterization of what is clinically transpiring is, in my mind, an open question (Dworkin 2019).

Another important reason for their increased acceptability is that respect for autonomy has become so dominant in modern medical ethics that other principles and virtues are often forgotten. As a matter of epistemology and logic, the moral power of autonomy is philosophically dependent on sovereign decision-making capacity (DMC). Some argue that access to assistance in dying for adults is a right that should be extended to infants and children or to those adults who have lost DMC (Brouwer 2018). However, infants and children do not have sovereign, autonomous, DMC. And "parental autonomy," often confused or conflated with parental authority, does not exist.

Others suggest that it is this very absence of DMC (or loss of it) that requires society to protect these individuals from being killed, even in the name of mercy (Mishara and Weisstub 2013). Of course, those opposed to ending the lives of patients with DMC are unlikely to support ending the lives of patients without DMC. While I am firmly opposed to physicians actively ending the lives of patients with DMC, my opposition to PAD in pediatrics is *independent* of my concern about the right to PAD for competent adults.

The Groningen Protocol

According to the Groningen protocol, there are five necessary criteria to establish ethical acceptability for the mercy killing of infants in the Netherlands (Verhagen and Sauer 2005). I will review what I consider to be major flaws in the second, fourth, and fifth criteria.

The second Groningen criterion requires that the infant be experiencing hopeless and unbearable suffering. It is, however, very difficult if not impossible to measure "unbearable suffering" even in the adult patient population; therefore, to speak of unbearable suffering in infants is *reductio ad absurdum.* When we visited Bernburg's former psychiatric hospital and learned how easily an institution initially dedicated to health care was converted to one of six Nazi killing or euthanasia centers, I immediately heard echoes of the argument that unbearable suffering could justify a patient's murder. Whether doctors in the early 1940s truly believed it, one of the arguments they put forth for "euthanizing" more than 8,000 human beings in Bernburg was unbearable suffering (Proctor 1988, 191; Lifton 1986, 50).

The fourth Groningen criterion requires parental consent, which is a non sequitur because parental permission is categorically different than consent from an autonomous person with DMC for clinical decisions, especially in regard to his or her own death. While we don't know how all of the parents of children killed in the children's euthanasia program reacted, there were some polls showing that a surprisingly high percentage of parents were in favor of mercy killing of their own disabled children (Proctor 1988, 94; Burleigh

1995, 23). Be that as it may, Nazi physicians used deception—falsified death certificates, for example—so that parents would believe their children died of natural causes. If a parent knew the truth of their child's murder, one would hope and expect he or she would be angry and bereaved, although it is likely that some parents would also feel some degree of relief.

Because human nature does not change, the conflicted emotions experienced by parents of children with disabilities in Germany in the twentieth century likely are similar to those of parents of children with disabilities in North America in the twenty-first century. Understanding parents' attitudes, values, hopes, fears, and life philosophy is an important aspect of decision-making for children with life-threatening conditions, but it need not be determinative. In fact, if it becomes determinative, then pediatricians and society would be abdicating their responsibility to protect vulnerable children and regressing to a time when children were considered property of their parents. And in some cases, we would be consigning children with congenital anomalies, cognitive impairment, or both, to medicalized murder.

The fifth Groningen criterion is that "the procedure must be performed in accordance with the *accepted medical standard* [italics mine]." Are the authors alluding to the technical expertise required to administer a lethal dose of medication? If so, the criterion is easily met, rendering the fifth criterion essentially meaningless. My argument is that the technical and the ethical must always be evaluated together, for the risks of component analysis in the morality of medical practice is too great. In this case, we must ask the hard question: is actively ending the life of an infant or young child (or an adult, for that matter) ever within the bounds of the accepted medical standard? After experiencing Bernburg, I say, absolutely not.

Is it possible to provide safeguards to prevent infanticide and the medicalized killing of children? As discussed above, parents cannot always be relied upon to protect their vulnerable children. It would also be a grave mistake to rely on the government to protect children, as demonstrated during the Third Reich. The best safeguard, then, is the professional integrity of individual pediatricians, and one of the best and easiest ways to instill in medical students and pediatric residents the qualities of a medical professional with integrity is to study medical history, especially medicine during the Holocaust. Learning about the murderous delusions of Nazi doctors during the Third Reich, the best doctors in the world at the time, may incline medical students and doctors to deeper introspection about their own moral premises and behavior, as I myself discovered.

In response to the Groningen Protocol, especially its concept of actively ending the life of a child "in accordance with the accepted medical standard," I called for resistance by pediatricians in my 2008 repudiation essay (Kodish

2008). I am now even more firmly committed to civil disobedience (Childress 1985). If an American state considers legalizing physician assistance in dying for children, pediatricians should actively oppose it; if a state legalizes the practice, pediatricians should oppose its implementation; if a hospital allows pediatric euthanasia, pediatricians should conscientiously object and, if necessary, boycott the hospital. Physician participation in the death penalty, reproductive conscientious objections, and bans on the discussion of gun safety in the pediatrician's office provide precedents for this kind of medical professional activism (Davis and Kodish 2014).

Civil Disobedience

Physicians and professional organizations have avoided taking a stand on some important ethical issues (Kheriaty 2019). Regarding pediatric euthanasia, I recommend that pediatricians and pediatric professional organizations take a stand against it rather than remain neutral. American pediatric professional organizations, such as the American Academy of Pediatrics with approximately 67,000 physician members, should initiate the resistance by protesting infant and child euthanasia, advocating for excellent palliative and hospice care, and banning pediatricians who euthanize infants or children from membership.

The American Board of Pediatrics (ABP) certifies "excellence in pediatrics—for a healthier tomorrow," primarily through governance of both pediatric board certification and recertification (American Board of Pediatrics website n.d.). If physicians participate in pediatric euthanasia, then the ABP should either revoke their certification or declare them ineligible for certification and recertification. If, catalyzed by the ethical objections of their physician members, these two powerful organizations take a clear stand, they would create a firewall against pediatric euthanasia in the United States.

Because pediatricians do not work in a vacuum, other medical professionals and professional organizations may become ethically complicit in pediatric euthanasia. For example, if a pediatrician orders a lethal dose of a drug for a child then, at a minimum, a pharmacist must prepare it, and a nurse must administer it, resulting in a cascade of complicity. If they are opposed to pediatric euthanasia, then neither the pharmacist nor the nurse should, in the name of independent practice and professional autonomy, accede to it. By conscientiously objecting, they honor their professional integrity.

I have been a resident of Ohio for more than 50 of my 58 years. What if Ohio considers legalization of PAS for competent adults, which is a much more likely first step than pediatric euthanasia? Now, because I have studied the slippery slope, I would vehemently oppose it, citing the Code of Ethics of the American Medical Association's decades-old prohibition of physician participation in state-sanctioned executions (Truog, Cohen, and Rockoff 2014). Because I am convinced that high quality palliative and hospice care are almost always able to provide excellent symptom relief and, moreover, that legalization of PAS could, paradoxically, prevent implementation of palliative and hospice care, I would actively protest against legalization. I would also encourage my physician colleagues to join me in protesting and resisting legalization of PAS for competent adults. What may start as a well-intentioned process with presumed safeguards could expand to the killing of infants, children, and other patients without decision-making capacity. My own sense of vulnerability as a Jew, which I confronted in Berlin, combined with an ethical obligation to protect my vulnerable pediatric patients, make it clear to me that Ohio should not legalize PAS.

Children are vulnerable, but they also represent our hopes for the future; the way we treat them is an important measure of the ethical quality of our society. While it may seem kind and merciful to put suffering children out of their misery, their vulnerability and inability to consent make such an action ethically abhorrent. In 1988, four prominent leaders in medical ethics published a paper in the *Journal of the American Medical Association* entitled "Doctors Must Not Kill" (Gaylin et al. 1988). My assessment 30 years later, reinforced by my experiences in Germany and in pediatrics, is that they were absolutely correct. Pediatricians must not kill.

BIBLIOGRAPHY

American Board of Pediatrics. n.d. Accessed October 13, 2019 https://www.abp.org.

Brouwer Marjorie, Christopher Kaczor, Margaret P. Battin, Els Maeckelberghe, John D. Lantos, and Eduard Verhagen. 2018. "Should Pediatric Euthanasia be Legalized?" *Pediatrics* 141, no. 2 (February): e20171343. DOI: https://doi.org/10.1542/peds.2017-1343.

Brudney, Daniel, and John Lantos. 2011. "Agency and Authenticity: Which Value Grounds Patient Choice?" *Theoretical and Medicine Bioethics* 32, no. 4 (April): 217–27.

Burleigh, Michael. 1995. *Death and Deliverance: "Euthanasia" in Germany c. 1900–1945*. Cambridge: Cambridge University Press.

Childress, James F. 1985. "Civil Disobedience, Conscientious Objection, and Evasive Noncompliance: A Framework for the Analysis and Assessment of Illegal Actions in Health Care." *Journal of Medicine and Philosophy* 10, No.1 (February): 63–84.

Davis, Dena S., and Eric Kodish. 2014. "Laws that Conflict with the Ethics of Medicine: What Should Doctors Do?" *Hastings Center Report* 44, no. 6 (February): 11–14. DOI: 10.1002/hast.382.

Dworkin, Gerald. 2019. "Suicide, Strictly Speaking." *3 Quarks Daily* (blog), July 22, 2019. https://www.3quarksdaily.com/3quarksdaily/2019/07/suicide-strictly -speaking.html.

Gaylin, Will, Leon Kass, Edmund Pellegrino, and Mark Siegler. 1988. "Doctors Must Not Kill." *Journal of the American Medical Association* 259, no.14 (April): 2139–40.

Kheriaty, Aaron. 2019. "First, Take No Stand." *New Atlantis*, no. 59 (Summer): 22–35.

Kodish, Eric. 2008. "Paediatric Ethics: A Repudiation of the Groningen Protocol." *Lancet* 371, no. 9616 (March): 892–93.

Lifton, Robert Jay. 1986. *The Nazi Doctors: Medical Killing and the Psychology of Genocide*. New York: Basic Books.

Mishara, Brian L., and David N. Weisstub. 2013. "Premises and Evidence in the Rhetoric of Assisted Suicide and Euthanasia." *International Journal of Law and Psychiatry* 36, no. 5–6 (September–December): 427–35. doi: 10.1016/j.ijlp .2013.09.003.

Proctor, Robert. 1988. *Racial Hygiene: Medicine Under the Nazis*. Cambridge, MA: Harvard University Press.

Robertson, Campbell, Christopher Mele, and Sabrina Tavernis. 2018. "Rampage Kills 11 at a Synagogue in Pittsburgh." *New York Times*, October 27, 2018.

Truog, Robert, Glenn Cohen, and Mark Rockoff. 2014. "Physicians, Medical Ethics, and Execution by Lethal Injection." *Journal of the American Medical Association* 311, no. 23 (June 18): 2375–2376. doi:10.1001/jama.2014.6425.

Verhagen, Eduard, and Pieter Sauer. 2005. "The Groningen Protocol: Euthanasia in Severely Ill Newborns." *New England Journal of Medicine* 352, no. 10 (March): 959–62.

Chapter Nineteen

"The Syringe Belongs in the Hand of a Physician"

Power, Authority, Control, Death, and the Patient-Physician Relationship

Daniel P. Sulmasy

"The syringe belongs in the hand of a physician." This was the motto of Viktor Brack, the administrator of the Nazi euthanasia program for mentally ill adults, *Aktion* T4 (Lifton 2017, 71). Mid-century German euthanasia was always done under medical supervision and considered a medical procedure, even when performed *en masse* and carried out by means of poison gas rather than lethal injection. In the concentration camps, physicians performed some lethal injections themselves (apparently scrupulously employing sterile technique), and the selection of those designated for mass killings was considered a medical task and carried out by physicians (Lifton 2017, 254–61).

"The syringe belongs in the hand of a physician." The phrase has a distinctive resonance. It is sufficiently noteworthy that it is quoted not only by Robert Lifton, but also by Robert Proctor (1988, 177) and Michael Burleigh (1994, 134). Its mantra-like quality seems to convey much more than the words themselves. What makes this phrase so evocative, so plausible, and, yet, so chilling?

The resonance of this phrase derives from its relationship to the notions of power, authority, and control. The argument supporting this thesis begins with a few sociological observations about medicine and its practitioners—observations that are widely applicable across the history of medicine but seem especially operative in a scientific age. These observations, in turn, ground a series of philosophical reflections on the use of medical power, on how authority differs from power, and about proper roles of the physician and the state. These philosophical reflections are not intended simply as an exercise in the history of ideas but should be relevant to medicine in all its temporal, cultural, and political instantiations.

Viktor Brack was a politically appointed bureaucrat, yet, as the son of a physician, he understood the culture of medicine and was put in charge of implementing a medical program championed and supervised by Hitler's personal physician, Dr. Karl Brandt (Burleigh 1994, 123). Brack was an enthusiastic supporter of the Nazi idea that politics should become applied biology and had no trouble recruiting equally enthusiastic physicians to carry out the program.

Euthanasia was an idea that had been at the forefront of medical thinking for years and had broad popular support among the general public in Germany and elsewhere (Burleigh 1994, 12–87; Proctor 1988, 177–94). The Nazi government did not force it upon physicians and the public—euthanasia was both a medical idea and a decades-old popular movement. This understanding is tellingly reflected in the discussion of euthanasia by Rudolf Ramm, a prominent Nazi physician, who, in his textbook of medical ethics, *Ärztliche Rechts und Standeskunde* (Medical Law and Professional Studies), wrote, "It is the task of the physician to be pioneering in this regard. It is the task of the state to give it the force of law" (Ramm 1943, 108). In carrying out euthanasia, physicians were empowered to advance to what they considered to be the forefront of medicine. Brack directed the bureaucratic apparatus by which the state gave their actions sanction. He put the needle in the physicians' hands. They, in turn, had no doubt that this was where it belonged.

The German euthanasia programs, described in detail in chapter 3 of this book, can best be considered a medical and philosophical movement that was given the force of law by the Nazis, not a totalitarian regime's alien ideology forced upon an unwilling profession. In defending the practice of euthanasia during the Nuremberg Medical Trial, Brack insisted:

> Just as the soul belongs in the helping hands of the priest, so the body belongs in the helping hands of the physician. Only so can the sick person really be assisted. In that case, however, this means that for the doctor that his duties, particularly in view of the person's spiritual life—it is his duty to free the person from his unworthy condition, so—I might even say—from his prison. (quoted in Proctor 1988, 296)

This chapter explores the hypothesis that the phrase, "the syringe belongs in the hand of a physician," denotes a complex interaction between power, authority, and control as played out in the patient-physician relationship. After describing how these concepts function in medicine's own self-conception, in popular expectations of medicine, and in the legal and social structures in which medicine operates, I will argue that these forces help to explain what happened in pre-Nazi and Nazi medicine, while also shedding light on the ethics of modern medicine.

TERMS AND DEFINITIONS

Power, authority, and control are related but distinct concepts. While these words can be used in slightly different ways, their usage in this chapter is precise and squares with the ordinary use of these terms. Importantly, the definitions used in this chapter differ from the definitions of Max Weber (1978) and Michel Foucault (2008).

Power. Power refers to pure potential, to the capacity to act or to affect something in the world. In this chapter, the word will be employed in this most general sense, encompassing both hydroelectric power and the power of a king. In this most general sense, power is not a moral term. It is obvious that human beings can use their various powers (physical, mental, verbal, political) rightly or wrongly, for good or otherwise. It is not power per se that is good or bad. Ethics is about the judgments we make regarding the free exercise of human power, and our ethical judgments depend upon such things as the kind of act, the kind of power that enables it, the results, the circumstances, and the intentions of the one who is exercising the power. Agency is power. As agents, for example, we have the power to speak. Speech is a result of our free choices and what we say, when we say it, how we say it, to whom we say it, and why we say it are subject to ethical examination. Yet the mere power to speak is not, itself, something we can judge to be right or wrong. Moral judgments depend on *how* power is used.

Authority. Authority is a form of interpersonal power. It is a power that one person has over at least one other person with the expectation of (or possibly the license to enforce) obedience or compliance. Authority is a power that is ideally mutually accepted by all parties—that is, those under the authority accept the legitimacy of the authority and freely comply. Obviously not all forms of power are forms of authority. Neither the power of nuclear fission nor the power of speech can be described as forms of authority. Authority refers to a relationship within the field of social power, requiring at least two persons. It is inescapably social. The authority one person exercises over another can be characterized as weak or strong; it can be differentiated in proportion to its scope (e.g., circumscribed or absolute); it can be classified according to its origin (e.g., Weber's distinction between charismatic, traditional, and rational-legal authority can be regarded as a classification of the *origin* of a given kind of authority). Authority, like other forms of human agency, is subject to moral scrutiny. Authority can be used rightly or wrongly and can be obtained rightly or wrongly. Various forms of authority can be abused or used well; can originate legitimately or illegitimately; can be exercised justifiably or unjustifiably. Systems of authority exist in all cultures and seem necessary for the coordinated action of social creatures like human beings. Authority, as such, is not intrinsically right or wrong. Moral judgments about authority depend on how the authority originates and is used.

Control. Control is the power to direct something (e.g., a body, a process, or another person) to carry out one's will. Control implies a use of power that can (though not necessarily must) steer a body, process, or person in a direction at odds with its natural tendency, inclination, or autonomous self-direction. Control implies a state of conformity between the controlling agent's intention and the state of affairs of a body, process, or person. Any deviation from the will of the agent implies deficient control. Control thus implies that the aim is for mastery. Not all power is control. That I have the power to throw a baseball does not imply that my control is such that it will end up in the strike zone. Not all authority is control. Often the one in authority and the one under authority cooperate toward a shared goal, so that the power and the aim are shared. Nor is all authority absolute in the way that control implies. Authority can be weak or circumscribed. Like the other terms, control is not, of itself, a moral term. Control can be good or bad. We can control a river to prevent it from flooding a town, or control someone's blood sugar to prevent kidney damage, or control an impulse to laugh when it would be hurtful or inappropriate. These are all good things. That we can control the course of a bullet so that it kills an innocent person, or control access to the internet to suppress dissident political speech, or control the ethnic makeup of a country through forced resettlement are all bad things. Control, as such, is not intrinsically right or wrong. Moral judgments depend on how the control is used.

MEDICINE AND POWER

Medicine is a power. The power of medicine has been increasing over the last several centuries and has increased geometrically in the last hundred years. The dawning of the scientific era and the application of science to understanding the human body has generated vast amounts of knowledge, unprecedented in human history. As Francis Bacon famously noted, "knowledge itself is power" (Bacon 1597). The growth of scientific knowledge about human biology has given us new capacities to act upon the human body in extraordinary and remarkably beneficial ways, and these new capabilities have made medicine powerful.

It is important to note, however, that the paradigmatic form of scientific medical power is control. A diseased body is one that is out of equilibrium and the task of the contemporary physician is best understood as an external exercise of control to restore the diseased body to homeostatic normality. Medicine has come to mean control over life, and, unless limited by philosophical conceptions, professional norms, or law, the asymptotic goal is absolute control. Control over life, in turn, requires control over death if it is to be absolute. Unless otherwise held in check by professional, ethical, social, and legal norms, medicine will tend toward an unstated goal of absolute control over both life and death.

History bears out this analysis. Beginning with Bacon and the scientific revolution in the seventeenth century, control over life has been the implicit (and sometimes explicit) aim of medicine (McCullough et al. 2008). As early as 1638, Francis Bacon wrote *The Historie of Life and Death, With Observations Naturall and Experimental for the Prolonging of Life*, urging the use of the new scientific method not only to treat disease but also to extend human life (Bacon 1638/1977). The control of life gives rise to the hope of controlling death. As the surgeon Xavier Bichat put it at the end of the eighteenth century, "Life is the assemblage of the functions which resist death" (Bichat 1827, 10).

These efforts have proven wildly successful, particularly in the last 100 years. Cardiac bypass, dialysis, ventilators, solid organ transplantation, effective chemotherapy for cancer, insulin for diabetes, the eradication of smallpox, and countless other successful therapies control or eliminate disease. Death is resisted by the power of medicine and life is prolonged.

Sometimes this success can go to the heads of physicians, who may be tempted to think that being a doctor really is about total control. In the 1990s, advertisements in medical journals for the Coumadin brand of the drug warfarin, touting more precise dosing, absorption, and anticoagulant effect with the brand name compared with generic forms, came with the message, in big print, "Control. Mastery" (Sulmasy 1997, 117). Such an advertisement speaks volumes about how marketers think they can appeal to physicians. Absolute control (i.e., mastery) is assumed to be the goal. I remember an oncology fellow when I was an intern who referred to a comatose, intubated, catheterized patient on vasopressors and dialysis with a pacemaker in place by saying, "That's how I like patients. Respiratory rate, heart rate, blood pressure, volume: I'm in control of everything. And they can't talk back." Now, certainly, this oncology fellow is not representative of *all* physicians. But he does stand out as representative of a temptation all physicians face. Physicians have great authority. They have great powers of control. Yet it seems that ethics demands the acceptance of limits on physicians' control over the body and limits on their authority over patients. A fundamental task for medical ethics, then, would seem to be the delineation of the proper limits of medical power.

From the late nineteenth century on, medicine deployed a two-track system to pursue control while subjecting its practice to ethical constraint. Physicians could pursue the technological goal of control over the body subject only to the limits of scientific progress while their authority over patients was con-strained by establishing the exercise of compassion as a professional ideal (Arney and Bergen 1984, 53–57). This approach prevented attitudes of the sort exhibited by the oncology fellow. Physicians could be "aggressive" in controlling disease while seeing patients as suffering human beings in need of medical power.

PATIENTS, PHYSICIANS, AND CONTROL OF THE BODY

Patients, particularly in the late twentieth century Western world, have come to admire the scientific power of medicine, sharing with physicians the need for knowledge and control. The autonomy movement has often been under-stood as pushing reluctant physicians into sharing their power with patients. Despite this conceptualization of the patient-physician relationship, it is only in very rare instances that the relationship becomes an adversarial clash between conflicting autonomous wills. Most often it is better described as a co-conspiracy. Physicians do not lose their power by sharing knowledge with patients. Rather, they become heroes. The shared goal of both physician and patient is control over the patient's body. In the interpersonal sphere, patients gladly grant physicians authority (rational-legal in origin) because, in the biological sphere, the knowledge that physicians possess is a power that can restore control over the body. That is what both patients and physicians want. Physicians gladly share their medical knowledge, which empowers the patient, and the empowered patient then authorizes the physician to use that powerful knowledge to control the body which is now out of control. Doing so actually enhances the standing of the physician. As one oncology patient wrote in the *New England Journal of Medicine* in 1981, "The very best doc-tors—and I have had the very best—share their power with their patients and try to give us the information we need to control our own treatment" (Trillin 1981). Physicians thus receive *authority* from patients to use the *power* of medical knowledge to exercise *control* over their patients' bodies.

Both the patient and the physician, under this conception, engage in an odd, dualistic relationship with the patient's body. The patient conceives of himself or herself not as an embodied being but as an autonomous will that exists apart from, and controls, the body. Disease threatens or interrupts that control. The assistance of the physician is therefore sought in order to reas-sert control. The physician brings the patient's body into conformity with the physician's will through the power of medical knowledge, for the sake of the patient and on the authority of the patient. From the perspective of each, the central issue is control. And the form of this control is a pair of independent wills autonomously engaged in a joint project to control the patient's body.

Contemporary biomedical technology has amplified this reconception of the patient-physician relationship as a joint venture to control the body. Heidegger's famous essay, "The Question Concerning Technology," helps to explain how technological developments have augmented medicine's drive for absolute control over the body (Heidegger 1977, 3–35). In that essay, Heidegger distinguishes between new and ancient forms of technology. Heidegger argues that ancient forms of *techne* (craft) were practiced as acts of *poiesis* (bringing into being). He interprets acts of the old *techne* as acts of *hervorbringen*, bringing forth the intrinsic capacities of the natural world. Ancient forms of technology were, in Heidegger's view, a kind of coaxing of elements of the natural world into allowing their intrinsic properties to serve human needs: for example, by bringing the wooden post out of the trunk of a living tree. Prescientific medicine was such a craft. Hippocratic physicians employed dietary interventions to coax the natural capacities of the embodied patient until the patient brought herself back into homeostatic equilibrium.

Contemporary scientific medicine, however, has a very different flavor. Contemporary medical technology consists of acts that Heidegger called *herausfordern*, acts of commanding forth, acts that enframe the natural world as undifferentiated, manipulable stuff, and forcibly bend this stuff into things that we find useful. For Heidegger, "Enframing (*Gestell*) means the gathering together of that setting-upon which sets upon man, i.e., challenges him forth, to reveal the real, in the mode of ordering, as standing-reserve" (Heidegger 1977, 20). The natural world has ceased to have independent value, and natural things have ceased to have their own integrity.

Contemporary medicine has adopted this form. The human body has become, like all of reality, standing reserve, manipulable stuff, a malleable ore, ready to be shaped by the will of the physician, as authorized by the patient, to carry out the patient's autonomously willed project. What has changed in the last few decades is the source of the physician's authority, not the centrality of controlling the body, which is one of the reasons why it is important to distinguish interpersonal authority from the notion of control. Ancient physicians derived their authority religiously, as conferred by a deity or deities. Until the late twentieth century, scientifically trained physicians derived their authority socially, through the norms of professionalism. Contemporary physicians, by contrast, increasingly derive their authority through the consent of the patient. Yet the patient is only willing to authorize the physician because the physician has power, the power of medical knowledge to control the body. Operating within the old model of paternalism (which is probably a caricature anyway), the physician commanded the body forth without consulting the patient. In the new model, the physician is given the authority to use his power to command the body by the patient, who also regards the body as standing reserve, enframed beforehand, to be shaped in a joint project of control. The autonomy model of the last few decades has done nothing to change this enframing. Medical knowledge is power. The physician still wields the authority to use that power, albeit as authorized by the patient's consent. Their joint project is the control of the body.

NAZI MEDICINE

The anlage of this contemporary approach to medicine, this techno-medical *Gestell*, preceded National Socialism by several centuries. It might have started with Bacon, yet it did not really become dominant until the turn of nineteenth into the twentieth century. While the pace of growth of the scientific power of medicine has steadily increased since then, this was the inflection point, the period of the first great blossoming of scientific medicine. Germany was widely regarded as the center of scientific medicine in this era. Virchow and Koch were the models. Osler went to Germany to study this model and bring it to the United States (Duffy 2011; Schulte-Bockolt, Soergel, and Stein 2016). Mendelian genetics and Darwinian evolution were the cutting edge of biology, and the Germans were the best at incorporating such biological advances into medicine. They were the exemplars of enframing medicine as a form of technology, the paragons of the techno-medical *Gestell* in which all of us now operate (Heidegger 1977, 20; Duffy 2011).

It was *these* physicians, the outstanding physicians of Germany, who joined the Nazi party in numbers disproportionately higher than any other profession; not a band of ignorant or inferior physicians (Ernst 2001). While opinions differ about why it is that so many German physicians so enthusiastically embraced National Socialism, one important factor seems to be that they saw in this political ideology opportunities for social authority and control that they believed medicine deserved and by which medicine could improve the lot of humankind (Haque et al. 2012; Proctor 1988, 69–70). Hitler did not invent Nazi medicine or impose it on German physicians. Rather, he permitted doctors to do what most of them thought they ought to be doing but were constrained from putting into practice under the strictures of a previous ethical and political system that they had come to regard as outmoded.

German physicians were considered beacons of medical progress—arguably the best in the world. For instance, they embraced preventive medicine as the rational alternative to treating patients only once they were sick. *Für-*

sorgen (care for the sick) became *Vorsorgen* (caring ahead, or prevention) (Reich 2001; Proctor 1988, 73). The emphasis of practice became teaching patients to care for themselves. The patient-physician relationship became almost like that between a player and a coach. For example, the subtitle of Ramm's textbook, is *"Der Arzt als Gesundheitszieher"* (The physician as "health guide" or "health coach").

German physicians also embraced what we now call population medicine. Under National Socialism, however, the primary object of care became the population, not the individual patient. The object they sought to control was now the *Volkskörper* (the body of the people). They were at the forefront of genetics, but thought they were falling behind the United States and the United Kingdom in eugenics. Under the Nazi banner, however, they soon shot past their international competitors in implementing the world's most advanced and systematic program of sterilization, reported on in admiring tones in the US medical literature in the 1930s (From Our Regular Correspondent 1933, and 1934; Peter 1934; Black 2012, 301). As the superintendent of a Virginia psychiatric hospital put it, "The Germans are beating us at our own game" (Black 2012, 277).

Within the German academy, medicine also gained greater prominence (Lifton 2017, 39). Physicians became university chancellors and rectors in unprecedented numbers (Proctor 1988, 93–94). In a way, as Lifton observed, National Socialism was politics as biology: a "biocracy" (Lifton 2017, 17). From 1933–1945, German physicians occupied perhaps the most powerful and prestigious social position that physicians have ever held in any society before or after.

WHAT CANNOT BE CONTROLLED

Control of the body has become the ideal of contemporary medicine. The body is standing reserve, commanded by the doctor, the patient, or both. Bacon's dream seems within our grasp. Both patients and physicians share this view. It is not that we see our bodies in this way or consciously use our bodies in this way. We simply implicitly inhabit these ideas. This is our techno-medical *Gestell*. I call it *Hyper-Medicine.*

The body is standing reserve to be manipulated at will. The patient autonomously authorizes the physician to control the body—to command it forth. On this view, medicine becomes a kind of transaction for the purpose of commanding forth a desirable product out of the standing reserve of the patient's body. If you don't like your nose, no problem. Medicine has the power to change it.

If control is the central issue, then, it is reasonable to ask what happens when one encounters something that cannot be controlled. The Baconian dream is the expectation of total control of the forces that resist death, but reality still intervenes. When medicine appears to reach a limit, what happens? To understand what happens when the controlling tendency of Hyper-Medicine confronts an insurmountable limit requires a shift in focus to explore the meaning of suffering.

Suffering

Suffering is, at its root, an encounter with finitude (Sulmasy 1999; 2018). Pain hurts, but pain becomes suffering when it imposes limits on us, when it forces us to confront our finitude. Arthritic joints are painful, but the suffering of arthritis arises from the way that painful joints prevent us from opening a jar or walking up the stairs. Illness, injury, and disability are all potential occasions of suffering. Despair, loneliness, and alienation also are all potential occasions of suffering—experiences of finitude. Those who would reach out to the suffering are not exempt. For physicians, the limits of medicine are always, also, inherently, occasions of suffering.

Earlier eras accepted this suffering. It was understood that the function of medicine is not to relieve the human condition of the human condition (Paul Ramsey cited in Campbell 1990). Etymologically, *compassion* means "suffering with." At the end of life, physician and family and friends and clergy and community could accompany the incurable and dying person, express compassion and solidarity, and do what they could to ease the physical occasions of the patient's suffering.

Control, Suffering, and the Limits of Medicine

Within the framework of Hyper-Medicine, however, the limits of medicine become unthinkable. What cannot be controlled, what cannot be cured, what cannot be brought into conformity with our autonomous, disembodied wills threatens the validity of that *Gestell* and becomes intolerable. In the enframing of Hyper-Medicine, in which the only sense that can be made is control, what cannot be controlled is rendered not just suffering, but *senseless* suffering. This situation is a crisis. It threatens the very structure of the techno-medical *Gestell* that grips both patient and physician. Ultimately, without proper checks, what is beyond one's control becomes so intolerable that it appears that there is only one solution—the elimination of that which obstinately defies control.

An unwillingness to understand or to tolerate what is beyond one's control is at the root of the contemporary drive to legalize physician-assisted suicide (PAS) and euthanasia. Autonomy, after all, is not a justification. All autonomy means is that the choice is freely made; it does not explain why it should be so decided. "Because I want to," is not an ethical justification. One can autonomously embrace or reject PAS or euthanasia. It is reasonable to ask the person who chooses assisted suicide or euthanasia, why did you make that autonomous choice? What justifies your action?

Empirical research suggests that patients choose PAS or euthanasia primarily for issues related to control, not because of intractable symptoms (Smith et al. 2015; Oregon Health Authority 2018; Malpas, Mitchell, and Johnson 2012). The source of the suffering they find intolerable is lack of control. It is the unwillingness to accept a lack of control over one's limbs, or bladder, or daily routine; the unwillingness to accept help from others; the refusal to wait for death to happen, that lead to the urge to *make* death happen.

Proponents argue, "I want to control the manner and timing of my death" (Rodriguez-Prat et al. 2016; Death with Dignity n.d.). Studies show that patients in the United States who actually use the PAS laws tend to have what is called, in attachment theory, a *dismissive* character style, with life-long, deep, overriding concerns for control and independence (Smith et al. 2015).

It is said that patients who seek PAS differ from psychiatrically ill suicidal patients not only in that they are rational, but in that they do not want to die. The interpretation I am proposing explains how those seeking PAS paradoxically can be said to want to live. They do want to live—as long as they are in control. It is when they can no longer control life, staving off death and disability, that the urge arises then to eliminate what is beyond control.

For physicians, the urge to assist patients with suicide or to provide active euthanasia may similarly stem from the intolerability of accepting that some forms of human suffering are beyond the control of medicine. When the patient asks, "Doctor, can't you do something?" some physicians simply find it intolerable to be forced to confront the limits of medicine and say, "No. I can't fix that. I can only walk with you and assure you that you do not have to face this alone." Psychologically, it is much easier for the physician to say, "Yes I can," and to reach into his or her black bag and pull out the syringe or the prescribing pen. In effect, the provider of PAS or euthanasia says of the syringe (or the pen), "It belongs in my hands. I have the authority. The patient has authorized me. I can be a pioneer in this regard. The state has given my action the force of law."

Data show that it is psychologically difficult for physicians to confront loss of control: a third of physicians self-identify as "control freaks," and many think that this character trait makes them better doctors (Lemaire and Wallace 2014, 616). Many physicians share the dismissive attachment style that characterizes patients who seek PAS and euthanasia (Dehning et al. 2013; Ciechanowski et al. 2004; Cherry, Fletcher, and O'Sullivan 2013; Kafetsios et al. 2016). It stands to reason that such physicians would be more likely to agree to a request for PAS or euthanasia.

This is not to say that these traits are associated with a malign motive. Physicians tend to operate in the "fix-it mode," seeking to control the body for beneficent ends. But this may make it even harder to confront the limits of medicine and admit that certain clinical situations are beyond control. As one oncologist described the situation of not being able to provide a patient with any more effective antineoplastic treatment, "It's an awful thing to come to the patient with your bag of tricks empty" (Sulmasy 2006). PAS and euthanasia provide "a way out" for the doctor as well as for the patient.

For all involved parties, then, the syringe belongs in the hand of the physician. The patient places it there, authorizing the physician to use it, because the physician has the knowledge and power to do so efficiently. The physician stands ready to accept the syringe or prescribing pen, sharing the *Gestell* of the patient. This *Gestell*, which subliminally enjoins the control of the body through medical knowledge, is so totalizing that it appears to all that the problem of death now has a solution (at least a solution of last resort). The state also benefits by placing the syringe in the hand of the physician, inasmuch as this strategy enables the state to accomplish many of its ancillary ends while simultaneously absolving the state of direct responsibility. For patients, physicians, and families, putting the syringe in the hand of the physician also validates acts that have been considered forbidden for several millennia. The task of the state is to give these acts the force of law. The physician is, thereby, socially authorized as the guardian of the powerful knowledge of medicine and its application—not just with the authority to extend life, but also with the authority to end life. The power required to accomplish the latter is actually much less than that required by the former, as Hippocrates well knew. It is much easier, technically, for a physician to end a life than to save it, and that is part of why Hippocrates thought it important that physicians be restrained from using lethal force (Cavanaugh 2017, 73–99). Through the legalization of PAS and euthanasia, that lethal power is unleashed.

This interpretation also partly explains why it is inevitable that legalized PAS will give way to euthanasia, as has been the case in the Netherlands, Belgium, and Canada. The *Gestell*, the enframing, by which PAS is legalized conceives of this action as a means of reasserting control over the body. Yet, it is well-known that PAS can go awry (Groenewoud et al. 2000; Oregon

Health Authority 2018; Sinmyee et al. 2019). The patient might lose capacity before taking the prescribed lethal pills. These drugs can cause nausea and the patient can vomit them up. It can sometimes take days to die. The patient might awaken, or never become completely comatose. Sometimes the patient does not die even after ingesting the pills. Euthanasia, which is done by the doctor, assures far better control than does PAS. Literally, on this view, the syringe belongs in the hand of a physician. In a recent review article by an international group of anesthesiologists advocating improved assisted dying, the argument has been made forcefully that direct physician involvement through euthanasia is medically and humanely necessary because of the frequent complications of PAS (Sinmyee et al. 2019).

THE PROBLEMS

This chapter thus far has given an interpretation of how the demand for PAS and euthanasia emerged in the twentieth century, an explanation for why these practices were adopted in the manner they were in Nazi Germany, and why they have subsequently been adopted as voluntary practices in several jurisdictions in the contemporary Western world. No arguments have been advanced about why this interpretation makes PAS or euthanasia ethically problematic. Yet it seems that this interpretation permits several new insights into why PAS and euthanasia might be judged as ethically misguided, even outside the Nazi context.

False Control

The first problem with these practices, based on this interpretation, is that the control over death sought by advocates of PAS and euthanasia, now understood as a consequence of the regnant techno-medical *Gestell*, is illusory. Death, ultimately, cannot be controlled. The Baconian project fails the test of metaphysics. The appearance of control that PAS and euthanasia offer is not really control over death. It is ironic to believe that one has defied death by bringing it upon oneself. One has not exerted effective control over one's fate by such actions, which may be likened to kicking apart a sandcastle in the face of an oncoming hundred-foot-tall tsunami. It is misguided for society to foster such an illusion.

Invoking respect for patient autonomy does not get one out of this bind. Authority is not the primary issue. Whether the physician is authorized by a deity, the state, or a patient who autonomously asks the physician to act on his or her behalf, the central issues remain the same: power, control, and limits.

Moreover, one can legitimately question just how autonomous these actions really are. As Kevin Yuill has pointed out, even PAS, despite being presented as an assertion of autonomous control, requires that the patient be placed in the hands of a physician, who must vet the request, determine the patient's eligibility by making judgments about his or her prognosis, suffering, freedom from coercion, rationality, etc. and write the prescription (Yuill 2013, discussed in chapter 2 and chapter 6). The physician, not the patient, holds the keys.

Countertransference is also a real worry (Sulmasy 2017, 49–64; see chapter 12 of this book). Many physicians seem to fear disability and death. Such fear may even be a primary motivation for some to become physicians. Further, the work of caring for dying or seriously disabled patients is hard. Dying bodies are not fully responsive to the physician's control. In the setting of a subconsciously internalized goal of total control, frustration with bodies that resist control can give rise to an urge (equally subconscious) to eliminate what cannot be controlled. It can be all too easy for patients to read such signals and then play back to their physicians (whom they often aim to please) the physicians' own subconscious frustrations at not being in control. The patient might make a request for PAS in words that superficially assume the form of an autonomous choice, but actually might be expressing his or her physician's subconscious preference to be done with him or her (Miles 1995).

Autonomy is also limited by the objectification that typifies the techno-medical *Gestell*. Although with good intentions, physicians increasingly view patients as data sets, and their autonomous preferences are characterized as additional data points, along with their genes, histories, lab values, and the socioeconomic determinants that comprise the complete set (Arney and Bergen 1984, 50–61). Even those clinicians who see themselves as champions of patient autonomy unconsciously view it from deep within the techno-medical *Gestell*, leading them to try to objectify the subjective. Today's medical culture demands measurable outcomes like patient satisfaction scores. Pain and the spiritual life are inherently subjective, and yet, these well-intentioned physicians tackle the problems by developing quantifiable pain scales (Price et al. 1983) and scales of spiritual distress (Monod et al. 2012, 13). Even in trying to foster empathy, medical educators remain caught in the techno-medical *Gestell*. Rather than calling forth (*hervorbringen*) their natural empathy, they train physicians to speak words that will sound empathetic to patients and, thereby, improve their satisfaction scores (S. Tayal, Michelson, and N. Tayal 2016; Hardee 2003). Preferences are objectified into measurable utilities. Autonomy itself is in danger of becoming a form of standing reserve for the enterprise of Hyper-Medicine, symptomatic of the move to objectify the subjective.

Dualism

The second problem is that the sort of dualism presupposed by the techno-medical *Gestell* is false. The body is not standing reserve to be disposed of at the autonomous will of the patient and/or physician. The patient *is* an embodied person, and there is no locus of non-embodied will that can freely dispose of the body as something other than the person. The elimination of one's embodied person through the precipitation of one's death is, therefore, not the act of a whole person, inasmuch as it falsely attempts to sunder person and body. By attempting to divide body and person, suicide and euthanasia do violence to the notion of the person as valuable in each embodied realization and, thus, can never be morally justifiable.

The Limits of Medicine

Third, good therapy adheres to what I have elsewhere called the Canon of Discretion (Sulmasy 2018). Medicine should, from an ethical perspective, hew to its traditional goals and respect the boundaries of its scope, not transgress them. Good clinicians, for instance, recognize their own individual limits in expertise and refer to colleagues who have that expertise. At the end of life, in particular, clinicians need to recognize when medical control over the body has reached its limits. The response of some clinicians is to deny this limit and continue to try to stave off death with futile treatment, which is ethically wrong. Yet it is equally wrong to deny that medicine has met its limits by reaching into the black bag for the syringe, falsely asserting that medicine is still in control and denying that medicine has met an insurmountable limit.

The interpretation proposed in this chapter gives further insight into the meaningfulness of the distinction between killing and allowing to die. Good medicine is humble, adhering to the Hippocratic dictum that one should refrain from treating patients who are "overmastered by disease, recognizing that in such cases medicine is powerless" (Hippocrates 1972, 193). Adherence to this dictum is the ethically appropriate approach that permits withholding or withdrawing of life-sustaining treatments when they become more burdensome than beneficial. To forego life-prolonging treatments that have become marginally effective and disproportionately burdensome in the face of impending death is to acknowledge the limits of medicine, to recognize when medicine has become powerless. By contrast, physicians practicing futile medicine, PAS, or euthanasia all transgress this limit by refusing to acknowledge that medicine has become powerless and by asserting false control over the metaphysically uncontrollable. Hippocratic forbearance is preferable to the illusion of Baconian power.

Justice and the Chronically Dependent

Fourth, the disabled, who already lack control over their bodies, are further disempowered and disenfranchised when the state permits patients to declare that dependency on others renders their lives no longer worth living and licenses physicians to assist them in killing themselves. If loss of control of bowel or bladder becomes sufficient to permit state-authorized suicide, then the lives of all incontinent persons are thereby demeaned. Once this legal option exists, the burden of proof shifts. Implicitly, if not explicitly, legalization of PAS and/or euthanasia forces chronically ill and disabled persons who require assistance with transfers, toileting, mobility, speech, eating, or other functions to explain why they would burden themselves or society by continuing to live lives that depend upon the assistance of others.

Hyper-Medicine and the Totalitarian State

Fifth, the most serious possible consequence is the ever-present danger of a marriage between Hyper-Medicine and the totalitarian state. Since both Hyper-Medicine and the totalitarian state are fixated on control, it is easy to see how the overreaching tendencies of much of the pre-war German medical community blended so seamlessly into the totalitarian Nazi state. Both Hyper-Medicine and the totalitarian state seek complete control. What escapes control becomes intolerable and must be eliminated. For the totalitarian state, the need for control culminates in the elimination of political dissidents, journalists, religious believers, and other nonconformists. For Hyper-Medicine, the need for control culminates in the elimination of incurable patients.

The justification for euthanasia is always based on an implicit assumption regarding the necessity of controlling the body via the power of medical knowledge. When Hyper-Medicine and the totalitarian state are wedded, there is a danger that the incurable become simply another group of nonconformists—those who might resist when the state gives medicine the power of control over life and death.

Nazi euthanasia and contemporary Western PAS and euthanasia differ in one salient way—the source of the physician's authorization to use lethal power. In the Third Reich, the source was the state; in the contemporary Western world, the source is the individual patient. That difference is significant, but one can ask whether informed consent is a sufficient protection against potential abuse. Changing who authorizes the use of lethal power may be far less significant than granting physicians license to use such power in the first place. Control is attracted to control. Those who are focused on control might begin by asserting more control over themselves, but they often end up asserting more control over others. Both the power of medicine and the power of the state need to be limited by ethics and law.

COUNTERARGUMENTS

First, it might be objected that the picture of medicine painted in this chapter is far too bleak. One might complain that it is unfair to characterize physicians as control freaks, and argue that there are plenty of compassionate physicians, especially in palliative care, who can carry out PAS or euthanasia with sensitivity and compassion, who really do elicit autonomous choices and preside over very peaceful deaths. Yet this chapter is not suggesting that all physicians are like the anti-heroes that Goethe (1808/1994) and Mary Shelley (1818/1974) depicted in their famous tales. All that is being suggested is that there is a dominant enframing (*Gestell*) that permeates the culture and from which even virtuous physicians will have difficulty escaping. We need to be honest that this *Gestell* can afflict even palliative care, which is, at least sometimes, susceptible to a kind of "palliative care triumphalism" that promises an orchestrated, happy, totally controlled death, free from all suffering (Barnard 2006). It is just such thinking that ought to worry us in legalizing PAS and euthanasia. The drive to make the end *look* peaceful will not end well.

Moreover, with legalization, these practices become open to any and all physicians, not just the caring, sensitive, respectful, deeply compassionate physicians of the world. If the syringe belongs in the hands of a physician, then it can wind up in the hands of *any* physician. If the data are right, that about one-third of physicians have a dismissive attachment style and are deeply invested in control, and if many physicians are not good at following practice guidelines, then this power will certainly be misused. Training might help, but it is often ineffective in promoting adherence to guidelines and is unlikely to change personalities.

Another objection might be that the views presented here are Luddite, counseling against the use of medical technology and opposed to medical progress. One might argue that it is precisely by *controlling* nature that we have made progress in extending life and improving the quality of life. One might also level the charge that opposition to that sort of control would be a grave mistake. The observations about the techno-medical *Gestell* put forward in this essay, however, should not be interpreted as a rejection of medical progress or as an attempt to restore Hippocratic dietetics and humoral medicine. Medical progress and biomedical research are both good: most people in the contemporary Western world benefit enormously from the control medicine exerts over the human body. The aim of this chapter is not to reject medical progress. Rather, the aims are to become conscious of contemporary medicine's constitutive drive for control, to urge vigilance lest that drive become an all-encompassing mindset, and to counsel adherence to the limits that metaphysics and good ethics should rightly impose on medical practice. For example, while we can (and often should) use psychopharmaceuticals or technologies like deep brain stimulation to restore psychiatrically ill patients to a healthy state of mind, we ought to reject the urge to use that technology to control the thoughts of other human beings or to enhance our individual mental capacities to gain competitive advantage over others. Similarly, a physician should be prepared to accept his or her patient's death, but not to precipitate it as part of a false and inevitably corrupting crusade for absolute control.

Others would argue that autonomy will protect us from behaving like the Nazi doctors who killed people against their wills. I have argued, however, that autonomy is not the central issue. There needs to be a justification for why one should autonomously choose to make oneself dead or why physicians ought to serve such autonomous requests. And if the answer is that we seek to control the human body and to eliminate those bodies that do not submit to our control, then the ethical issues raised here are salient whether the act is PAS or euthanasia, and whether it is voluntary, nonvoluntary, or involuntary. Moreover, one should bear in mind that many early advocates for euthanasia in Germany, such as Jost (1895) and Gerkan (1913), called for voluntary euthanasia. Haeckel (1904) and Binding and Hocke (1920) did argue for nonvoluntary euthanasia for eugenic purposes, but they also argued for voluntary active euthanasia for incurably ill adults. These calls for voluntary euthanasia and for nonvoluntary euthanasia (with family concurrence or with the presumptive consent of the incapacitated patient) happened well before the Nazis came to power. Pre-war surveys among parents of mentally disabled German children showed broad popular support for euthanizing their children (Burleigh 1994, 23; Proctor 1988, 94). The actual practice began with parents freely requesting mercy-killing (*Gnadentod*) for their disabled children (Lifton 2017, 49–51). It is the mindset that directs one to eliminate what cannot be controlled, insisting that one still is in control, that propelled these ideas into practice. Respect for autonomy does not seem a strong enough bulwark against that urge and its consequences.

Another critique might be that assisted suicide and euthanasia have been lumped together unfairly, and that the syringe, literally, is only in the hand of the physician in euthanasia. In assisted suicide, one might argue, the pills are in the hand of the patient (who is, therefore, in control), and this fact provides a protection against potential abuse.

There are at least three responses to this objection. First, the argument of this chapter is that both PAS and euthanasia are driven by the ideal of absolute control over the body and a dualistic conceptualization of the patient's own body as standing reserve, ideas which constitute the *Gestell*, or enframing, that both the patient and the physician inhabit. Second, as noted above, legal access to PAS is under the control of the physician. The prescribing pen can be readily understood as standing in for the syringe, just as the carbon monoxide gas valve can be understood as standing in for the syringe in Nazi medical euthanasia. This chapter is not literally just about syringes. Third, while space does not permit a fully developed argument here, I agree with Singer (2011, 155–190) and Brock (1992), both notable PAS proponents, that the arguments that justify PAS are the same ones that justify euthanasia, and that the distinction between the two carries no substantive moral weight. Political expediency, not ideology, seems to drive a preference for PAS, but the same techno-medical *Gestell* drives both practices. It seems implausible to hold that legalized euthanasia will not come to pass in the United States if PAS becomes widely legalized, even if the time course before that happens might differ from that seen in other nations (Keown 2018; Gorsuch 2006; Jones 2011).

A further objection is that both the techno-medical *Gestell* and the subsequent program of medically precipitated death will serve us well if only we adhere to our pluralistic, liberal, democratic principles and protect them from the ever-present threat of reactionary politics. Such thinking, however, seems naïve. The history reviewed in this chapter, and in more detail elsewhere in this volume, teaches us that the impetus for euthanasia came from within the German medical community: euthanasia was not a practice imposed upon liberal physicians by the National Socialist government. Euthanasia was, even before the rise of the Nazis, one of several cutting-edge ideas that physicians themselves were espousing. The government had only to give these ideas the force of law. Moreover, history teaches us that it is the reigning Zeitgeist and not the government that typically propels such movements. German medical students and physicians who opposed euthanasia were pushed aside in the 1930s, were unable to publish because editors considered their views reactionary and outmoded, and were shouted down by students convinced of the political correctness of their own views (Lifton 2017, 39). Today, similar situations are developing regarding bioethical issues on campuses in the Western world (Somerville 2017; Cohen-Almagor 2015; Somerville 2013; McAdams v. Marquette University 2018). Suppression of opposing ideas and speech is also a kind of totalitarianism, whether led by boorish thugs or cultural elites (Noonan 2019).

Finally, some of those who reject the view presented here may do so not because they believe the account is false, but because they find it uncomfortably true. It can be difficult to hear that one's fundamental orientation toward medicine has deviated from its Hippocratic origins. Good people become physicians, yet most cannot help being caught up in the techno-medical *Gestell*. If one is enmeshed in the *Gestell*, it can be difficult to hear that the primary justification for PAS or euthanasia springs (implicitly) from understanding the end of medicine as absolute control over the human body and from understanding the body as manipulable standing reserve. The *Gestell* is not typically questioned. It is simply lived. It is only with great effort that one can emerge from within the *Gestell* to see it from the outside as problematic. For many, the ideas presented in this chapter might represent an intolerable affront to the dominant *Gestell* and must, therefore, be rejected without further argument.

ALTERNATIVES

One might wonder if there are alternative visions, or whether the picture depicted here is inevitable. One might worry that some horrific moral catastrophe would need to occur before society could admit that legalizing PAS and euthanasia had been a mistake and could muster the strength to reverse course. Yet, widespread PAS and euthanasia are not a foregone conclusion. It remains possible that the social forces propelling these practices might be restrained and that laws permitting PAS and euthanasia might be reversed before the advent of such a moral crisis. Changing course on PAS requires, however, changes both in medicine and in society at large.

These changes include first, physicians standing back from their typical patterns of practice and research long enough to recognize the techno-medical *Gestell* that dominates their operations and to recognize the totalizing tendencies of Hyper-Medicine. Only by seeing itself for what it has become can medicine be prevented from venturing where this enframing otherwise leads. Such introspection requires the cultivation of Hippocratic humility and a respect for limits—ethical, social, and metaphysical. Nothing is more uncontrollable than death. Whether one throws futile care at the dying human body or eliminates the dying body because it will no longer submit to one's control, death wins. Dying is a condition of being alive and the Baconian dream of forestalling death indefinitely through science is false.

Second, society needs to reject the form of dualism that views the human person as an autonomous locus of preferences, owning and directing the body. We humans are embodied beings, flesh and blood, not disembodied wills that subject the flesh to the whims of autonomous choice, commanding forth what we will from the standing reserve of our own corporeality. We need to return not just to a fuller, neo-Aristotelian view of healing as a calling forth of the body's own powers, but also to a neo-Aristotelian form of hylomorphism, by which mind and body are viewed as inseparable. From a hylomorphic perspective, the patient is as an embodied person, not an autonomous chooser who owns a body that is susceptible to the commanding forth of medical power.

Third, society needs to embrace a political philosophy that sees the importance of keeping the powers of profession, state, market, academy, religion, and its various institutions and voluntary association distinct—de Toqueville's prescription for a flourishing, pluralistic, liberal, representative democracy (1835/2012). The state ought not exert too much power over medicine, nor grant medicine powers that it ought not to have. We ought to reject politics as applied biology. The power to kill is not a power that wise physicians should want, nor a power that a wise society ought to grant its physicians.

Whether the West can correct its vision in these three ways before disaster strikes is an open question. But unless our culture can come to appreciate what is going on beneath the surface of debates about PAS and euthanasia, neither patients nor physicians will understand what is really at stake, or how society might change course. The real moral and social issues will not be answered by reading exceedingly "thin" reports issued by state monitoring commissions and arguing about what such numbers mean. Based on the arguments presented in this chapter, it should be clear that physicians ought to resist the urge to take the syringe into their hands, and that no reasonable society ought to place it there.

BIBLIOGRAPHY

Arney, William Ray, and Bernard J. Bergen. 1984. *Medicine and the Management of Living: Taming the Last Great Beast.* Chicago: University of Chicago Press.

Bacon, Francis. 1597. *Meditationes sacrae.* Londini: Excusum impensis Humfredi Hooper.

Bacon, Francis. (1638) 1977. *The Historie of Life and Death, With Observations Naturall and Experimental for the Prolonging of Life.* New York: Arno Press.

Barnard, David. 2006. "The Skull at the Banquet." In *Death in the Clinic*, edited by Lynn Jansen, 66–80. Lanham, MD: Rowman and Littlefield.

Bichat, Xavier. (1800) 1827. *Physiological Researches on Life and Death. (Recherches physiologiques sur la vie et la mort).* Translated by F. Gold. Boston: Richardson and Lord, 1827 [1800].

Binding, Karl, and Alfred Hoche. (1920) 1992. *Die Freigabe der Vernichtung lebensunwerten Lebens: ihr Mass und ihre Form.* Leipzig: Felix Meiner Verlag, 1920; 2nd Edition 1922. Available in English translation as: Karl Binding and Alfred Hoche, "Permitting the Destruction of Unworthy Life: Its Extent and Form." *Issues in Law and Medicine* 8, no. 2 (Fall): 231–65.

Black, Edwin. 2012. *War Against the Weak: America's Campaign to Create a Master Race*, 2nd ed. Washington, DC: Dialog Press.

Brock, Dan W. 1992. "Voluntary Active Euthanasia." *Hastings Center Report* 22, no. 2 (Mar–Apr): 10–22.

Burleigh, Michael. 1994. *Death and Deliverance: 'Euthanasia' in Germany: 1900–1945.* New York: Cambridge University Press.

Campbell, Courtney S. 1990. "Religion and Moral Meaning in Bioethics." *Hastings Center Report* 20, no. 4 (Summer): 4–10.

Cavanaugh, Thomas A. 2017. *Hippocrates' Oath and Asclepius' Snake: The Birth of the Medical Profession*. New York: Oxford University Press.

Cherry, M. Gemma, Ian Fletcher, and Helen O'Sullivan. 2013. "Exploring the Relationships among Attachment, Emotional Intelligence and Communication." *Medical Education* 47, no. 3 (March): 317–25.

Ciechanowski, Paul S., Joan E. Russo, Wayne J. Katon, and Edward A. Walker. 2004. "Attachment Theory in Health Care: The Influence of Relationship Style on Medical Students' Specialty Choice." *Medical Education* 38, no. 3 (February): 262–70.

Cohen-Almagor, Rafael. 2015. "Medical Ethics and Academic Freedom—My Dutch Experience." In *Autonomy, Altruism and Authority in Medical Ethics–Essays in Honor of Professor Shimon Glick*, edited by Alan Jotkowitz and Shifra Shvarts, 11–29. New York: Nova.

Death with Dignity. n.d. "Stories." Accessed February 20, 2019. https://www.death withdignity.org/stories/.

Dehning, Sandra, Sarah Gasperi, Daniela Krause, et al. 2013. "Emotional and Cognitive Empathy in First-Year Medical Students." *ISRN Psychiatry* (October): 801530. http://doi.org/10.1155/2013/801530.

Duffy, Thomas P. 2011. "The Flexner Report–100 Years Later." *Yale Journal of Biology and Medicine* 84, no. 3 (September): 269–76.

Ernst, E. 2001. "Commentary: The Third Reich—German Physicians between Resistance and Participation." *International Journal of Epidemiology* 30, no. 1 (February): 37–42.

Foucault, Michel. 2008. *The Birth of Biopolitics: Lectures at the College de France, 1978–1979.* Translated by Graham Burchell. New York: Palgrave Macmillan.

From Our Regular Correspondent. July 31, 1933. "Berlin." *Journal of the American Medical Association* 100 (July): 866–67.

From Our Regular Correspondent. January 8, 1934. "Berlin." *Journal of the American Medical Association* 102 (January): 630–31.

Gerkan, Roland. 1913. "Euthanasie," *Das Monistische Jahrhundert*. (May 17): 169–73. https://babel.hathitrust.org/cgi/pt?id=njp.32101078252911;view=1up;seq=177.

Goethe, Johann Wolfgang von. (1808) 1994. *Faust I & II.* Translated by Stuart Pratt Atkins. Princeton, NJ: Princeton University Press.

Gorsuch, Neil. 2006. *The Future of Assisted Suicide and Euthanasia.* Princeton, NJ: Princeton University Press.

Groenewoud, Johanna H., Agnes van Der Heide, Bregje D. Onwuteaka-Philipsen, Dick L. Willems, Paul J. van Der Maas, and Gerrit van Der Wal. 2000. "Clinical

Problems with the Performance of Euthanasia and Physician-Assisted Suicide in the Netherlands." *New England Journal of Medicine* 342, no. 8 (February): 551–56.

Haeckel, Ernst. 1904. *The Wonders of Life: A Popular Study of Biological Philosophy.* Translated by Joseph McCabe. London: Watts.

Haque, Omar S., Julian De Freitas, Ivana Viani, Bradley Niederschulte, and Harold J. Bursztajn. 2012. "Why Did So Many German Doctors Join the Nazi Party Early?" *International Journal of Law and Psychiatry* 35, no. 5–6 (Sep–Dec): 473–79.

Hardee, James. 2003. "An Overview of Empathy." *Permanente Journal* 7, no. 4 (Fall): 51–54.

Heidegger, Martin. 1977. "The Question Concerning Technology." In *The Question Concerning Technology and Other Essays*, edited and translated by William Lovitt. New York: Harper and Row.

Hippocrates. 1972. "The Art." In *Hippocrates, volume II*. Translated by W. H. S. Jones. Cambridge, MA: Harvard University Press.

Jones, David. 2011. "Is There a Logical Slippery Slope from Voluntary to Nonvoluntary Euthanasia?" *Kennedy Institute of Ethics Journal* 21, no. 4 (December): 379–404.

Jost, Adolf. 1895. *Das Recht auf den Tod: Sociale Studie.* Göttingen: Dieterich. Accessed December 7, 2019. http://hdl.handle.net/2027/chi.086229789.

Kafetsios, Konstantinos, Konstantina Hantzara, Fotios Anagnostopoulos, and Dimitrios Niakas. 2016. "Doctors' Attachment Orientations, Emotion Regulation Strategies, and Patient Satisfaction: A Multilevel Analysis." *Health Communication* 31, no. 6: 772–77.

Keown, John. 2018. *Euthanasia, Ethics, and Public Policy: An Argument Against Legalisation*, 2nd ed. Cambridge: Cambridge University Press.

Lemaire, Jane B., and Jean E. Wallace. 2014. "How Physicians Identify with Predetermined Personalities and Links to Perceived Performance and Wellness Outcomes: A Cross-Sectional Study." *BMC Health Services Research* 14 (November): 616. doi: 10.1186/s12913-014-0616-z.

Lifton, Robert J. (1986) 2017. *The Nazi Doctors: Medical Killing and the Psychology of Genocide.* New York: Basic Books.

Malpas, Phillipa J., Kay Mitchell, and Malcolm H. Johnson. 2012. "'I Wouldn't Want to Become a Nuisance under Any Circumstances"—A Qualitative Study of the Reasons Some Healthy Older Individuals Support Medical Practices that Hasten Death." *The New Zealand Medical Journal* 125, no. 1358 (July): 9–19.

McAdams v. Marquette University. 2018. 383 Wisc. 2d 358, 914 N.W.2d 708.

McCullough, Laurence B., John Caskey, Thomas R. Cole, and Andrew Wear. 2008. "Scientific and Medical Concepts of Nature in the Modern Period in Europe and North America." In *Altering Nature, Volume One: Concepts of 'Nature' and 'The Natural' in Biotechnology Debates*, edited by B. Andrew Lustig, Baruch A. Brody, and Gerald P. McKenny, 137–198. Dordrecht, Netherlands: Springer.

Miles, Steven H. 1995. "Physician-Assisted Suicide and the Profession's Gyrocompass." *Hastings Center Report* 25, no. 3 (May–Jun): 17–19.

Monod, Stephanie, Estelle Martin, Brenda Spencer, Etienne Rochat, and Christophe Büla. 2012. "Validation of the Spiritual Distress Assessment Tool in Older Hospitalized Patients." *BioMed Central Geriatrics* 12 (March): 13.

Noonan, Peggy. 2019. "Get Ready for the Struggle Session." *Wall Street Journal*, March 9–10, 2019, A13.

Oregon Health Authority. 2018. Public Health Division, Center for Health Statistics. "Oregon Death With Dignity Act: Data Summary 2017," February 9, 2018. https://www.oregon.gov/oha/PH/PROVIDERPARTNERRESOURCES/EVALUATION RESEARCH/DEATHWITHDIGNITYACT/Documents/year20.pdf.

Peter, W. W. 1934. "Germany's Sterilization Program." *American Journal of Public Health and the Nation's Health* 24, no. 3: 187–191.

Price, Donald D., Patricia A. McGrath, Amir Rafii, and Barbara Buckingham. 1983. "The Validation of Visual Analogue Scales as Ratio Scale Measures for Chronic and Experimental Pain." *Pain* 17, no. 1 (September): 45–56.

Proctor, Robert N. 1988. *Racial Hygiene: Medicine Under the Nazis.* Cambridge, MA: Harvard University Press.

Ramm, Rudolf. 1943. *Ärztliche Rechts und Standeskunde: Der Arzt als Gesundheitszieher.* 2nd ed. Berlin: Walter de Gruyter.

Reich, Warren T. 2001. "The Care-Based Ethic of Nazi Medicine and the Moral Importance of What We Care About." *American Journal of Bioethics* 1, no. 1 (Winter): 64–74.

Rodriguez-Prat, Andrea, Cristina Monforte-Royo, Josep Porta-Sales, Xavier Escribano, and Albert Balaguer. 2016. "Patient Perspectives of Dignity, Autonomy and Control at the End of Life: Systematic Review and Meta-Ethnography." *PLoS ONE* 11, no. 3 (March): e0151435. https://doi.org/10.1371/journal.pone.0151435.

Schulte-Bockolt, Arnd, Konrad H. Soergel, and Juergen Stein. 2016. "Internal Medicine in the United States and Germany: Mutual Influences from 1870 to Today." *Wiener Medizinische Wochenschrift* 166 (November): 479–86.

Shelley, Mary. (1818) 1974. *Frankenstein; or, The Modern Prometheus*, edited by James Rieger. Indianapolis: Bobbs-Merrill.

Singer, Peter. 2011. *Practical Ethics.* 3rd ed. New York: Cambridge University Press.

Sinmyee, S., V. J. Pandit, J. M. Pascual, et al. 2019. "Legal and Ethical Implications of Defining an Optimum Means of Achieving Unconsciousness in Assisted Dying." *Anaesthesia* 74, no. 5 (May): 630–37. doi: 10.1111/anae.14532.

Smith, Kathryn A., Theresa A. Harvath, Elizabeth R. Goy, and Linda Ganzini. 2015. "Predictors of Pursuit of Physician-Assisted Death." *Journal of Pain and Symptom Management* 49, no. 3 (March): 555–61.

Somerville, Margaret. 2017. "Shutting Up by Shouting Down: When an Anti-Euthanasia Speaker at a Doctors' Conference is Prevented from Speaking, You Know that Something is Very Wrong." *MercatorNet*, March 17, 2017. https://www.mercatornet.com/features/view/shutting-up-by-shouting-down/19508.

Somerville, Margaret. 2013. "'Brave New Ethicists': A Cautionary Tale." In *The Public Intellectual in Canada*, edited by Nelson Wiseman, 212–32. Toronto: University of Toronto Press.

Sulmasy, Daniel P. 1997. *The Healer's Calling: A Spirituality for Physicians and Other Health Care Professionals.* Mahwah, NJ: Paulist Press.

Sulmasy, Daniel P. 1999. "Finitude, Freedom and Suffering." In *Pain Seeking Understanding: Suffering, Medicine, and Faith*, edited by Mark J. Hanson and Margaret E. Mohrmann. Cleveland, OH: Pilgrim Press.

Sulmasy, Daniel P. 2006. "Spiritual Issues in the Care of Dying Patients: '. . . It's Okay Between Me and God.'" *Journal of the American Medical Association* 296, no. 11 (September): 1385–92.

Sulmasy, Daniel P. 2017. "Ethics and the Psychiatric Dimensions of Physician Assisted Suicide: A View from the United States." In *Euthanasia and Assisted Suicide: Lessons from Belgium*, edited by David Jones, Chris Gastmans, and Calum MacKellar, 49–64. New York: Cambridge University Press.

Sulmasy, Daniel P. 2018. "The Last Low Whispers of our Dead: When Is it Ethically Justifiable to Render a Patient Unconscious until Death?" *Theoretical Medicine and Bioethics* 39, no. 3 (June): 233–63.

Tayal, Suzanne C., Kristen Michelson, and Neeraj H. Tayal. 2016. "Listening with Empathy: Save Time, Communicate More Effectively and Improve Patient and Provider Satisfaction." Accessed March 14, 2018. https://edhub.ama-assn.org/steps-forward/module/2702561.

Tocqueville, Alexis de. (1835) 2012. *Democracy in America.* Edited by Eduardo Nolla and James T. Schleifer. Indianapolis: Liberty Fund, 2012.

Trillin, Alice Stewart. 1981. "Of Dragons and Garden Peas: A Cancer Patient Talks to Doctors." *New England Journal of Medicine* 304 (March): 699–701.

Weber, Max. 1978. *Economy and Society: An Outline of Interpretive Sociology.* Edited by Guenther Roth and Claus Wittich. Berkeley: University of California Press, 1978.

Yuill, Kevin. 2013. *Assisted Suicide: The Liberal, Humanist Case Against Legalization.* New York: Palgrave Macmillan.

Index

About the Contributors

Florian Bruns, MD, MA, is a medical doctor and historian at the Institute of History and Ethics of Medicine at Martin Luther University Halle-Wittenberg, Germany. He currently is a visiting professor for the history of medicine at Charité Berlin. His research areas include medicine under National Socialism, health care in the communist German Democratic Republic, history of medical ethics, clinical ethics, and the patient's perspective in the history of medicine.

LaVera Crawley, MD, MPH, is the director of Hospital Chaplaincy and Clinical Pastoral Education at the California Pacific Medical Center in San Francisco. Dr. Crawley received her medical degree from Meharry Medical College; her residency in Family Medicine at UC San Francisco; an MPH from the University of California at Berkeley; and completed two fellowships in Ethics and Palliative Care Education and Research at Stanford and Harvard, respectively. A former family physician on the Navajo Reservation and empirical bioethicist at Stanford, she has focused her life work on understanding and eliminating health inequities at the end of life. She continues this work as a Certified Chaplain Educator and hospital chaplain.

James Downar, MD, MHSc, graduated from McGill Medical School and completed residency training in Internal Medicine, Critical Care, and Palliative Care at the University of Toronto, where he also received a master's degree in bioethics from the Joint Centre for Bioethics. He is head of the Division of Palliative Care at the University of Ottawa, associate professor in its Department of Medicine, co-chair of the Pan-Canadian Palliative Care Research Collaborative, chair of the Ethical Affairs Committee of the Canadian Critical Care Society, and a former Associated Medical Services Phoenix Fellow. His research interests include communication and decision-making for seriously ill patients and their families, and palliative care for the critically ill and for noncancer illnesses.

Alan Elbaum, MS, is a medical student in the UC Berkeley-UC San Francisco Joint Medical Program. Prior to medical school, he worked as a disability advocate at the AlManarah Association in Nazareth. He completed a master's degree at UC Berkeley on the subjectivity of illness among the Jews of medieval Egypt, based on Hebrew and Arabic manuscripts from the Cairo Genizah. He is among the first medical students in the United States to have completed a unit of hospital chaplaincy training (Clinical Pastoral Education). He is interested in the psychological aspects of serious illness and plans to pursue a career in psychiatry and palliative care.

Ashley K. Fernandes, MD, PhD, is the Director of Competency for Professionalism and associate director of the Center for Bioethics at The Ohio State University College of Medicine, and an associate professor of pediatrics at Nationwide Children's Hospital. He received his MD from The Ohio State University and his PhD in philosophy from Georgetown University. He directs ethics education for pediatric residents at Nationwide Children's Hospital, has been active in clinical ethics committees throughout his career, and is an elected member of the American Academy of Pediatrics' Executive Committee on Bioethics. Dr. Fernandes has taught Medical Ethics and the Holocaust to medical and graduate students and presented and published on this topic.

Gerrit Hohendorf, MD, is a psychiatrist, medical historian, bioethicist, and adjunct professor and head of the Research Unit for the History of Medicine at the Institute for History and Ethics of Medicine at Technical University of Munich. His research interests include the prerequisites, the reality, and the aftermath of medicine in National Socialism, the history and ethics of psychiatry, and the ethics at the beginning and end of life. He contributed to the historical information at Berlin's Memorial and Information Point for the Victims of National Socialist Euthanasia Killings and the editing of the Memorial Book for the Munich euthanasia victims. Dr. Hohendorf helps to identify the victims of unethical neuropathological research at institutes of the former Kaiser-Wilhelm-Society.

Scott Kim, MD, PhD, is a psychiatrist and a philosopher, and a senior investigator in the Department of Bioethics, National Institutes of Health, and former co-director of Center for Bioethics and Social Sciences in Medicine, University of Michigan. Dr. Kim combines philosophical, clinical, and empirical approaches to study ethical issues, including assessment of decision-making capacity, surrogate consent for incapacitated patients, and physician-assisted death. He served on the Council of Canadian Academies Expert Panel on Medical Assistance in Dying.

Eric Kodish, MD, is an ethicist, pediatric hematologist, professor of pediatrics at Lerner College of Medicine/Case Western Reserve University, and former F. J. O'Neill Professor and Chair of Bioethics at Cleveland Clinic. He has published more than 130 peer-reviewed papers and is the editor of *Ethics and Research with Children: A Case-Based Approach*. Dr. Kodish is an elected Fellow of the Hastings Center and received the Distinguished Service Award from the Children's Oncology Group (2005) and the American Society for Bioethics and Humanities (2016). After decades of focus on clinical care, research, and leadership, Dr. Kodish is currently dedicated to teaching the next generation.

Barron H. Lerner, MD, PhD, is a professor of medicine and population health at the New York University School of Medicine. He has written on the history of medicine for the *New England Journal of Medicine*, the *Annals of Internal Medicine* and the *Lancet* as well as *The New York Times*, the *Washington Post*, *The Atlantic*, and *Slate*. Dr. Lerner is the author of five books, including *The Breast Cancer Wars*, named a notable book of 2001 by the American Library Association and Booklist. He has appeared on numerous television and radio programs, including NPR's "Fresh Air" and "All Things Considered." Dr. Lerner teaches internal medicine, bioethics, and the history of medicine.

Diane E. Meier, MD, is CEO of the Center to Advance Palliative Care. Under her leadership, the number of US palliative care programs has more than tripled. She is co-director of the Patty and Jay Baker National Palliative Care Center; professor of geriatrics and palliative medicine; Catherine Gaisman Professor of Medical Ethics; and the founder and director of the Hertzberg Palliative Care Institute, 1997–2011, all at the Icahn School of Medicine. Dr. Meier was elected to the National Academy of Medicine in 2013. She has over 200 peer-reviewed publications; her most recent book, *Meeting the Needs of Older Adults with Serious Illness: Challenges and Opportunities in the Age of Health Reform*, was published in 2014.

H. Christof Müller-Busch, MD, PhD, is a retired consultant for palliative medicine, pain therapy, and anesthesiology at Gemeinschaftskrankenhaus

342 *About the Contributors*

Havelhöhe Berlin and other institutions. He was president of the German Association for Palliative Medicine and is a member of the German Medical Association's ethics and medicine committee. In 2008, he launched the Charter for the Care of the Critically Ill and The Dying in Germany and is a volunteer expert for palliative medicine in the Shandong province (China) and Morocco. He has authored about 150 articles and book chapters and *Abschied braucht Zeit*, his reflections on death and dying. He received the Federal Cross of Merits of Germany and the National Prize for Palliative and Hospice Care.

Kenneth Prager, MD, a pulmonologist for 46 years, is professor of medicine, director of medical ethics, and chair of the Medical Ethics Committee at Columbia University Medical Center. He teaches pulmonology and lectures widely on medical ethics. His writings on medicine and medical ethics have appeared in medical journals, textbooks, as well as the op-ed pages of the *New York Times* and the *Wall Street Journal*. Dr. Prager has received numerous honors for his patient care, clinical expertise, teaching, and contributions to organ donation, including The Leonard Tow Humanism in Medicine Award and the Columbia University Presidential Award for Excellence in Teaching.

Robert A. Pearlman, MD, MPH, is a health care ethicist and senior evaluation consultant with the National Center for Ethics in Health Care (Veterans Health Administration) and a professor of medicine, health services, and bioethics and humanities at the University of Washington. For over 35 years, he has conducted empirical research and evaluations of clinical and organizational ethics concepts and practices, such as quality of life in decision-making, end-of-life treatment preferences, advance care planning, shared understanding of patient suffering through figurative language, and ethics consultation quality. Dr. Pearlman also teaches trainees in palliative medicine. He is the author of three books and over 150 publications.

Timothy E. Quill, MD, is distinguished professor in palliative care and professor of medicine, psychiatry, medical humanities, and nursing at the University of Rochester Medical Center (URMC). He was founding director of the URMC Palliative Care Division and past president of the American Academy of Hospice and Palliative Medicine. He is acting director of the URMC Schyve Center for Biomedical Ethics. He was the lead physician plaintiff in the New York State legal case challenging the law prohibiting physician-assisted death heard in 1997 by the U.S. Supreme Court (*Quill v.*

Vacco). Dr. Quill is a fellow in the American Academy of Hospice and Palliative Medicine and a master in the American College of Physicians.

Volker Roelcke, MD, PhD, is professor and chair of the Institute for the History of Medicine, Giessen University, Germany, and a member of the Leopoldina—German National Academy of Sciences. His fields of expertise include: medicine during the Nazi period; the impact of Nazi medical atrocities on post–World War II debates in medical ethics; relations between eugenics and medical genetics in the twentieth century; history and ethics of human subjects research; history and epistemology of the animal model of human disease; history of psychiatry and psychosomatic medicine. His recent books include: *Silence, Scapegoats, Self-Reflection: The Shadow of Nazi Medical Crimes on Medicine and Bioethics* (2014, co-editor) and *Vom Menschen in der Medizin: Für eine kulturwissenschaftlich kompetente Heilkunde* (2017).

Sheldon Rubenfeld, MD, is clinical professor of medicine at Baylor College of Medicine. For the past 20 years, Dr. Rubenfeld studied Jewish medical ethics with a small, dedicated group led by Rabbi Yossi Grossman. He taught Jewish Medical Ethics and continues to teach *Healing by Killing: Medicine in the Third Reich* at Baylor. In 2010, he founded the Center for Medicine after the Holocaust (CMATH). Among his four books are *Medicine After the Holocaust: From the Master Race to the Human Genome and Beyond* and *Human Subjects Research after the Holocaust*. He practiced endocrinology and internal medicine for 36 years until he retired in 2014 and became CMATH's executive director.

Stephan Sahm, MD, PhD, studied medicine and philosophy, trained in internal medicine, gastroenterology, and palliative medicine, and qualified as professor in medical ethics. He is director of Medical Clinic I at Ketteler Hospital and head of the Gastrointestinal Cancer Center in Offenbach. He is also professor at the Senckenberg Institute of History and Ethics of Medicine at Frankfurt University Medical School. His research interests include ethics of end-of-life care, digital medicine, and organ transplantation. He is a member of ethics committees, has served as an expert in German Parliament hearings, writes for the *Frankfurter Allgemeine Zeitung* on bioethical issues, and is a member of multiple national and international scientific societies and academies.

Avraham Steinberg, MD, is the director of the Medical Ethics Unit and senior pediatric neurologist at Shaare Zedek Medical Center in Jerusalem and head of the editorial board of the Talmudic Encyclopedia. He has authored

30 books and 240 scientific articles and chapters related to medical ethics. Dr. Steinberg has received numerous awards, among them the Israel Prize in 1999 for his *Encyclopedia of Jewish Medical Ethics*.

Daniel P. Sulmasy, MD, PhD, is the André Hellegers Professor of Biomedical Ethics in the Departments of Medicine and Philosophy and the acting director of the Kennedy Institute of Ethics at Georgetown University. A practicing internist and a philosopher, he serves as editor-in-chief of the journal *Theoretical Medicine and Bioethics* and has written extensively on ethics and care at the end of life. Among his previous six books are *Methods in Medical Ethics* (2010) and *The Rebirth of the Clinic* (2006).

Eduard Verhagen, MD, JD, PhD, worked in Curaçao for five years before becoming professor of pediatrics and the department chair at the University Medical Center Groningen and clinical director of the Beatrix Children's Hospital/UMCG. He received his MD and JD from the University of Utrecht and completed his pediatric specialty training in Amsterdam. His PhD thesis was on neonatal end-of-life decisions in Dutch NICU's. He has written numerous scientific papers about ethical decision-making and end-of-life care, co-authored the "Groningen Protocol" for newborn euthanasia, leads several national research and pediatric palliative care initiatives, and is a member and chair of several national and governmental medical-ethical and legal advisory councils.

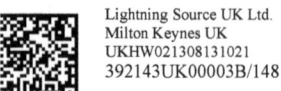